Integrated Approach to
Obstetrics and Gynaecology

Revised and Updated

Integrated Approach to
Obstetrics and
Gynaecology

Revised and Updated

Edited by

Kuldip Singh
National University Health System, Singapore

World Scientific

NEW JERSEY · LONDON · SINGAPORE · BEIJING · SHANGHAI · HONG KONG · TAIPEI · CHENNAI · TOKYO

Published by

World Scientific Publishing Co. Pte. Ltd.

5 Toh Tuck Link, Singapore 596224

USA office: 27 Warren Street, Suite 401-402, Hackensack, NJ 07601

UK office: 57 Shelton Street, Covent Garden, London WC2H 9HE

Library of Congress Cataloging-in-Publication Data
Names: Singh, Kuldip, 1953–   editor.
Title: Integrated approach to obstetrics and gynaecology / editor, Kuldip Singh.
Description: New Jersey : World Scientific, [2016] | Includes index.
Identifiers: LCCN 2016022161| ISBN 9789813108547 (hardcover : alk. paper) |
    ISBN 9813108541 (hardcover : alk. paper) | ISBN 9789813108554 (pbk. : alk. paper) |
    ISBN 981310855X (pbk. : alk. paper)
Subjects: | MESH: Gynecology--methods | Obstetrics--methods | Genital Diseases, Female |
    Pregnancy Complications
Classification: LCC RG110 | NLM WP 100 | DDC 618--dc23
LC record available at https://lccn.loc.gov/2016022161

British Library Cataloguing-in-Publication Data
A catalogue record for this book is available from the British Library.

First published 2016
Revised and updated 2019

DEDICATION

- **All the generation of students and doctors** — past, and present for their enthusiasm, and encouragement that has kept my passion to teach and mentoring prevail despite the many obstacles in life.
- **My late mother, Madam Nihal Kaur,** for teaching me to persevere and succeed in the wake of all adversities in life. Without her, I would not have been able to be where I am today.

Kuldip Singh

CONTENTS

FOREWORD

by
Tan Chorh Chuan
President, National University of Singapore

Integrated Approach to Obstetrics and Gynaecology is a unique text that is specifically targeted to serve the needs of our local medical undergraduates, residents and family medicine doctors. Previously, there had not been a textbook that covers the extensive practical experience and management protocols used in Singapore, and particularly at the National University Hospital. The publication of this comprehensive resource is thus timely.

The chapters in the textbook cover the essentials in Obstetrics and Gynaecology, namely, Maternal Foetal Medicine, Benign Gynaecology, Reproductive Endocrinology and Gynaecological Oncology. Throughout the book, the clinical management advocated is founded on a rigorous evidence-based approach and on international guidelines which are well referenced.

The authors have established reputations in undergraduate and postgraduate medical education and assessment. Professor Kuldip Singh, the editor, is a passionate educator whose expertise and teaching excellence has been consistently recognised by his peers and students.

I am confident that *Integrated Approach to Obstetrics and Gynaecology* will become the authoritative reference for our medical undergraduates and residents in Singapore. It may also serve as a useful source of information for others in the region and internationally. The key outcomes of a text such as this will be that the medical practitioners will be strengthened in their knowledge, exam preparations and eventual practice, and that most importantly, the safe and proper care of our patients will be enhanced.

FOREWORD

by
Yeoh Khay Guan
Dean, Yong Loo Lin School of Medicine
National University of Singapore
Deputy Chief Executive, National University Health System

Integrated Approach to Obstetrics and Gynaecology is a compilation of the collective clinical experience, knowledge and wisdom of the clinical and teaching faculty of the Department of Obstetrics and Gynaecology at the NUS Yong Loo Lin School of Medicine. This book is a labour of love from the Department that has championed the health and wellbeing of Singaporean women for nearly a century.

Edited by Professor Kuldip Singh, eminent scholar and Senior Consultant in Obstetrics and Gynaecology, this textbook is designed to address the needs of our residents and medical undergraduates. It is a compilation of the extensive practical experience and management protocols used at the National University Hospital and in Singapore.

Throughout the book, the clinical management protocols described are founded firmly on evidence–based approaches and international guidelines. The contents encompass the essentials of Maternal Foetal Medicine, Benign Gynaecology, Reproductive Endocrinology and Gynaecological Oncology. It is essential reading for residents and medical students.

I congratulate Professor Kuldip Singh, all the authors and the Department on producing the first locally authored Obstetrics and Gynaecology textbook that comprehensively documents local protocols and management practices at the NUH and other hospitals in Singapore. It is yet another milestone for the Department, which has a long and distinguished history as an international centre of excellence for teaching and research.

FOREWORD

by
Sir Sabaratnam Arulkumaran
Past President of the Royal College of O&G
British Medical Association & International Federation of O&G

The field of obstetrics and gynaecology (O&G) has evolved beyond recognition over the last few decades. This is due to new discoveries like assisted reproduction, advances in knowledge and modern technology like 3D and 4D ultrasound, endoscopic surgery and molecular biology that has made possible the non invasive pre-natal diagnosis. Early years saw each area of O&G practice became a subspeciality. The undergraduates and postgraduates were exposed to four main subspecialties in our field: Maternal Foetal Medicine, Reproductive Medicine, Gynaecological Oncology and Benign and Urogynaecology. Now we recognise the need to treat women's health as a continuum, as nutrition, life styles, health issues, genetic susceptibility and environmental exposure have impact on the developing girl, which continues into adolescence and into reproductive age and postmenopausal years. The department of obstetrics and gynaecology (O&G) at the National University of Singapore has recognised the importance of keeping the integrity of women's health as a life cycle approach than talking about technology and isolated problems.

Accordingly, the O&G Department has come out with an excellent text book *Integrated Approach to Obstetrics and Gynaecology* authored by the staff members. The authors of individual chapters are internationally known experts in women's health. The book consists of chapters in six stages of women's health. The preventive and treatment issues at various age groups are discussed clearly under the topics of the Early Years; Reproductive Years; Pre-conception; Early Pregnancy; Pregnancy (antepartum, intrapartum and postpartum); and Mature Women Functional Aging. This is a comprehensive approach with equal importance paid to all areas. With increased life expectancy, care to improve "healthy aging" is an important aspect as the burden shifts to noncommunicable diseases. All the chapters are well written with clear tables and "boxes" that consists of important messages which makes it easy to read. The management of the O&G problems are based on the guidelines from international bodies and the latest evidence available in the literature. The synthesis of the literature in O&G presented in the book is most suited for medical students and postgraduates starting to specialise in the specialty of Obstetrics and Gynaecology. In comparison to other available undergraduate texts one could consider this book to provide a "concise and complete" knowledge for undergraduates in a life cycle approach and to treat women's health as a continuum. The book is highly recommended for students who should have their personal copies in addition to the library copies.

Sir Sabaratnam Arulkumaran

PREFACE

This textbook has been produced to meet the needs of our medical undergraduates and residents. The authors are mainly our current medical specialists and faculty of our Department of Obstetricians and Gynaecology, National University Health System.

In this book, we have selected clinical problems which the medical students, houseofficers or residents are most likely to encounter in the course of their work.

This book is unique in that we have taken an integrated approach and dwelt with the six phases in the life of a woman, namely the

  (i) Early Years of Growing Up
 (ii) The Reproductive Years
(iii) Conception — Where Life Begins
 (iv) Early Pregnancy
  (v) Pregnancy Care: Antepartum, Intrapartum and Postpartum
 (vi) The Mature Woman and Functional Aging

The style of writing mostly follows on background instructions of history, examination and investigations to establish a diagnosis and then treatment and management. However, this may have been modified as deemed appropriate for a particular topic.

Emphasis has been focussed mainly on information that constitutes essential "core knowledge" in the blueprint of our medical undergraduate curriculum. We have restricted the amount of details on basic reproductive sciences to those aspects that are essential to the understanding the rationale for the diagnosis and management of the common clinical problems in Obstetrics and Gynaecology. Where appropriate, knowledge that is "good to know" has been incorporated beyond the essential "core knowledge."

This book would not have been possible without the invaluable help of our numerous faculty who have written the chapters in the book. I also want to specially acknowledge the timeless and dedicated effort of my administrative officer, Ms Kong Lee Chiu, who, with assistance from Mdm Triffany Tang Sow Fong, my management assistant, has spent long hours and assisted me in countless ways from start to finish. Without them, this book would not have been possible.

I am greatly indebted to:

- Professor Tan Chorh Chuan, President National University of Singapore for graciously writing a Foreword for us.
- Associate Professor Yeoh Khay Guan, Deputy Chief Executive of the National Health System (NUHS) and Dean of the Yong Loo Lin School of Medicine, National University of Singapore for his support and writing a Foreword.
- Associate Professor Aymeric Lim, Chairman, Medical Board of the National University Health System (NUHS) for encouraging me to embark on this project and supporting me throughout the long journey.
- Professor Sir S. Arulkumaran, former President of the Royal College of Obstetricians and Gynaecologists, United Kingdom who has reviewed this book, gave his most useful comments and graciously written a Foreword to us.
- Professor Yong Eu Leong, Head of Department of Obstetrics and Gynaecology, National University Health System (NUHS) for supporting the writing of this book.
- Last but not the least, I would like to thank Ms Lim Sook Cheng from World Scientific Publishing for her help in publishing this book.

The authors and I hope you will find this book useful to read and welcome your feedback.

Professor Kuldip Singh
Senior Consultant and Director of
Undergraduate Medicine Education
Department of Obstetrics and Gynaecology
National University Health System
Singapore

LIST OF CONTRIBUTORS

From the Department of Obstetrics and Gynaecology, National University Health System, Singapore

A. Ilancheran

Anita Kale

Anupriya Agarwal

Arijit Biswas

Arundhati Gosavi

Chan Shiao-Yng

Chong Yap Seng

Chua Tsei Meng

Citra Mattar

Clara Ong

Claudia Chi

Fong Yoke Fai

Harvard Lin

Huang Zhong Wei

Ida Ismail-Pratt

Jeffrey Low

Jeslyn Wong

Joseph Ng

Kuldip Singh

Lim Min Yu

Mahesh Choolani

Mary Rauff

Naushil Randhawa

Ng Kai Lyn

Ng Kwok Weng Roy

Ng Ying Woo

Pearl Tong

Pradip Dashraath

Shakina Rauff

Stephen Chew

Su Lin Lin

Susan Logan

Tan Eng Kien

Vanaja Kalaichelvan

Wong Peng Cheang

Wong Yee Chee

Yong Eu Leong

From the Department of Urology, National University Health System, Singapore

Joe Lee

Part I

THE EARLY YEARS/GROWING UP

Introduction

Adolescent gynaecology is perhaps one of the less familiar areas of gynaecology, traditionally under the remit of paediatricians and poorly taught in the Obstetrics and Gynaecology syllabus. However, with the move towards a life course approach to women's health, gynaecological care of adolescents has evolved into an area of special interest, addressing the health needs of girls aged 10–19 years.

The "Early Years/Growing Up" section starts with discussion of history and examination as this cannot simply be transferred from that undertaken in adult women. Fundamental differences lie in the fact that there are usually two stakeholders — the teenager and her parent (usually mother or another responsible female but sometimes the father). The health needs and concerns of both should be addressed for a successful consultation. Confidentiality, informed consent and the legal aspects relating to sex can be challenging. Sometimes, you may have to see each party separately to get the full picture and assess child protection. Finally, as the majority will not be sexually active, traditional vaginal examination is not possible and alternative approaches, usually in the form of non-invasive imaging, are required.

Following history and examination, puberty and adolescence are discussed, firstly with an outline of normal development and function, focusing on the significant endocrinological, anatomical and psychosocial changes which occur. A comprehensive review of common and less common adolescent problems follows. These may be temporary or may debut long-term issues and may present to the out-patient department or as acute, life threatening emergencies. Abnormal puberty (too early, too late and slow), abnormal uterine bleeding (absent, too little, too much, too painful), the pelvic mass and sexual health (contraception, teenage pregnancy, sexual assault and abuse, sexually transmitted infection) are highlighted owing to their common presentation or importance for future sexual and reproductive function.

1

GYNAECOLOGY HISTORY TAKING AND EXAMINATION

Stephen Chew

History

A careful and detailed history is the first necessary step in any good gynaecological assessment of a patient. Questions should be directed to obtain information on the following.

General. Name, age, years of marriage and parity. This can be conveniently represented as a four box gynaecological code. The first box on the left being for the age of patient, the next box the years of marriage, the third box the number of miscarriages or abortions and the last box for the number of livebirths.

History of presenting illness. This should focus on the presenting problem/complaint that brings the lady to see you. This may be a menstrual problem, infertility or an issue of urinary incontinence. Duration, severity and time course of her illness should be sought.

Menstrual History

Age of menarche. Usually around 12 years, but can range from 9–16 years.

Interval between periods. Classically, the first day (Day 1) of her period is when she has her first heavy flow (vaginal spotting doesn't count). Her menstrual cycle is thus the interval between Day 1 of two menstrual bleeds. As such, most women will report a regular 28 day cycle but this can range between 21–35 days.

Menstrual flow. The amount of menstrual flow should be assessed. Most have 3–4 days of heavy flow followed by another 3 to 4 days of spotting. Presence of blood clots and flooding should be recorded.

Last menstrual period. This refers to Day 1 of heavy flow of the last menstrual period.

Intermenstrual bleeding, post-coital bleeding, postmenopausal bleeding should be specifically sought as these may point to possible gynaecological malignancy.

Dysmenorrhoea. Severity and duration are important as this may point to endometriosis or adenomyosis.

Sexual and Contraceptive History

Information on sexual activity, dyspareunia and the use of any contraception must be obtained in a sensitive manner.

Past History

Previous medical conditions (e.g. diabetes) or previous surgery must be asked about.

Obstetric History

Previous pregnancies, especially miscarriages, ectopic pregnancies and deliveries by caesarean section are important.

Drug History and Allergies

Failure to recognise known drug allergies can lead to serious mistakes with medico-legal consequences.

Family History

Information on diabetes, hypertension and cancers in family members should be sought.

Social History

Occupation, smoking and alcohol intake should be elicited.

Physical Examination

Any examination should be carried out with the patient's consent and in the presence of a chaperone.

General Examination

- General condition
- Vital signs — pulse, blood pressure
- Peripheral signs — anaemia, peripheral oedema, leg swelling
- Neck for any enlarged supraclavicular node
- Heart
- Lungs

Breast Examination is also important, as missing a malignant breast lump has clinical implications for fertility treatment and management of any subsequent pregnancy. Remember, too, that breast cancer can spread to the ovaries (Krukenberg tumours) and may initially present as suspicious ovarian cysts for gynaecological assessment.

Abdominal Examination

The patient should be lying comfortably on her back with the area between xiphisternum and symphysis pubis exposed. Remember to empty the bladder before examination.[1-5]

Inspection

Look out for surgical scars and hernias that may be "hidden" until she is made to cough.

Palpation

Palpation of the abdomen is critical in the assessment of any pelviabominal mass. Hepatomegaly and the presence of shifting dullness are important abdominal signs of malignancy. Generally speaking, one may be able to get below an ovarian mass whereas a uterine mass will rise up above the symphysis pubis, defying all efforts to "get below" it.

Abdominal palpation is also critical in the assessment of a gynaecological patient presenting with pain. Guarding and rebound tenderness are important signs of peritoneal irritation and are present in pelvic inflammatory disease, twisted ovarian cysts, bleeding ectopics/corpus luteums and acute appendicitis.

Percuss for any free fluid in the abdomen.

Auscultation

Auscultation of bowel sounds is also important as gynaecological patients can also present with postoperative ileus.

Pelvic Examination

The pelvic examination must be conducted in a sensitive manner with a chaperone present throughout. The bladder is best emptied unless she complains of stress incontinence.

Inspection

The external genitalia should be inspected and the labia parted to visualise the urethra and introitus.

- Distribution of pubic hair
- Presence of any vaginal discharge, any accompanying skin irritation suggesting a genital tract infection
- Coughing to check for stress incontinence
- Straining to elicit any genital prolapse

Speculum examination

The Cusco or bivalve speculum is the instrument most commonly used to visualise the cervix and vagina. Increasingly, plastic disposable speculums are used and come in standard small/medium and large sizes. However, longer metallic speculums are still useful, especially in cases where the cervix is deep in posteriorly.

Standard lubricants can be used except when a Pap smear is needed; then water may be preferable.

Gently part the labia to expose the introitus before inserting the speculum. Exert gentle pressure posteriorly on the perineum to "create space and distance" from the sensitive urethra. As the speculum is advanced inwards, "horizontalise" the blades such that they now lie transversely in the three o'clock/nine o'clock position. So where is the cervix usually hidden? Generally speaking, for the anteverted uterus (seen in the majority of cases), the cervix is located posteriorly ... so advance in and direct the speculum posteriorly/downwards. Using the plastic speculums, you can sometimes even see the cervix through the clear plastic material.

For the retroverted uterus, the cervix is usually located anteriorly and less deep in compared to the above-mentioned anteverted uterus. It is also useful in this situation to place a firm pillow/support beneath to raise the patient's buttocks. This will enable you to more easily angle the speculum upwards/anteriorly and for you to "lower your head" in order to see the cervix at this awkward angle. Remember, also, that sometimes you may have to withdraw the speculum slightly as the cervix is also less deep in compared to the anteverted uterus.

Once the cervix is visualised, do note its:

- Size
- Shape
- Os (multiparous or nulliparous)
- Transverse slit in nulliparous
- Presence of abnormal polyps, growths, Nabothian cysts and ectropion

A Pap smear should then be taken.

Vagina

The vagina wall should be inspected for:

- Its colour — pink, pale
- Rugae
- Moisture

A well-oestrogenised vagina should be pink, have rugae and be moist.

Bimanual examination

With the labia parted by the left hand, the gloved and lubricated right index finger is inserted into the vagina. By pressing down posteriorly, space will then be created that will allow the right middle finger to be inserted without disturbing the sensitive urethral meatus. The two fingers are then advanced with the palm facing upwards (figure) and the cervix palpated for firmness, masses and tenderness ("cervical excitation").

Cervix

- Position e.g. anterior, posterior, axial
- Consistency
- Mobility
- Tenderness

Uterus

- Position — anteverted, retroverted, axial
- Size of the uterus from normal size to about 12 weeks size
- Mobility
- Tenderness

Adnexae

To assess the right adnexae, the fingers of the left hand are placed in the right lateral fornix and directed down. Meanwhile, the abdominal hand will sweep down to guide any ovarian cyst present towards the waiting vaginal fingers. In fact, it will be the fingers in the vaginal fornix that will be the first to detect any adnexal masses present. The same is done to examine the adnexae on the left.

Examination of the posterior fornix may sometimes reveal the presence of induration suggestive of endometriosis, but classically, thickened and nodular uterosacral ligaments seen in endometriosis are best examined per rectally.

Rectal examination

The rectal examination is sometimes used in patients who have not had sexual intercourse before. The examination is more uncomfortable than the usual vaginal assessment but may be superior in assessing the uterosacral ligaments (in endometriosis) and the parametrium (in cervical cancer).

Reference

1. Monga A, Dobbs S. (2011) *Gynaecology by Ten Teachers*, 19th edn.
2. Hacker NF, Gambore JC, Hobil CJ. (2010) *Essential of Obstetrics and Gynaecology*, 5th edn.
3. Oats JN, Abraham S. (2010) *Llewellyn Jones Fundamentals of Obstetrics and Gynaecology*, 9th edn.
4. Hart DM, Norman J. (2000) *Gynaecology Illustrated*, 5th edn.
5. Edmonds K. (2012) *Dewhurst's Textbook of Obstetrics and Gynaecology*, 8th edn.

2

PUBERTY AND ADOLESCENCE

Susan Logan

Introduction

In this chapter, we aim:

- To understand the normal physiological and endocrinological changes that occur during puberty and adolescence
- To understand common disorders that occur in puberty and adolescence, and the management of these disorders

Puberty is the stage of development through which a child becomes an adult. Puberty is characterised by the following:

- Maturation of the hypothalamic-pituitary-ovarian (HPO) axis and secretion of gonadal hormones (Fig. 2.1)
- Maturation of gametogenesis
- Development of secondary sexual characteristics
- Establishment of fertility

Adolescence comprises the cognitive, emotional, behavioural and psychosocial changes that occur during puberty, from 10–19 years.

Most patients attend with a caregiver, usually Mum, and you may have to see each separately to get the full picture and assess child protection.

Many menstrual disorders that originate in adolescence perpetuate into adulthood.

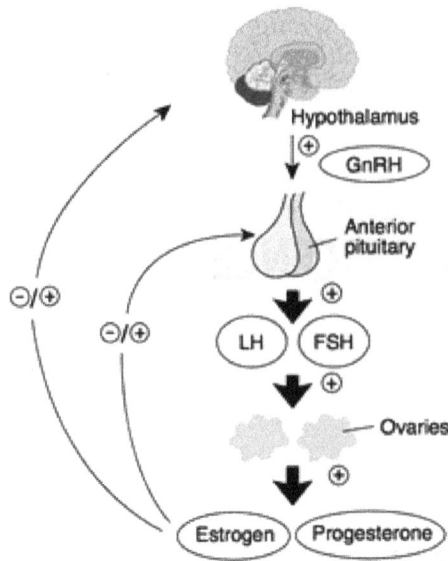

FIGURE 2.1 ■ Female hypothalamic-pituitary-ovarian axis.

Normal Puberty

Puberty in the female comprises a number of stages, usually over four to five years. How puberty starts is unknown but genetics, race, ethnicity, health, nutrition, body fat, hormones, bone maturation and growth factors all play a role. The onset occurs between the ages of 7–13 years and globally appears to be decreasing.[1,2]

Adrenarche starts one to two years before maturation of the HPO axis with the production of adrenal androgens from the zona reticularis of the adrenal gland in response to adrenocorticotrophic hormone (ACTH) secreted by the anterior pituitary. The main hormones are dihydroepiandrosterone sulphate (DHEAS) and dihydroepiandrosterone (DHEA) which rise to a sufficient level to produce pubic hair early in puberty.

Gonadarche comprises ovarian function and the release of sex hormones, which produce secondary sexual characteristics.

Thelarche comprises the initial stage and signifies the onset of breast development. It may be unilateral and each breast may develop at a separate rate.

Pubarche is the development of sexual pubic hair in response to androgens.

Menarche follows thelarche by 0.5–3 years and reflects the endometrial response to the sex hormones. The average age is between 12–13 years. While the HPO axis is maturing, approximately 50% of menses cycles are anovulatory in the first two years following menarche.

Pubertal Stages

Tanner staging or sexual maturity rating are used to evaluate puberty clinically. In females, there are five stages of breast and pubic hair maturity (Fig. 2.2).

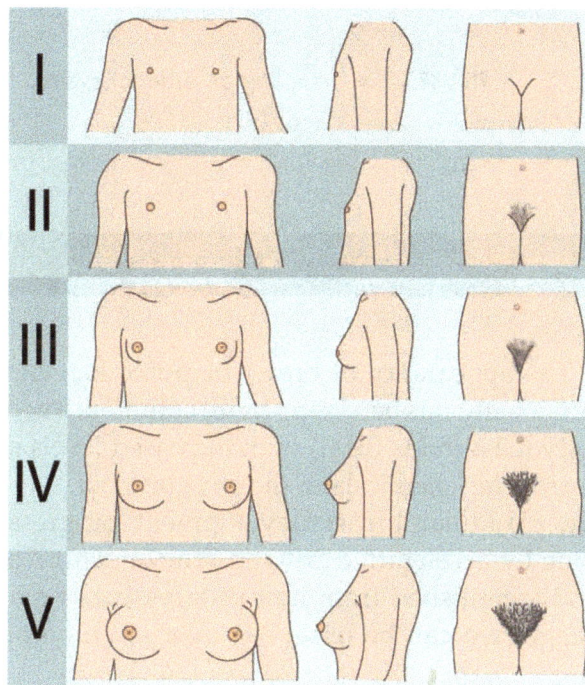

FIGURE 2.2 ■ Stages of breast and pubic hair maturity.

Growth

The pubertal growth spurt usually begins shortly before stage two breast development with peak height velocity (7–9 cm per year) reached within two years. Menarche tends to occur 6–12 months following peak height velocity. Adult height is achieved after complete maturation of the secondary sex characteristics.

Age in years

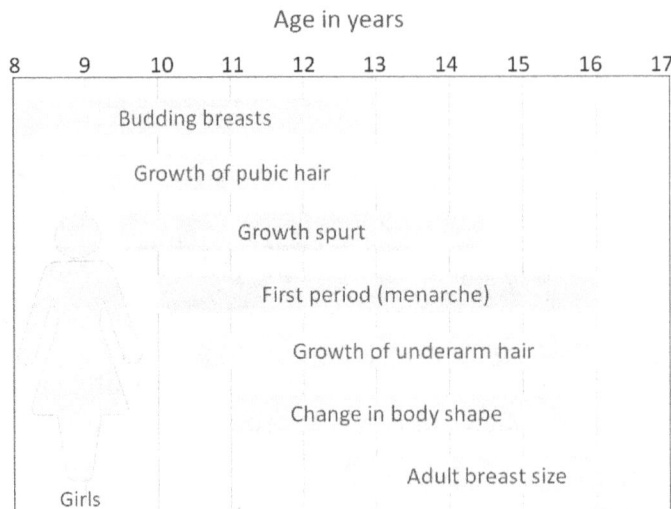

FIGURE 2.3 ■ Time line of pubertal events.

Precocious Puberty

Definition. The appearance of breast or pubic hair development prior to eight years of age. Globally, it is becoming more common. Theories include the influence of higher body mass index (BMI) with increased levels of leptin, derived from fat cells and oestrogenic chemicals in the environment.

Typically, glandular breast development progressively increases with an accompanying by-accelerative growth. True or central precocious puberty (CPP) needs to be distinguished from non-progressive or slowly progressive. Breasts at Tanner stage two can be observed over six months. If already stage three, investigate.

Note: Palpation will distinguish breast development from fat in obese girls.

Investigations

- A random luteinising hormone (LH) test will distinguish between prepubertal and pubertal girls. Oestradiol will also be in the pubertal range. Measurement of adrenal steroids or thyroid hormones is not usually necessary. If the results are equivocal, refer to a paediatric endocrinologist for dynamic testing — measurement of LH following administration of a gonadotrophin-releasing hormone (GnRH) analogue.

- Rapid progression of signs, accompanied by central nervous system symptoms (headaches, visual disturbances) merit a brain magnetic resonance imaging (MRI).
- A pelvic ultrasound is merited in cases of very high oestradiol and suppressed LH, suggestive of an ovarian tumour or large ovarian cyst. While ovarian tumours in this age group are rare, the granulosa cell tumour is the most common and merits treatment surgically by unilateral salpingo-oophrectomy. Large functional cysts can regress without intervention and conservative management should be first line.

McCune Albright syndrome is characterised by rapid breast development and/or a single large ovarian cyst, café-au-lait pigmentation and/or polyostotic fibrous dysplasia (cystic bone lesions).

Management

Patients may present to paediatricians or gynaecologists and are usually managed by paediatric endocrinologists using GnRH analogs. Treatment aims to prevent short stature due to early closure of the epiphyses. The evidence for improved psychological outcomes from delaying physical maturation is less clear. The majority of slowly progressive types achieve normal adult height without treatment.

Variants of Normal

Premature adrenarche comprises an early increase in adrenal androgen secretions which can result in pubic and/or axillary hair and body odour as early as 3–4 years of age. Bloods show an increase in dihydroepiandrostenedione sulphate (DHEAS). No treatment is necessary but girls, particularly those who are overweight, are at increased risk of developing polycystic ovarian syndrome (PCOS). Other rare causes include virilising ovarian or adrenal tumours (associated with clitoromegaly, acne and a pronounced growth spurt) and mild non-classical congenital adrenal hyperplasia (CAH).

Premature thelarche constitutes early breast development, as early as two years of age. Follow-up finds little increase, though it may persist/fluctuate. Unilateral development is common. It can be associated with small ovarian cysts.

Premature menarche is vaginal bleeding in a girl with no breast development when a vaginal foreign body, vaginal tumour and sexual abuse have been ruled out. The cause is unknown and most resolve over a few months. Ultrasound, examination under anaesthesia and vaginoscopy may be required.

Delayed Puberty and Primary Amenorrhoea

This group of girls present with lack of breast development with or without short stature or primary amenorrhoea. While race and ethnic differences are present, investigations should be instigated if there is a lack of breast development by 13 years or absent menarche by 15 years. Lack of progression to the next Tanner stage within a year, or no menarche three years after the onset of breast development, also need investigation. Growth acceleration will also be lacking. Two thirds will have underlying pathology.

Note: The presence of pubic hair, axillary hair and body odour do not reflect a functioning hypothalamic-pituitary-ovarian (HPO) axis as growth is stimulated by androgens from the adrenal gland.

History should include questions about past medical history (chronic medical conditions, hormonal issues, chemotherapy and radiotherapy), family medical history, galactorrhoea, vision issues, sense of smell, eating habits, exercise, stress and changes in height and weight.

Physical examination should include height, weight, BMI, general survey, pubertal staging of breasts and pubic hair. Consider visualisation of the vaginal opening and clitoris.

Poorly executed intimate examinations in adolescence can have long lasting negative effects into adulthood. Consider whether the examination is necessary. Keep Mum or accompanying relative close, minimise observers, let the girl decide the pace and never undertake a speculum/vaginal examination in a girl that has not been sexually active.

Investigations. Check LH and follicle stimulating hormone (FSH). If elevated (hypergonadotrophic), check karyotype and perform a pelvic ultrasound. If low, consider full blood count (FBC), electrolytes, liver panel, thyroid panel, prolactin +/− other pituitary hormones, brain MRI and pelvic ultrasound scan/MRI (presence/absence/size of ovaries and uterus, morphology of ovaries, haematocolpos/vaginal abnormalities) and abdominal USS. Hand and wrist X-rays determine "bone age" and growth potential.

Classification of management of Primary Amenorrhoea is discussed in detail in chapter on Amenorrhoea.

Hyperandrogenism

Hyperandrogenism is characterised by hirsutism, acne and androgenic (male pattern) baldness. In adolescence, while most are idiopathic or caused by PCOS, it may be the first sign of precocious puberty.

History. Ask about menstrual pattern, location/onset/family history/treatment of hirsutism, weight, acne, hair loss. Ask Mum about premature adrenarche. Check height, weight, BMI and BP.

Physical examination. Hirsutism can be assessed using the Ferriman–Gallwey score, although Chinese people are less hairy than Caucasians, who the scoring is based on. A score of over four is suggestive of hirsutism in Chinese girls. Look for signs of Cushing's (striae, buffalo hump/truncal obesity). Look for clitoromegaly.

Investigations. Check total testosterone. If raised, check an early morning 17 OH progesterone, and if raised refer for an ACTH stimulation test to rule out late onset congenital adrenal hyperplasia (CAH). Check DHEAS and if raised, perform a CT scan of the adrenals to rule out CAH. A pelvic ultrasound can assess the ovaries for tumour.

Management

Reduce weight if overweight or obese.

Acne — Facial washes, antibiotics, Roaccutane and combined hormonal contraception improve acne. Remember Roaccutane is teratogenic. Diane35® contains ethinyl oestradiol and cyproterone acetate (an anti-oestrogen) and is licensed for use in cases of moderate to severe acne and mild hirsutism.

Hirsutism — General cosmetic measures such as plucking, waxing, bleaching and permanent hair removal (laser and electrolysis) are encouraged. Combined hormones reduce hyperandrogenism by suppressing secretion of LH and ovarian androgen, while increasing sex hormone binding globulin. Diane35® takes six to twelve months to work. Spironolactone and anti-androgens such as finasteride are also used but take a similar length of time before a clinical difference is appreciated. An adrenal or ovarian tumour requires surgical excision.

Eating Disorders

Eating disorders in adolescent girls are common in Singapore. They often present to a gynaecologist with secondary amenorrhoea or menstrual irregularity, without an appreciation by the girl or her mother that the primary issue is her eating habits.

Classification

(1) Anorexia nervosa (AN)
(2) Bulimia nervosa (BN)
(3) Eating disorder not otherwise specified

Anorexia is associated with potentially life threatening medical and psychiatric morbidity, with mortality rates of 2–8%. It is characterised by refusal to maintain normal weight, an intense fear of weight gain, body image distortion and amenorrhoea. It may be of restrictive type or binge-eating/purging type.

Bulimia is characterised by recurrent episodes of binge-eating, occurring at least twice a week for three months, compensatory behaviour (diet pills, vomiting, laxatives, etc.) and preoccupation with body weight and shape.

History. Primary or secondary amenorrhoea, cold intolerance, dizziness, fatigue, faints, reflux, poor concentration, anxiety and depression, seizures, self-harm and suicide attempts, excessive exercise, preoccupation with calories, weight control measures, and body image concerns.

Note: There are validated questionnaires that can screen for eating disorders (e.g. SCOFF)
S — Do you make yourself **S**ick because you feel uncomfortably full?
C — Do you worry you have lost **C**ontrol over how much you eat?
O — Have you recently lost more than **O**ne stone (6.35 kg) in a three-month period?
F — Do you believe yourself to be **F**at when others say you are too thin?
F — Would you say **F**ood dominates your life?

An answer of "yes" to two or more questions warrants further questioning and a more comprehensive assessment.

Physical examination. Dry skin, hair loss, tooth erosion, parotid enlargement, fractures, bradycardia, hypotension, self-harm scars.

Russell's sign is calluses on knuckles or back of hand due to self-induced vomiting.

Investigation. Height, weight, BMI, BP and pulse. Laboratory tests to exclude other causes of weight loss and amenorrhoea and identify electrolyte disturbances. An ECG may report arrhythmias and a DXA scan can report bone mineral density (BMD) lower than expected for age with a Z score of less than –2.0.

Management. Patients suspected of having an eating disorder should be referred to paediatric specialists comprising a multidisciplinary team of physicians, dieticians, psychiatrists, psychologists and therapists. Most patients will be managed as out-patients but a minority will require in-patient care. A hypotensive, bradycardic girl is potentially a medical emergency and should be discussed with the on call team to assess the need for admission. Most treatment strategies are aimed at the family. Menses resume when weight reaches 90% of median body weight with oestriodiol levels greater than 30 pg/mL. The use of combined hormonal contraception or estrogen hormone replacement to induce menses has not been shown to consistently improve BMD. Judicious use may lull the family into a false sense that all is well and direct the focus away from the eating disorder. Fluoxetine and cognitive behavioural therapy are used to treat BN. Recovery rates for both vary, with high relapse rates.

Obesity

In some countries, adolescent obesity has reached epidemic levels. The World Health Organisation defines obesity as a BMI of 30 kg/m^2 but in Singapore, a BMI of 27.5 kg/m^2 or more represents a higher risk for cardiovascular disease and diabetes.

Obesity in adolescents is associated with the following morbidity (see Table 2.1).

Examination. Abdominal and intimate examinations can be challenging in the obese adolescent.

TABLE 2.1   Obesity Related Morbidity in Adolescents

Reproductive	Irregular menses
	PCOS
	Subfertility
	Unplanned pregnancy
	Pregnancy complications
Non-reproductive	Type II diabetes (NIDDM)
	Hypertension (HT)
	High cholesterol
	Gallstones
	Fatty liver
	Sleep apnoea
	Joint issues
	Poor wound healing
	VTE

Investigations. Consider screening for hypertension, diabetes, hyperlipidaemia and non-alcoholic fatty liver.

Management. Chronic obesity often affects the entire family and specialist units that take a multidisciplinary approach may improve outcomes. Approaches include dietary intervention, increased physical activity and behaviour modification. In adolescents, bariatric surgery is reserved for those with severe obesity (BMI > 50 or 40 with co-morbidity).

Pubertal Abnormal Uterine Bleeding

Normal menarche occurs between 12 and 13 years of age. Cycle length (from 1st day of bleeding to next 1st day of bleeding) usually ranges from 21–45 days. Bleeding lasts from 2–7 days, with 3–4 pad changes. Early cycles are anovulatory, becoming regular after two years.

History. Ask about menarche, cycle length, length of bleeding, number of pads used, blood clots, accidents and pain. Weight change, neurological symptoms (headache, visual field changes), coagulation symptoms (nose bleeds, gum bleeds, bruising easily), hirsutism and acne. The family history may reveal coagulation disorders such as Von Willebrand's disease. Social history may suggest risks of pregnancy or sexually transmitted infection (STIs). Drugs associated with menstrual disturbance include the following: warfarin, anti-psychotics, antidepressants, anti-epileptics and hormones. Traditional medicines may also contain hormones.

Physical examination. In the non-acute setting, check height, weight, BMI and BP. Record staging of secondary sexual characteristics. Does the girl have acne, hirsutism, striae, acanthosis nigrans, petechiae, bruising, goitre, pelvic mass or self-harm scars? Examine the external genitalia but reserve a speculum examination for those who are sexually active. If tumour, foreign body, abuse or trauma is suspected, consider examination under anaesthesia.

Investigations. Ask her to complete a menstrual calendar to document bleeding patterns. A pelvic ultrasound will assess the ovaries and uterus. Pelvic MRI can be used second line where positive findings need further delineation. Common laboratory tests include urinary pregnancy test, haemaccue/FBC, coagulation studies, amenorrhoea panel and sexually transmitted infection testing, where appropriate.

Management

The most common cause of abnormal uterine bleeding (AUB) in an adolescent is anovulation due to immaturity of the HPO axis. This is a diagnosis of exclusion.

Acute

Pubertal AUB can cause significant menorrhagia, with Hb levels below 5 g/dl not uncommon. The girl and her parents often leave bleeding for weeks, expected that it will stop "the next day". As in all cases of bleeding, the girl requires assessment for haemodynamic instability and resuscitation if confirmed. Control of bleeding is achieved using high doses of oestrogen (oral combined hormones or intravenous if oral is not tolerated). Nausea and headaches are common side effects. For those unable to take oestrogen for medical reasons, high dose progestogens are used. If a clotting disorder is suspected, liaise with haematology as haemostatic agents may be required. Severe cases may require an intrauterine balloon tamponade, dilatation and curettage or hysterectomy.

Chronic

In the out-patient setting, AUB can be managed by hormonal and non-hormonal preparations. Combined hormones and cyclical progestogens provide cycle control and reduction in bleeding. Tranexamic acid is an antifibrinolytic which is taken during bleeding. Non-steroidal anti-inflammatory (NSAIDS) drugs will reduce bleeding and pain. Deciding which one to use depends on the diagnosis, whether cycle control, bleeding reduction or both is required and medical contraindications. Treatment should be given over a few months and then stopped to assess whether it is still required.

Sexual Health

Adolescence is a time when girls and boys start to explore sexual feelings and behaviour. In Singapore, it is illegal to have sex (penetration of the penis into the vagina, mouth or anus) with a person under the age of 16, with or without the young person's consent. A girl under the age of 14 years cannot consent to sex. Sex in this case is statutory rape.

Doctors working with sexually exploring and sexually active adolescents need to balance the young person's right to confidentiality against child protection. Health issues including addressing safety, injury, prevention of unplanned pregnancy and sexually transmitted infection must always take precedence, but working within the law. A child protection assessment usually requires the young person to be seen alone and addresses such issues as age at sexual debut, age of partner, type of sexual activity and where it takes place, gifts, school attendance, home circumstances, safety, social media use, medical and mental health issues, self-harm, eating disorders, alcohol, smoking and drugs. Certain groups of adolescents — learning and physically disabled, children of teenage mothers, those with mental health issues, looking after and accommodating children, and LGBT (lesbian, gay, bisexual and transgender) are particularly vulnerable to sexual ill health.

Sex Education

Evidence from elsewhere supports early education in sex and relationships. There is no evidence that this approach encourages early sexual debut. Globally, abstinence programs have failed to reduce unplanned pregnancy rates. Within Singapore, sex and relationships education is provided in school and by outreach programs delivered by community workers. Reputable websites are also a source of reliable information.

Teenage Pregnancy

Most teenage pregnancies are unplanned. Teenage delivery is associated with poorer outcomes for both the mother and the baby. The mother is less likely to finish school and be in employment, more likely to live in substandard housing and is at higher risk of postnatal depression. The child is at higher risk of low school achievement and dropping out of school and becoming a teenage parent herself. In Singapore, the number of babies born to teenage girls is currently at its lowest level in two decades. In 2014, 404 were born to girls aged 19 and below. An alternative to delivery is termination of pregnancy and the number of abortions by girls aged below 20 fell from a high of 1,483 in 2003 to 578 in 2013. This decrease in teenage pregnancy is thought to be due to increased contraception awareness and use of alternative sex acts.

Contraception needs to be discussed and age is not a restriction to any method of contraception.[3–5]

Sexual Assault

Most sexual assault is unreported and involves alcohol rather than drugs. Vulnerable adolescents (see earlier) are at particular risk and most victims will know their assailant. Those wishing to progress a police report should not be examined and told to avoid showering, brushing teeth and washing clothes until a forensic medical examination takes place. These examinations are undertaken in Emergency & Gynaecology departments, depending on the timing of the assault — within 72 hours and > 72 hours, respectively. Standard operating procedures are followed to ensure consistency of history and examination and to preserve the chain of evidence when specimens are taken for analysis. This process is meant to facilitate prosecution of the assailant.

Regarding healthcare, the following areas need to be addressed:

- **Injury** — this takes precedence over forensic medical examination, particularly if life threatening. Depending on the history and apparent violence used, a whole body assessment, including mouth, vaginal and anus may be required
- **Pregnancy** — the risk of pregnancy can be estimated from LMP. It is good practice to offer emergency contraception — the IUD (most effective), LNG (up to three days) or Ella One (up to five days). In about 10% of sexual assaults, pregnancy results. Patients should be followed up to ensure emergency contraception hasn't failed
- **Infection** — the decision to test and give post exposure prophylaxis (PEP) in order to prevention the acquisition of a STI or blood borne virus (BBV) depends

on the type of assault. For example, unprotected assault comprising multiple assailants and trauma in a country with >10% HIV prevalence, means the girl is at risk of bacterial and viral STIs and blood borne viruses, including HIV. *Chlamydia* and gonorrhoea can be tested by endocervical/vaginal swabs or first void urine and *Trichomonas vaginalis* (TV) by high vaginal swab. Syphilis and HIV should be tested routinely. Testing for Hepatitis B and C depends on the history of immunisation, type of assault (traumatic with bleeding) and whether the assailant is known (substance misuser). Consideration can be given to prescribing antibiotics that cover *Chlamydia*, gonorrhoea and syphilis if prevalence rates or history suggests a high risk of transmission. Those at risk of HIV can be given PEP. As this involves giving HIV drugs over a month, is it only recommended in certain circumstances. While there is nothing to prevent Hepatitis C transmission (rare by isolated sexual intercourse), those not protected by natural immunity or vaccination to Hep B can undergo vaccination preferrably within 24 hours or by 2 weeks of the assault. *Chlamydia* and gonorrhoea can be retested three weeks later, HIV and syphilis at three months and the hepatoses at six months to take into account the incubation periods of the bacterial and viral infections

- **Safety** — is it safe for her to return home? Social work and the police may need to assess, and she may need to stay in temporary accommodation until safety can be assured
- **Psychological sequelae** — sexual assault can have short and long lasting effects. Psychosomatic complaints such as headaches, abdominal and pelvic pain are common. Depression, anxiety, and emotional post-traumatic stress disorder may be exacerbated if there were injuries or infection/pregnancy resulted. Volunteer organisations providing post sexual assault counselling and support should be offered to all victims

References

1. Oats JN, Abraham S. (2010) *Llewellyn Jones Fundamentals of Obstetrics and Gynaecology*, 9th edn.
2. Garden A, Hermen M, Topping J. (2008) *Paediatric & Adolescent Gynaecology for the MRCOG and Beyond*, 2nd edn.
3. Clinical Effectiveness Unit of the Faculty of Sexual & Reproductive Healthcare. Contraceptive Choices for Young People, March 2010. http://www.fsrh.org/pdfs/ceuGuidanceYoungPeople2010.pdf
4. BritSPAG: British Society of Paediatric & Adolescent Gynaecology. http://www.britspag.org/
5. NASPAG: North American Society for Paediatric & Adolescent Gynaecology. http://www.naspag.org/

3

MENSTRUAL DISTURBANCES

Stephen Chew

Menstrual Cycles

What's Normal and What's Not?

Menstrual cycles are measured from Day 1 of flow (spotting not counted) to the start of the next period. Most women have 28 day cycles with a range of 21–35 days. In addition, normal menstrual flow usually lasts 3–4 days (up to a week), with blood loss of less than 80 ml.

So What Happens When the Cycle Length Starts to Vary by Shortening or Lengthening?

Generally speaking, menstrual intervals that are longer than 35 days are usually associated with anovulation (e.g. patients with polycystic ovarian syndrome). In contrast, older women (e.g. >40 years) may report shortening menstrual cycles (less than 25 days) and this is caused by a shorter follicular phase.

How About Menstrual Flow?

The often quoted normal menstrual loss of 80 ml is quite useless in daily clinical practice. Which woman, or for that matter, which gynaecologist can accurately ascertain a 80 ml volume of menstrual loss in any patient in a busy clinic. So the key to menstrual blood loss is to ascertain the baseline loss for each woman and to check if her description of her menstrual loss has increased over time. For example,

Madam A reports her normal menstrual flow of four days, but has noticed that it has now increased to six days with clots over the last six months. If you can corroborate this with the fact that her haemoglobin is low at 8 gm%, then her heavier menses (menorrhagia) is clinically significant, requiring investigation, intervention and treatment. In contrast, a patient complaining of heavy periods for the last two years but has a haemoglobin of 13 gm% is less likely to have significant gynaecological pathology.

Abnormal Bleeding Patterns

Some common abnormal bleeding patterns seen in clinical practice include the following:[1-4]

(1) *Menorrhagia:* Regular but heavy and/or prolonged menstrual bleeding. The most common causes are fibroids, adenomyosis and dysfunctional uterine bleeding.
(2) *Post-coital bleeding*: Bleeding seen after intercourse and classically cervical lesions (polyps/pre-cancer/cancer) must be excluded.
(3) *Intermenstrual bleeding*: Bleeding present in between menstrual periods. Oftentimes it may just be post-ovulatory mid-cycle spotting but it is crucial that endometrial pathology (hyperplasia/carcinoma) be ruled out.
(4) *Post-menopausal bleeding*: Any bleeding occurring in the post-menopausal period must be taken very seriously. Cancers (endometrium/cervix) must be ruled out.
(5) *Irregular bleeding*: Irregular episode of vaginal bleeding (**metorrhagia**) is a common gynaecological complaint. It is critical that the so-called irregular menses be properly described and is best seen when it is charted onto a menstrual calendar. A menstrual chart will paint a better clinical picture than a thousand words! Oftentimes the irregular menstrual bleeding may also be heavy and be described as **menometrorrhagia**.

We will be covering only menorrhagia and irregular vaginal bleeding, as post-coital/intermenstrual/postmenopausal bleeding are closely associated with gynaecological cancers which will be addressed in other chapters.

Menorrhagia

Causes

- Uterine fibroids
- Adenomyosis

- Dysfunctional uterine bleeding
- Thyroid dysfunction
- Von Willebrands disease may also present as menorrhagia, as too with disease conditions associated with low platelet counts (idiopathic thrombocytopenia/dengue fever)
- Patients on warfarin or with intrauterine contraceptive devices can also present with menorrhagia

Physical Examination

- Signs of pallor
- Abdominal exam to detect possible pelviabdominal masses
- Speculum to exclude cervical pathology (polyp/cancer)
- Bimanual assessment of the uterine size and shape are also important

Classically, an irregularly enlarged uterus would suggest fibroids, whereas a regularly enlarged womb would point to adenomyosis.

Investigations

- Full blood count to check her haemoglobin
- Thyroid stimulating hormone (if you suspect any thyroid dysfunction) may be done
- A pelvic ultrasound scan would be useful to confirm the presence of fibroids (especially if submucous) and for adenomyosis

Clinical Management

Stopping the bleeding

This is necessary if the patient is presently actively bleeding and already anaemic. This is fairly common in clinical practice, as many patients will delay their visit to the doctor until the bleeding or anaemia becomes physically intolerable. We commonly use the progestogen Norethisterone (10 mg b.d./t.d.s.) and the bleeding should start to reduce within 24–36 hours. Haematinics should also be given to replace her now severely depleted iron stores.

The patient should be kept amenorrheic with continuous Norethisterone (NE) 10 mg b.d./t.d.s until her haemoglobin (Hb) recovers. As a rough guide, the Hb should increase at a rate of around 1 gm% per week. Once a normal Hb is reached, the Norethisterone can then be stopped, to allow her period to return in 3–4 days' time. We are now ready to prescribe medications to reduce her monthly flow.

Reducing the monthly menstrual flow

The following medical treatments can be used to reduce a patient's monthly flow.

Non-steroidal anti-inflammatory drugs (NSAIDS)

Can reduce menstrual blood loss by 20–30% and is best started 1–2 days before the heavy flow is expected. Once the flow is tailing off, the medication can be stopped. A cheap and effective NSAID would be mefenamic acid 500 mg taken 8 hourly.

Tranexamic acid

Can reduce blood loss by 50% when started on the first day of heavy flow. A dose of 1 gram every six hours is commonly used, and taken only during the days with heavy flow.

Combined oral contraceptive pill

Can reduce blood loss as well as provide effective contraception. However, the medication needs to be taken regularly for three weeks and is associated with a risk of thromboembolism.

Mirena (Levonorgestrel intrauterine system)

This intrauterine system releases 20 mg of levonorgestrel daily and provides effective blood loss reduction (> 90%) and contraception for five years. However, it is associated with irregular episodes of breakthrough bleeding.

Dysfunctional Uterine Bleeding (DUB)

Dysfunctional uterine bleeding is a diagnosis of exclusion. It is defined as bleeding from the female genital tract, for which no cause can be found on physical examination and investigations.[1–5]

Causes/Types

Anovulatory DUB

Adolescence (< 20 years of age)

Here the hypothalamic-pituitary-ovarian (HPO) axis is still immature while the ovaries are full of follicles.

The adolescent female presents with irregular cycles or periods of amenorrhoea followed by intermittent/continuous heavy vaginal bleeding that may last for weeks. However, with time as the HPO axis matures, she begins to ovulate and settle down to normal regular cycles.

Perimenopausal woman (> 40 years of age)

Generally, here the ovaries being depleted of follicles despite a mature HPO axis.

These women have irregular bleeding until they reach menopause.

Important that cancer (cervix/endometrium) be actively excluded as a possible diagnosis.

Childbearing years (20–40 years of age)

Irregular anovulatory cycles are less common, but can be commonly encountered in women with polycystic ovarian disease. Alternately, any severe stress or significant weight gain can also cause a woman to start having irregular menstrual cycles.

Ovulatory DUB

Most often seen in the childbearing years and is often due to early degeneration or prolonged function of the corpus luteum. The typical history is often of premenstrual spotting or prolonged spotting after a menstrual flow.

Irregular Vaginal Bleeding

Causes

Common causes of irregular vaginal bleeding are shown in Table 3.1.

Pregnancy must always be excluded right from the outset, as missing an ectopic pregnancy can result in serious morbidity or even death.

Cancers and polyps arising from the cervix and uterus are also important causes.

Irregular vaginal bleeding caused by anovulation is also commonly encountered in clinical practice as described under dysfunctional uterine bleeding (DUB).

TABLE 3.1   Causes of Irregular Vaginal Bleeding

Causes of Irregular Vaginal Bleeding
- Pregnancy (miscarriage/ectopic pregnancy)
- Cancer: cervix/endometrial
- Polyps: cervical/endometrial
- Anovulatory causes: Adolescent period

                                Childbearing period: Polycystic ovarian disease

                                               Stress/weight gain

                                               Thyroid dysfunction

                          Perimenopausal period

Investigations

- A urine pregnancy test is critical in ensuring we don't miss a pregnancy complication or an ectopic pregnancy
- Ensure a Pap smear is done and the cervix well visualised during the speculum examination to avoid missing a large polyp or cervical cancer
- Endometrial sampling using either the Pipelle or at dilatation and curettage is important to exclude endometrial pathology (hyperplasia/cancer). This is generally recommended for women > 40 years old with heavy irregular vaginal bleeding. However, younger women, especially patients with polycystic ovarian disease may also need endometrial sampling. This is because their chronic anovulatory state with its unopposed oestrogen tends to put these women at higher risk of endometrial hyperplasia and cancer
- Blood tests

Follicle stimulating hormone (FSH), luteinising hormone (LH), and prolactin are useful in uncovering possible hormonal causes of anovulation. Thyroid stimulating hormone (TSH) is done if thyroid dysfunction is suspected.

- The pelvic ultrasound scan is useful in diagnosing polycystic ovaries, as well as detecting thickened endometrial linings with cystic changes suggestive of endometrial hyperplasia

TABLE 3.2   Useful Investigations for Irregular Vaginal Bleeding

Urine pregnancy test

Pap smear

Pipelle/Dilatation and curettage

Blood: Full blood count
        Thyroid stimulating hormone
        Follicular stimulating hormone
        Luteinising hormone
        Prolactin

Pelvic ultrasound scan

Clinical Management

The clinical management of patients presenting with irregular vaginal bleeding can be summarised in **3 key steps:**

(1) Ensure you **exclude** any **pregnancy** (urine pregnancy test) and **cancer** (cervical/ endometrium) by carrying out the appropriate tests (Pap smear/endometrial sampling).

(2) **Stop the acute bleeding.** As in the management of menorrhagia as described earlier, patients will need progestogens (Norethisterone) and haematinics. Occasionally, blood transfusions may be necessary if Hb levels are excessively low (e.g. 4 gm%) and the patient very symptomatic. As described earlier, the patient should be kept amenorrheic with continuous Norethisterone (NE) 10 mg d.s./t.d.s. until her haemoglobin (Hb) recovers.

(3) **Medical treatment** (cyclical progestogens/oral contraceptive pills/ovulatory drugs).

For the **adolescent** patient with anovulatory irregular cycles, cyclical progestogens, e.g. Norethisterone (NE) can be used. Doses of 5–10 mg daily taken for 12–21 days can be used. A simple plan would be to take the medication from Day 1 to Day 12 of each calendar month. Alternatively, she can take the medication from Day 5 to Day 25 of her menstrual cycle, but this often causes much confusion to patient and parent alike! A menstrual calendar is also given to track her subsequent menstrual pattern.

For the patient of **childbearing age** with irregular anovulatory cycles, management would depend on her fertility wishes.

For example, if an anovulatory woman has polycystic ovarian disease but is keen on childbearing, ovulatory drugs will correct her anovulation, regulate her cycles and increase her chances of conceiving.

If instead she is keen for contraception, then the oral contraceptive pill would not only provide effective contraception, but will also ensure regular withdrawal bleeds in the future.

For **perimenopausal** women complaining of irregular bleeding, cyclical progestogens can be used, once hyperplasia and cancer have been excluded. As before, a simple regime of NE 5–10 mg daily for the first 12 days of each calendar month will nicely regulate her cycles. This can be continued until she reaches menopause if required.

References

1. Marshburn P, Bradly Hurst. (2011) *Disorders of Menstruation.*
2. Edmonds K. (2012) *Dewhurst's Textbook of Obstetrics and Gynaecology*, 8th edn.
3. Mong A, Dobb S. (2011) *Gynaecology by Ten Teachers*, 19th edn.
4. Hart DM, Norman J. (2000) *Gynaecology Illustrated*, 5th edn.
5. Ehrenthal D, Hillard P, Hoffman M. (2006) *Menstrual Disorders: A Practical Guide.*

4

AMENORRHOEA AND OLIGOMENORRHOEA

Yong Eu Leong

Introduction

- To understand the physiology of normal menstruation
- To recognise amenorrhoea and correlate the clinical presentation with the underlying causes
- To be familiar with principles of investigation and the various modalities of treatment

Physiology of the Normal Menstrual Cycle

- The human menstrual cycle is remarkable in that, instead of homeostasis, the normal condition is a 28–29 day cyclical rhythm
- The menstrual cycle is regulated by hormones from the hypothalamic-pituitary-ovarian (HPO) axis[1,2]
- Environmental influences act on the cerebral cortex, resulting in chemical cues that act on the hypothalamus, resulting in pulsatile secretion of gonadotrophin-releasing hormone (GnRH) (Fig. 4.1A). These 90 minute pulses of GnRH stimulate the secretion of the pituitary gonadotropins, luteinising hormone (LH) and follicular secreting hormone (FSH)
- LH and FSH act in a coordinated pattern to turn on the production of the sex steroids oestrogens and progestogens in a sequential manner to form the follicular and the luteal phases in the ovary cycle (Fig. 4.1B)
- Oestrogens and progesterone induce the proliferative and secretory phases of the endometrium respectively. In the absence of pregnancy, progesterone levels

drop precipitously, the endometrium sheds, and menstruation results. Low levels of oestrogens stimulate FSH secretion to start the next menstrual cycle

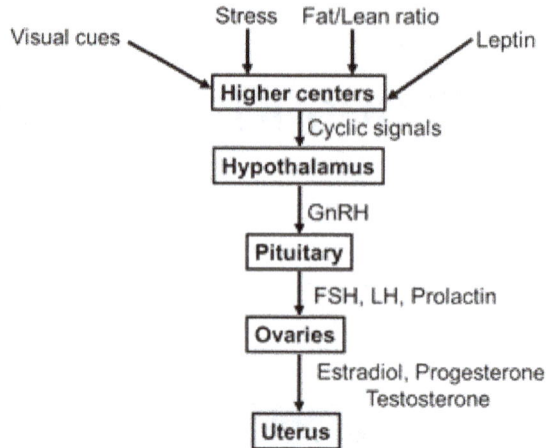

FIGURE 4.1A ■ Regulation of the menstrual cycle by the hypothalamic-pituitary-ovarian axis.

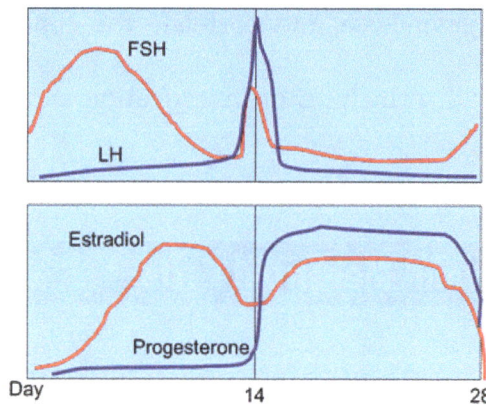

FIGURE 4.1B ■ Hormonal factors regulating the human menstrual cycle. FSH increases oestradiol production in the follicular phase (Day 1–14). The mid-cycle LH surge triggers progesterone production and marks the start of the luteal phase (Day 14–28).

Phases of the Menstrual Cycle

Follicular Phase (14 Days)

- The first day of menstruation marks the start of the follicular phase. In the early follicular phase, oestradiol levels are low, causing FSH secretion to increase through negative feedback (Fig. 4.1B)

- The rise in FSH causes increasing oestradiol production from the dominant follicle
- Oestrogen secretion reaches a peak in the late follicular phase, resulting in a mid-cycle LH surge which causes ovulation and formation of the corpus luteum
- Oestrogens cause proliferation of the endometrium

Luteal Phase (14 Days)

- The LH surge marks the start of the luteal phase. The oocyte is released.
- The dominant follicle is luteinised and progesterone is secreted (Fig. 4.1B)
- Progesterone causes endometrial proliferation to halt and the start of the secretory phase of the endometrium in preparation for implantation
- In the absence of pregnancy, the corpus luteum regresses, endometrium sheds and menses start

Clinical Approach to Amenorrhoea

- A complete menstrual history gives vital clues on the function of the HPO axis. A normal 28 days cycle attests to the health of the HPO axis
- Menstrual history is critical for diagnosis of amenorrhoea and oligomenorrhoea. Points in the history taking, clinical examination and investigation of patients with amenorrhoea and oligomenorrhoea are summarised in Table 4.2
- Measurement of the gonadotropins (FSH and LH) and their target steroid hormones (oestradiol and progesterone) allow classification of the conditions into hypo- or hypergonadotrophic or eugonadotrophic amenorrhoea (Fig. 4.8)
- Management pathways naturally follow once a clear diagnosis is made and these are summarised in (Fig. 4.8)

Primary Amenorrhoea

Primary amenorrhoea is when no menses have occurred by 16 years of age.

Clinical approach. Primary amenorrhoea may be the result of disruption of the hypothalamic pituitary ovarian axis at any of the levels indicated in Fig. 4.1A. Genetic causes have to be considered. The level of HPO axis disruption is indicated by serum FSH and LH levels. The following syndromes, although rare, are worth understanding because they are illustrative of the consequences when the HPO axis malfunctions due to specific genetic mutations.[3,4]

Hypothalamic-pituitary failure (low FSH, low LH, low oestradiol): Kallman's syndrome

The patient exhibits primary amenorrhoea, has poorly developed breasts and secondary sexual characteristics. Anosmia can be present and is pathognomonic. Mutations of the X' chromosomal KAL1 (encoding anosmin), or the fibroblast growth factor receptor 1 genes, results in agenesis of, which indicates isolated hypogonadotrophic hypogonadism wherein other pituitary hormones (TSH and ACTH) are normal. Treatment is by GnRH or hormone replacement.

Ovarian failure (high FSH, high LH, low oestradiol): Turner's syndrome

The patient has only one X chromosome (45, XO). Patients have poor secondary sexual development and may have varying degrees of web neck, wide carrying angle, broad chest with widely spaced nipples, colour blindness, coarctation of the aorta and short metatarsals. They have streak ovaries.

Treatment: Puberty needs to be induced with oestradiol initially, followed by maintenance of secondary sexual characteristics with oestrogen/progestin combination. Genetic counselling with regard to infertility and the possibility of oocyte donation or adoption need to be discussed.

Sex reversal (normal FSH, high LH only, high testosterone): Androgen insensitivity syndrome

Here, chromosomally normal (46, XY) male individuals develop as females. In the complete form, subjects are tall, exhibit female external genitalia, have good breast development (Fig. 4.3). Examination shows the pathognomonic absence of pubic and axillary hair, absence of uterus and a blind ending vagina.

Patients have defects in their androgen receptor gene causing non-functional androgen receptor protein. Complete, partial (Fig. 4.4), and minimal forms (male infertility) exist. They have normal male levels of testosterone, raised LH. In the complete form the sex of rearing is usually female.

Like all sexual reversal syndromes, sensitive counselling of infertility and sexual status need to be undertaken.

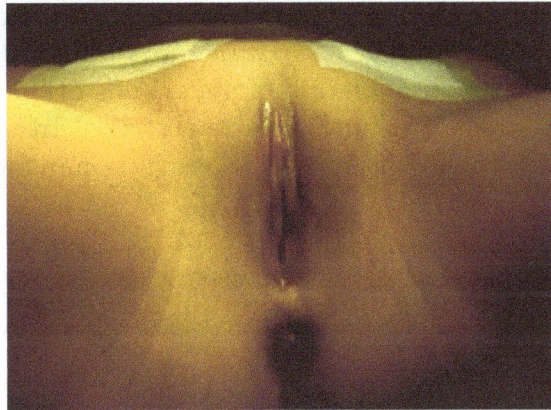

FIGURE 4.3 ■ Androgen insensitivity syndrome (complete type).

Male 46 XY phenotype with female external genitalia: note inguinal incisions where testes have been removed to prevent malignant transformation.

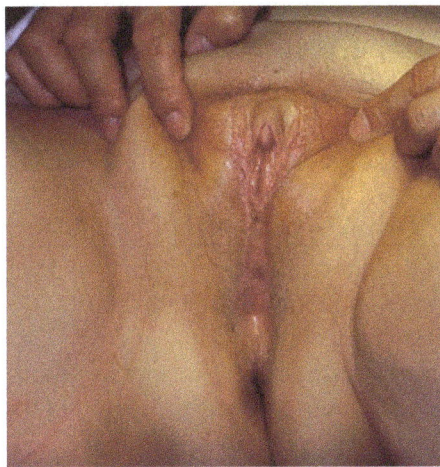

FIGURE 4.4 ■ Androgen insensitivity syndrome (partial type).

Male 46 XY phenotype with ambiguous external genitalia: partial lower labial fusion has occurred and clitoromegaly is present. Surgery to restore female anatomy can be performed.

Outflow tract abnormalities (normal FSH, normal LH)

If the menstrual outflow tract is congenitally undeveloped, primary amenorrhoea results despite a normally functioning HPO axis. *Imperforate hymen* results in monthly pelvic pain at puberty. Examination reveals a pelvic mass cause by blood retained in the vagina (hematocolpos). Acute retention of urine may result.

Treatment with incision of hymen relieves the hematocolpos and restoration of normal menstrual bleeding. *Mullerian agenesis or vaginal atresia* in its various forms result in lack of canalisation of the caudal ends of the mullerian duct. Clinically shallow or no vaginal openings may be observed. Treatment may include passive dilatation of the shallow vagina or reconstruction in more severe cases.

Secondary Amenorrhoea and Oligomenorrhoea

Diagnosis. Disruption of the tightly coordinated menstrual cycle (Fig. 4.1A) results in infrequent menstruation or oligomenorrhoea (defined as menses more than 35 days apart) or amenorrhoea (absence for more than six months) in those who have been menstruating.

Clinical approach. The common causes of secondary amenorrhoea are shown in Table 4.1. Like primary amenorrhoea, secondary amenorrhoea may be the result of disruption of the hypothalamic-pituitary-ovarian axis at any of the levels indicated in Fig. 4.1A. The level of disruption may be usefully diagnosed by measuring serum FSH and oestrogen levels.

TABLE 4.1   Causes of Secondary Amenorrheoa

Hypothalamic-pituitary failure (low FSH, low oestradiol):
   Hypogonadotropic amenorrhoea
   Hyperprolactinaemia
Ovarian failure (high FSH, low oestradiol)
   Ovarian failure: surgery, chemotherapy, radiation
   Menopause: premature ≤40 years
Eugonadotrophic (normal FSH, normal oestradiol)
   PCOS

Hypothalamic-Pituitary Failure (Low FSH, Low Oestradiol)

Hypogonadotropic amenorrhoea can occur in subjects with severe weight loss, or excessive exercise causing a BMI < 19 or body weight < 45 kg. Psychiatric stress, such as anorexia nervosa or those undergoing examinations, may also cause shut down of the pituitary. Pharmacological agents active on hypothalamic-pituitary system include steroidal preparations, psychoactive drugs (antidepressants, anti-psychotics), narcotics, metoclopramide and antihypertensives (methydopa).

Treatment is directed at resolving the underlying cause of the stress. Add back therapy usually in the form of combined oral contraceptive pills may be given to reduce the risk of osteoporosis. Fertility restoration may require the use of ovulation induction with gonadotropins or pulsatile GnRH.

Hyperprolactinaemia due to a prolactin secreting benign tumour of the pituitary may cause up to 20% of all cases presenting with secondary amenorrhoea. Severe cases may be associated with headaches and visual disturbances such as bilateral hemianopia, due to disruption of the visual neuronal pathways by the enlarging pituitary tumour. Breastfeeding and pregnancy have to be excluded. Galactorrhoea may be present. *Diagnosis* is made if persistently high serum prolactin levels are found in those not pregnant or breastfeeding. CAT or MRI scan may indicate the presence of pituitary micro- or macroadenoma (>1 cm diameter) (Fig. 4.5).

Treatment in the first instance is the use of the oral dopamine agonists bromocriptine or longer acting carbegoline. Bromocriptine may initially cause nausea. Persistence with drug therapy usually results in amelioration of adverse symptoms and restoration of menstrual cyclicity within six weeks. Surgery is only very rarely required. Follow-up is with serum prolactin.

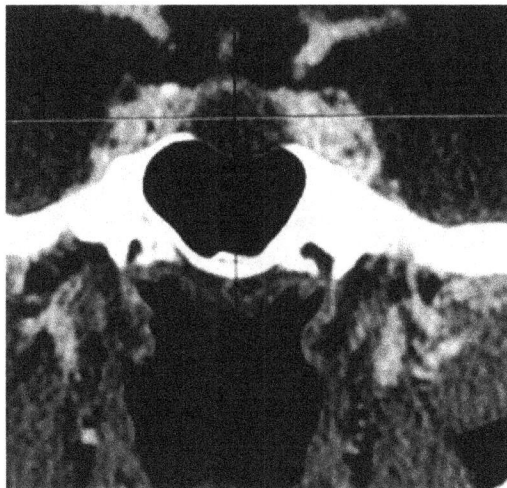

FIGURE 4.5 ■ MRI of pituitary fossa in patient with macroadenoma and hyperprolactinaemia.

Ovarian Failure (High FSH, Low Oestradiol)

Premature ovarian failure is defined as ovarian failure before the age of 40 years. Here, the lack of oestrogen stimulation results in high FSH production due to negative feedback to the pituitary. A common cause of ovarian failure is the surgical removal of the ovaries. Chemotherapy or radiotherapy for breast and other cancers may also result in ovarian failure. Chromosomal disorders like Turner's syndrome, although usually presenting as primary amenorrhoea (see above), may also manifest later (Turner's mosaic: mixture of XX and XO karyotypes).

Treatment with oestrogen and progestin replacement therapy is required to reduce the risk of osteoporosis.

Eugonadotrophic (Normal FSH, Normal Oestradiol)

Polycystic ovarian syndrome (PCOS) is the most common condition in this category. PCOS occurs in 5–8% of women of reproductive age.[5]

Diagnosis. The full condition is defined by the triad of oligomenorrhoea and anovulation, the polycystic ovarian morphology (Fig. 4.6), and hyperandrogenism (clinical or biochemical). Two of the triad is sufficient for the diagnosis. Secondary causes of PCOS including congenital adrenal hyperplasia (late onset), Cushing's disease, adrenal and androgen secreting tumours need to be excluded.

The condition is most common around puberty. The syndrome is named after the ovaries which are enlarged by multiple small follicles that do not develop into dominant follicles but are arrested at antral follicle stage (Fig. 4.7). Increased

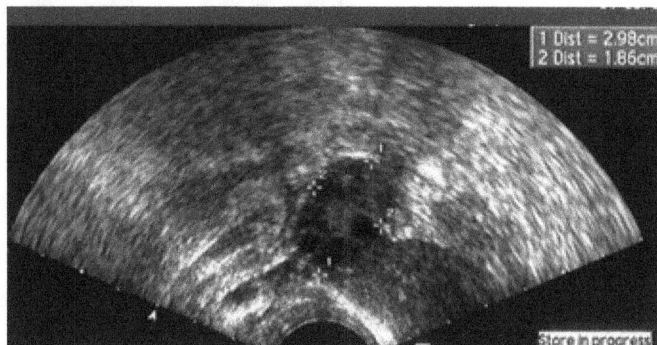

FIGURE 4.6 ■ Transvaginal ultrasound showing polycystic ovarian morphology. Multiple small cysts (>12) with increased ovarian volume (>10 ml) were observed.

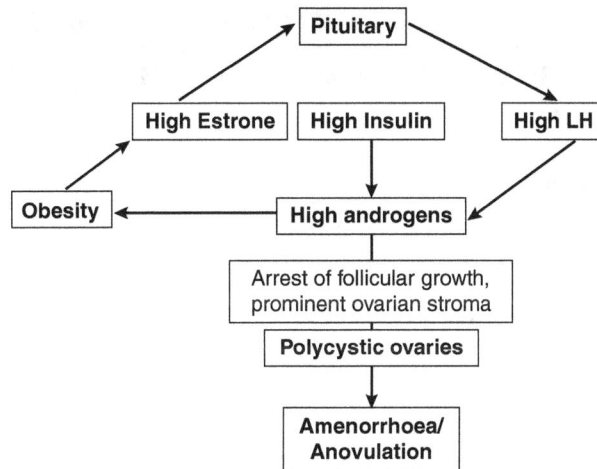

FIGURE 4.7 ■ Pathophysiology of PCOS.

TABLE 4.2

HISTORY TAKING IN CASES WITH AMENORRHOEA
Pregnancy
Primary or secondary amenorrhoea
Developmental milestones
Congenital abnormalities
Menstrual cycle: menarche, regularity, cyclical symptoms suggestive of ovulation
Excessive weight gain or loss, exercise
Menopausal symptoms
Drug history
Virilisation or hirsutism
Galactorrhoea, smell
Recent stressful events
Chronic illness

PHYSICAL EXAMINATION IN CASES WITH AMENORRHOEA
Height, weight/BMI
Visual field defect
Stigmata of chromosomal disorders
Thyroid disease/Cushings's
Blood pressure
Hirsutism/virilisation
Galactorrhoea
Secondary sexual characteristics
External genitalia
Outflow tract abnormalities
Uterus
Ovaries
Adnexal masses

(Continued)

TABLE 4.2 *(Continued)*

INVESTIGATIONS IN CASES WITH AMENORRHOEA
Beta-hCG
FSH, LH
Oestradiol
Prolactin
Testosterone
Thyroid function
Ultrasound pelvis
Primary amenorrhoea:
  Karyotype
  Bone age
  MRI brain

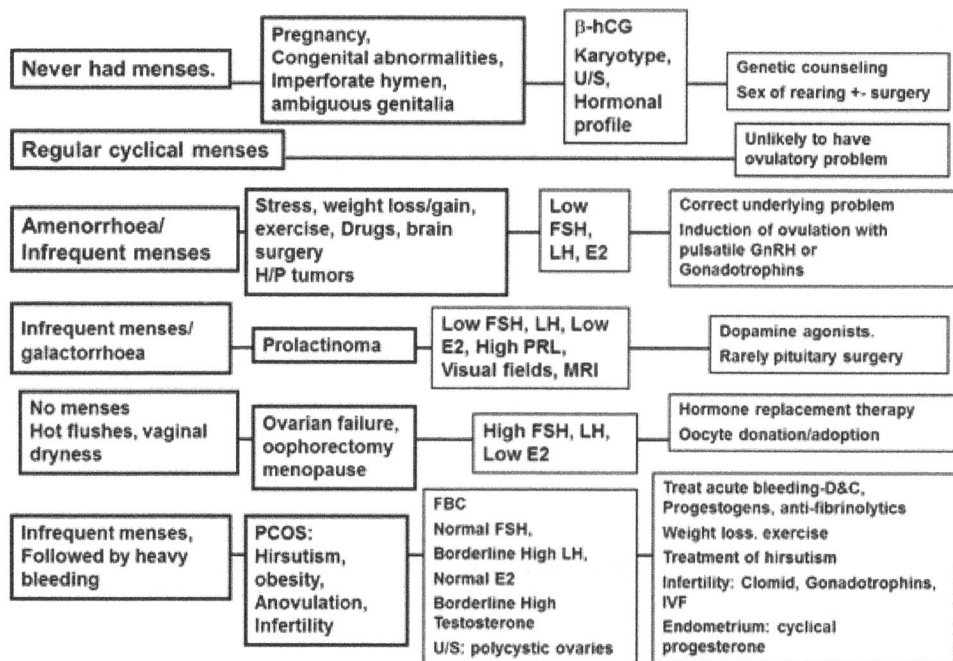

FIGURE 4.8 ■ Summary of Management of Amenorrhea/Oligomenorrhoea.

secretion of LH stimulates testosterone secretion from the theca cells of the ovary. Clinical hyperandrogenism may manifest as hirsutism, but these vary with ethnic group and may not be evident in subjects of East Asian descent. Milder forms of the syndrome, with two of the three conditions can be observed. PCOS is made worse with obesity and its resultant metabolic syndrome, hyperinsulinaemia and insulin resistance syndromes. The aetiology of the syndrome remains unclear but a situation of homeostasis exists wherein borderline high intraovarian androgen levels result in arrested follicular development.

Clinical significance is due to anovulation and associated infertility. Restoration of ovulation may be obtained with ovulation inducing agents such as clomiphene, metformin or injections of gonadotropins. Some subjects require assisted reproduction technologies such as *in vitro* fertilisation and embryo transfer for successful pregnancies. The risk of ovarian hyperstimulation syndrome with the use of ovulation inducing agents is higher with PCOS. Surgical ovarian resection and drilling to reduce stroma may reduce endogenous testosterone and restore ovulation. These, however, may result in tubal adhesions. Those pregnant have a higher risk of miscarriages and gestational diabetes (Fig. 4.5).

Anovulation and resultant lack of progesterone can also result in endometrial hyperplasia, and it is necessary to induce cyclical secretory changes with cyclical progesterone preparations for at least four months a year. Oral contraceptive agents containing progestogens may be used to suppress LH production and restore menstrual cyclicity.

Hyperandrogenism may result in troublesome facial hirsutism which can be resolved with anti-androgens such as cyproterone acetate or by cosmetic removal of unwanted hair.

In the longer term, PCOS patients have higher risk of adult onset diabetes, obesity, metabolic syndrome and diabetes. Exercise, weight loss, and the anti-diabetic medication metformin are effective therapies.

References

1. Mong A, Dobb S. (2011) *Gynaecology by Ten Teachers*, 19th edn.
2. Edmonds K. (2011) *Dewhurst's Textbook of Obstetrics and Gynaecology*, 8th edn.
3. Fritz MA, M Speroff Leon. (2011) *Clinical Gynaecologic Endocrinology and Infertility*, 8th edn.
4. Fourman LT, Fazeli PK. (2015) Neuroendocrine causes of amenorrhea — an update. *J Clin Endocrinol Metab*. **100**(3):812–824.
5. Yong EL. (2016). Polyycystic ovarian syndorome: Best Practice & Research: Clinical Obstetrics and Gynaecology. **30**:8.

5

DYSMENORRHOEA

Yong Eu Leong

Introduction

- To understand the definition of dysmenorrhoea and the common cause(s)
- To be able to provide initial treatment for primary dysmenorrhoea
- To understand the approaches in the management of the common causes of secondary dysmenorrhoea
- To be able to counsel on basic side effects and complications of the different modes of treating endometriosis and adenomyosis

Physiology

- Most women suffer some menstrual cramps during their menstrual periods. Such cramps may precede menstruation by several days or may accompany it, and it usually subsides as menstruation tapers off
- It is usually caused by uterine contractions, dilatation of the cervix and expulsion of menstrual blood. Prostaglandin release is the cause of menstrual cramping and discomfort
- Interestingly, mild menstrual cramps are a feature of normal ovulatory cycles and usually appear within 6–12 months of menarche

Dysmenorrhoea is the medical condition whereby pain during menstruation interferes with daily activities.

- About 50% of women are affected by dysmenorrhoea, and 10% have severe symptoms that necessitate time off work
- Symptoms of dysmenorrhoea can begin after ovulation and last until the end of menstruation
- The use of certain types of oral contraceptive pills can prevent the symptoms of dysmenorrhoea, because the birth control pill stops ovulation from occurring

Pathophysiology

- During the secretory phase of the menstrual cycle, the endometrium thickens in preparation for potential pregnancy
- In the absence of pregnancy, progesterone drops and the built-up endometrial lining is not needed and sheds as strips of decidual tissue
- During this process of decidual shedding, prostaglandins and other inflammatory mediators are released
- Prostaglandins cause uterine contractions which squeeze the decidual tissue through the cervix and out of the body through the vagina. These contractions, cervical dilation and the resulting temporary oxygen deprivation to nearby tissues are responsible for the pain or "cramps" experienced during menstruation
- Compared with other women, women with primary dysmenorrhoea have increased activity of the uterine muscle, with increased contractility and frequency of contractions. In dysmenorrhoic patients, magnetic resonance imaging can show features on cycle days 1–3 that correlate with the degree of pain

Definitions

Primary dysmenorrhoea is painful menstruation where there is no underlying pathology.

Secondary dysmenorrhoea is associated with organic pathology, usually appearing several years after menarche.

Primary Dysmenorrhoea

Clinical Features

Most women begin to have pain within two years of menarche with the commencement of ovulation. Cramping usually begins a few hours before the onset of menstrual bleeding. It may persist for some hours or days. Pain is centred at the lower abdomen and may radiate to the back. Severe cases may have nausea and headache. Clinical and pelvic examination is normal.[1-3]

Treatment is conservative with oral analgesia and contraceptive pills.

Nonsteroidal anti-inflammatory agents (NSAIDS) such as ibuprofen (400 mg 6H), naproxen sodium (250 mg 6H), and mefenamic acid (500 mg 6H) are highly effective. For more severe cases, NSAIDS can be combined with paracetamol (500 mg 8H).

Oral contraceptives reduce the amount of menstrual bleeding and pain. Injectable progestogens such as Norplant or depot medroxyprogesterone acetate (DMPA) are also effective, since these methods often induce reduced menstrual bleeding or even amenorrhoea. The intrauterine system (Mirena IUD) has been cited as useful in reducing symptoms of dysmenorrhoea.

Psychotherapy, hypnotherapy and heat therapy may also be helpful.

Secondary Dysmenorrhoea

Menstrual pain may be secondary to other causes. Common causes are:

- Endometriosis.
- Adenomyosis.
- Uterine fibroids, especially the sub-mucous variety (refer to Menstrual Disturbances chapter).
- Chronic pelvic inflammatory disease (refer to STI and PID chapter)
- Intrauterine contraceptive device, IUCD (refer to "Contraception and Family Planning" chapter).

Endometriosis and adenomyosis will be discussed in detail in this chapter. For other conditions please refer to indicated chapters.

Diagnostic Features

A careful menstrual history and examination in many cases will suggest the diagnosis. A history of fever with smelly discoloured vaginal discharge may suggest chronic PID. A history of IUCD insertion is important. Progressively severe dysmenorrhoea may indicate endometriosis. Past surgical history, including previous laparoscopies or laparotomies, will indicate pre-existing pelvic disease.

Endometriosis

Dysmenorrhoea and infertility are common presenting complaints for endometriosis (defined as endometrium outside its normal location within the lining of the uterus).[4]

- Endometriosis is a common condition that affects ~6–7% of all females and may be encountered in up to 20–25% of women undergoing laparoscopic tubal ligation
- 30–40% of women with endometriosis are subfertile. Surprisingly, severe dysmenorrhoea may be associated with milder disease
- Endometriosis-associated infertility can be related to scar formation and anatomical distortions due to the endometriosis.
- On the other hand, large endometriotic cysts (> 5 cm in diameter) can be observed in those with progressive disease. These "chocolate" cysts of the ovaries contain thick viscid brown-coloured altered blood that is intensely inflammatory when in contact with the peritoneum
- Rupture of these chocolate cysts causes acute abdomen necessitating emergency surgery, peritoneal lavage and cystectomy
- Lesser degrees of leakage of chocolate material may result in formation of peritoneal and omental adhesions, resulting in bowel and ureteral obstruction in the most severe cases

Ectopic endometrium may also manifest as cyclical pain outside the pelvis, such as in LSCS scars, umbilicus and other sites in the abdomen and chest. For example, pleural implantations are associated with recurrent right pneumothoraces at times of a menstrual period, termed catamenial pneumothorax.

Pathophysiology. The main theories for the formation of ectopic endometrium are retrograde menstruation, coelomic metaplasia and transplantation.[5]

Physical examination for endometriotic involvement of the uterosacral ligaments is important. Vaginal and rectal examination may reveal thickened and tender utero-sacral ligaments. Tender nodules in the recto-vaginal septum may represent deep infiltrating endometriosis which is very difficult to treat. Pelvic abdominal masses may be palpable on abdominal examination and represent large endometriotic cysts.

Investigation with pelvic sonography might show typical ovarian cysts filled with low echoes, suggesting the presence of altered blood. The presence of multiple loculated cysts and the presence of solid areas should alert us to the possibility of ovarian neoplasm and merit further investigation and biopsy for histological examination. Endometrioid cancer of the ovary can occur in endometrial cysts. Tender nodules shown on ultrasound may represent endometriotic deposits in the pelvis or elsewhere (Fig. 5.1).

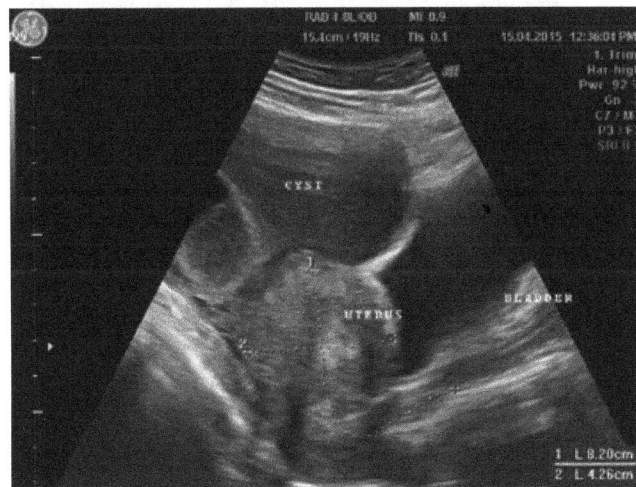

FIGURE 5.1 ■ Ultrasound of low-echo endometriotic cyst.

Treatment

Medical treatment of menstrual pain with oral analgesia and oral contraceptives do not differ from that of primary dysmenorrhoea (described above).

- Progestogens administered orally, or injected such as DMPA, creates a pseudo-pregnancy state that prevent growths of endometriotic deposits and reduces pain
- Dienogest (trade name Visanne) is a progestogenic agent, used continuously, that has been approved for endometriosis
- GnRH depot preparations create an artificial menopause. These are effective, but bone loss is an issue with long-term use

Diagnostic laparoscopy may be needed in those with severe chronic pelvic pain in order to confirm the disorder. Match-head deposits of endometriosis in the pelvic peritoneum may be observed, and when ablated by cautery may resolve dysmenorrhoea.

Surgical treatment:

- Surgical ablation and excision of endometriosis (laparoscopic/open) (Fig. 5.2)
- Cysts larger than 5 cm in diameter are unlikely to respond to conservative therapy and may need to be surgically removed
- Hysterectomy to prevent recurrence
- Pelvic clearance for frozen pelvis associated with intractable chronic pelvic pain

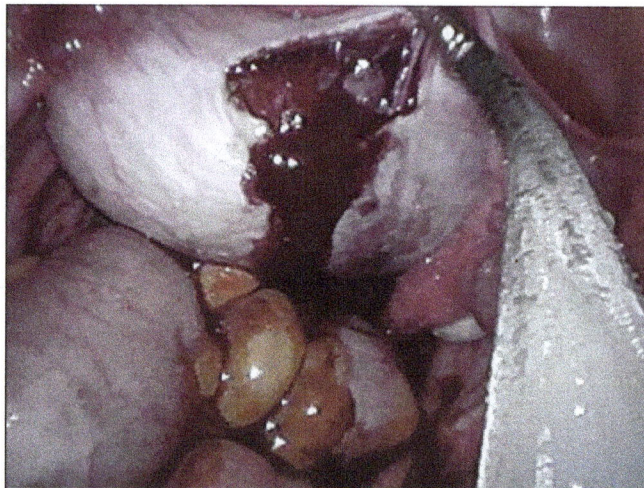

FIGURE 5.2 ■ Laparoscopic view of chocolate cyst.

Adenomyosis

- Adenomyosis refers to endometrial implants in the myometrium, located outside its normal site in the lining of the uterus
- These endometrial implants respond to oestrogen stimulation and progesterone withdrawal to bleed
- Since these endometriotic implants cannot be discharged through the vagina, they result in uterine enlargement
- The increased surface area and vascularity of the uterus affected by adenomyosis result in excessive menstrual bleeding and dysmenorrhoea

Although both adenomyosis and endometriosis are due to ectopic endometrium, the pathophysiology of these two conditions differs significantly. Adenomyosis affects ~20% of women. The majority of patients are between 40 and 50 years old, parous (80%), but incidence does not correlate with increasing parity. Adenomyosis also has high association with other uterine disorders (fibroids 50%, endometriosis 11%, endometrial polyps 7%).

The presence of dysmenorrhoea with increasingly heavy menstrual bleeding strongly suggests adenomyosis, the other differential being sub-mucosal polyps or fibroids. Enlarged uterus may also produce bladder symptoms. Subfertility may also result.

Examination reveals an enlarged, globular uterus that is tender. This is distinct from uterine fibroids, which tend to produce an irregular, lumpy uterus.

Transvaginal ultrasound shows an enlarged uterus. The presence of subendometrial linear striations has the highest diagnostic accuracy for adenomyosis. (Fig. 5.3)

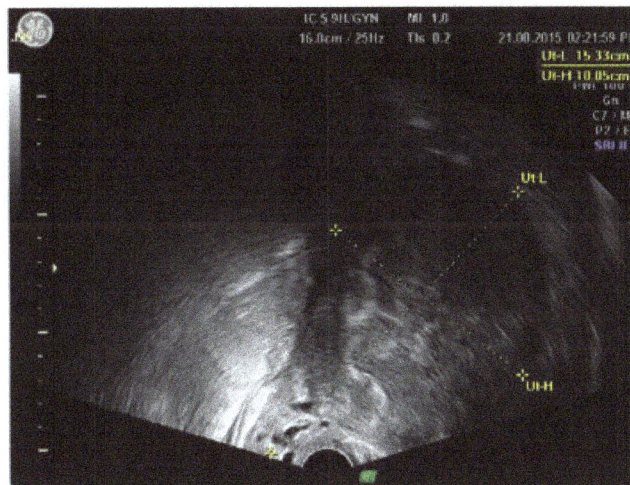

FIGURE 5.3 ■ Ultrasound view of adenomyosis.

Conservative treatment often consists of analgesics such as ibuprofen or other NSAIDs. Hormonal manipulation may include combined or progestin-only oral contraceptives, as well as other options such as transdermal patches and progesterone-releasing intrauterine devices. Hormonal suppression may be used in the form of danazol or a gonadotropin-releasing hormone agonist. These medications simulate menopause, a period in which adenomyosis often resolves naturally.

Based on one's desire for future fertility and the size of the lesion, surgical options may include endometrial ablation, laparoscopic myometrial electrocoagulation and adenomyomal excision.

Unlike fibroids, adenomyosis does not have a capsule and cannot be easily shelled and removed surgically. Although wedge resection may be done for those who wish conservative surgery, the operation is technically difficult, with closure of the uterine wound an issue. Hysterectomy is the definitive treatment, if pain management with analgesics is not effective.

Chronic Pelvic Pain

Chronic pelvic pain refers to pain of more than six months' duration. Careful evaluation is necessary to differentiate gynaecologic conditions from gastrointestinal, orthopaedic, urological and neurological pain. Abnormal bowel movements (gastrointestinal), one-sided lower abdominal pain radiating to lower limbs (spinal and orthopaedic), dysuria and frequency (urological) need to be carefully evaluated and may indicate relevant investigations. Nonetheless, chronic pelvic pain can be very debilitating and needs specialist referral and evaluation.

References

1. Edmonds K. (2012) *Dewhurst's Textbook of Obstetrics and Gynaecology*, 8th edn.
2. Fritz MA, M Speroff Leon. (2011) *Clinical Gynaecologic Endocrinology and Infertility*, 8th edn.
3. Lacovides S, Avidonn I, Baker FC. (2015) What we know about primary dysmenorrhoea today: A critical review. *Hum Reprod Update.* **21**(6):762–778.
4. Hansen SO, Knudsen UB. (2013) Endometriosis, dysmenorrhoea and diet. *Eur J Obstet Gynecol Reprod Biol* **169**(2):162–171.
5. Ju H, Jones M, Mishra G. (2014) The prevalence and risk factors of dysmenorrhoea. *Epidemiol Rev* **36**:104–113.

Part II

REPRODUCTIVE YEARS

Introduction

Reproductive gynaecology is a more familiar area to medical students, addressing the health needs of women aged 20–50 years. Within a woman's life course, gynaecological issues often become the sole reason for personal contact with healthcare professionals at this stage. Many women will be fit and healthy, seeking advice on disease prevention and health promotion. Sexual relationships are usually established during this time and can play an important role in a woman's physical, emotional, mental and social well-being. However, due to the personal and sensitive nature of sex, woman may delay bringing concerns to the attention of healthcare staff, with life ruining and even life threatening consequences. Doctors can reduce this risk by taking a sexual history routinely as part of holistic care. The more you ask, the more comfortable you will get at asking questions of a personal nature. Finally, as this stage covers some 30 years, the social trends of increased marital delay and breakdown and smaller numbers of pregnancies give rise to the development of a variety of gynaecological conditions which would have previously been protected by pregnancy and breastfeeding.

The topics in this section — contraception, cervical screening, abnormal smear, vaginal discharge, vulval itch, sexually transmitted infections and family planning have been chosen based on the frequency of presentation, importance for future sexual and reproductive function and potential life threatening emergencies. Basic science input lays the foundation for key points to elicit in the history and examination. Investigations, be it radiological, cyto-pathological, viral or bacteriological, play an important role in confirming the diagnosis. The issues highlighted may be seen in a well woman, one with signs or symptoms but ambulatory or one who is acutely ill. Being able to recognise an ill woman with a gynaecological complaint is a key skill to attain. Management must be sensitively approached taking into account the woman's cultural and religious beliefs, past and family medical history, drug history, sexual history and reproductive plans. Key points covering psychological, medical and surgical aspects of care are discussed.

6

ABNORMAL SMEAR AND CERVICAL SCREENING

Ida Ismail-Pratt and Jeffrey Low

Introduction

Worldwide, cervical cancer is the fourth most common cancer in women, with 528,000 new cases diagnosed in 2012. Around 85% of these new cases occur in developing countries, leading to 266,000 deaths. This accounts for 7.5% of all female cancer deaths globally.[1]

The incidence and mortality of cervical cancer in developed countries is much lower. In most developed countries such as United Kingdom, an organised cervical cancer screening programme has led to significant reduction in cervical cancer incidence and mortality.

Screening for cervical cancer is a recognised method of cervical cancer prevention. The disease has a long natural history with a well-established pre-malignant phase. The cervix is also easily accessible and detection of pre-malignant disease is possible using a simple test. These criteria fit the WHO definition for screening (Table 6.1) making cervical cancer a suitable cancer for mass screening.

TABLE 6.1   WHO Criteria for Disease Screening

(1) Important health problem
(2) Accepted treatment for recognised disease
(3) Facilities for diagnosis and treatment
(4) Suitable latent and symptomatic stage
(5) Suitable test or examination
(6) Test acceptable to population
(7) Natural history of condition understood
(8) Agreed on policy on whom to treat
(9) Cost of finding economically balanced with overall health
(10) Case finding should be continuous process

In Singapore, cervical cancer is the 10th most common female cancer (Fig. 6.1). The incidence rate of cervical cancer in Singapore has steadily declined over the years, from 16.8 per 100,000 in 1974–1978 to 6.9 per 100,000 in 2009–2013.[2]

In terms of mortality rates, cervical cancer is the 8th cause of death in Singaporean women.

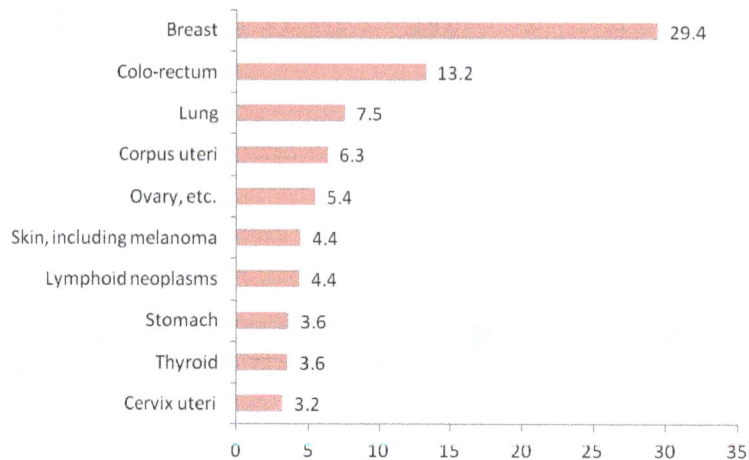

FIGURE 6.1 ■ Ten most frequent cancers in Singapore females (%) in 2009–2013.[2]

The aim of this chapter is to provide basic knowledge and outline the principles of cervical cancer prevention and screening, including the important role of human papillomavirus (HPV), not only in the aetiology of cervical cancer but also in how it has influenced the modern approach to cervical cancer prevention and screening worldwide.

Aetiology

Human Papillomavirus (HPV)

Professor Harald zur Hausen, a German physician, was the first to discover the association of HPV infection and cervical cancer.[3] This very important finding is now the base of the current development in cervical cancer prevention and screening that will be discussed in this chapter.

The papilloma virus is a small DNA virus that has a double stranded, tightly coiled circular genome of about 8,000 Da. It is species specific. The human papillomavirus (HPV) is specific only to humans, and currently more than 100 types of HPV virus have been identified.

All viruses, including the HPV, are obligate intracellular parasites, which means that they cannot survive outside their target cells. Because of this, a HPV virus will always be trying to infect a susceptible host through skin, mucosa of the eye, oral cavity, urogenital tract or respiratory tract, to name a few. About 30–40 types are associated with anogenital tract infection. They can further be divided into two sub-types: (1) high risk types/oncogenic (causes cervical cancer) and (2) low risk types/non-oncogenic (non-cancer causing).

HPV infection is very common in sexually active people. It is reported that 9 out of 10 sexually active people will have a HPV infection at some point in their life. In the majority of cases, the body's immune system will eradicate the virus. Some HPV infection will cause genital warts. Only a small percentage of these viruses will cause abnormal Pap smear and cervical cancer.

There are more than 100 types of HPV virus. The majority are harmless and asymptomatic. The most common manifestation of HPV infection is genital warts. HPV 6 and 11 cause 90% of genital warts. Most genital warts are also harmless, but some can grow and become cosmetically unsightly and occasionally cause bleeding and pain.

Approximately 14 types of HPV virus are related to cervical cancer and are also known as oncogenic viruses. Out of these 14 types, HPV 16 and 18 cause 70% of cervical cancer. Other HPV types related to cervical cancer are seen in Table 6.2.

It is important to understand that not all HPV infection will lead to cancer. In fact, cervical cancer is an uncommon manifestation of a very common infection.

TABLE 6.2   Different Manifestations of HPV Infection

Harmless — No warts or cancer	
Genital warts	• HPV 6 and 11 make 90% of genital wart infections
Cancer related	• Most clear up
Type 16, 18 (70% of cervical cancer)	• Some persist, but no abnormalities on the cervix
Type 31, 33, 35, 39, 45, 51, 52, 56, 58, 59, 68	• Some persist and cause low grade and high grade abnormalities of the cervix
	• A much smaller number progress and become cervical cancer

Anatomy of the cervix

In order to fully understand the mechanism of HPV infection, and management of preinvasive disease and cervical cancer, a sound understanding of the anatomy of the cervix is crucial.

The cervix is a cylindrical fibromuscular organ that connects the vagina to the uterus. It can be divided into the ectocervix and the endocervix.

The **ectocervix** is a readily visible portion of the cervix situated at the top of the vagina. It is lined by stratified squamous epithelium, consisting of multiple layers of cells. It is a tough epithelium, as it needs to withstand the harsh acidic environment of the vagina. On direct visualisation, it gives the cervix a smooth appearance.

The **endocervix** is not readily visible and makes up the endocervical canal portion of the cervix. It is lined by a thin, single layer columnar epithelium.

The junction where the stratified squamous epithelium and single layer columnar epithelium meet is called the squamocolumnar junction (SCJ). The position of the SCJ in relation to the external os varies depending on various factors such as age, menstrual status, pregnancy and oral contraceptive use. Under the influence of oestrogen, such as following menarche and pregnancy, eversion of the columnar epithelium onto the ectocervix happens. On direct visualisation, the cervix can appear to be "raw looking" and is commonly incorrectly known as cervical erosion. This condition is a normal physiological change of the cervix called cervical ectropion.

The everted columnar epithelium will undergo changes, with a progressive change to the tougher stratified squamous epithelium taking place. This is called squamous metaplasia and is due to exposure of columnar epithelium to the acidic environment of the vagina.

The region where squamous metaplasia occurs is called the transformation zone.

The transformation zone is an area between the old and new SCJ. This is an important area in terms of cervical cancer prevention because almost all preinvasive disease and cervical cancer occurs in the transformation zone.

Risk factors for HPV infection

The risk factor for HPV infection leading to cervical cancer depends on the degree of exposure to the infection and the body's ability to combat infection. Women who are sexually active, have multiple partners, have partners who have had multiple sexual partners and early onset of sexual intercourse have a much greater exposure to HPV infection that those who have never been sexually active.

Likewise, a person with a strong immune system or defense against infection will have a better ability to prevent HPV infection than those who have a lower immunity. Cigarette smoking is an independent factor that also increases the risk of women getting an HPV infection that can lead to cervical cancer in the future (Table 6.3).

The mechanism of HPV infection is also known as the *"Seed and Soil Theory"*. Like any plant, for it to grow and spread, it will start from a seed which will need to land on the transformation zone of the cervix. Having only a seed and soil will not be sufficient to get the seed to grow. Other cofactors such as sun, water, nutrients and sunlight will also be required.

Similar to this analogy, the HPV virus itself on the transformation zone is not sufficient to cause pre-cancerous cells or cervical cancer. Other cofactors (risks of HPV infection as per Table 6.3) will be needed to encourage the HPV virus to grow and effect changes (Table 6.4).

TABLE 6.3   Risk Factors for HPV Infection

Increase Exposure to HPV Infection	Decrease Immunity/ Defense Against HPV Infection
• Onset of sexual intercourse at an early age • Multiple sexual partners (either partner)	• Cigarette smoking • HIV infection • History of sexually transmitted infection • Immunosuppression

TABLE 6.4   The Seed and Soil Theory

Seed	HPV
Soil	Cervical transformation zone
• Cofactors • Water • Nutrients • Sunlight • CO_2 • O^2	• Cofactors • HIV infection • Cigarette smoking • Immunosuppression • History of sexually transmitted infections • Multiple sexual partners (either partner) • Onset of sexual intercourse at an early age

Cervical Cancer Prevention

Cervical cancer prevention comprises of three aspects.

- **Primary prevention**: Preventing the initial infection by HPV virus. This can be done through HPV vaccination, sexual abstinence and a healthy lifestyle.
- **Secondary prevention**: Preventing the HPV infection that has already happened from progressing further. This will be by detection and treatment of preinvasive state. For example, cervical cancer screening.
- **Tertiary prevention**: Detection and treatment of early stage cancer.

Primary Prevention of Cervical Cancer

Primary cancer prevention can be achieved through prevention and control of genital HPV infection. Health promotion strategies such as a healthy sex life, minimising exposure to HPV infection and cofactors, such as stopping smoking, minimising the number of sexual partners and HPV vaccination can help to prevent cervical cancer.

HPV vaccination

The HPV vaccine is a viral like protein (VLP). It is not a virus but reassembled viral capsid proteins without the viral genome. Hence, it is non-infectious but can induce increased immunity when injected, by generating high levels of HPV IgG antibodies that can provide type specific protection.

The HPV vaccine is designed for protection against the HPV 16 and 18 infections that cause 70% of cervical cancers. It is not 100% protective and women must still be reminded to go for their cervical cancer screening when they reach the required criteria for screening.

There are two types of HPV vaccine on the market: the quadrivalent and bivalent HPV vaccines. The characteristics of each vaccine are shown in Table 6.5 below. Both vaccines protect against HPV 16 and 18 infection, but the quadrivalent vaccine also protects against HPV 6 and 11 which cause 90% of genital warts. Genital warts are the commonest clinical manifestation of an HPV infection, especially in the young.

The HPV vaccine is given by intramuscular injection in three doses within the span of six months. The efficacy of the HPV vaccine is well established, with studies reporting protection against high grade CIN by up to 99% protection.

The best protection is seen in women who have never been exposed to HPV infection, such as those who have not been sexually active before. In view of these, increasing number of countries including United Kingdom, Australia, Malaysia and Brunei have incorporated HPV vaccination into the school vaccination programme. The most recent study from Australia, following its national school HPV vaccination programme using the quadrivalent HPV vaccine, showed a significant decrease in the incidence of high grade CIN and genital warts.

The HPV vaccine is a prophylactic vaccine i.e. it protects against future infection by HPV 16 and 18. It does not cure current HPV infection. To date, no therapeutic HPV vaccine is clinically available.

The HPV vaccine safety profile is well established. As it has no genetic material, it provides increased immunity to its recipient without inducing infection itself. The most common adverse side effect reported by women receiving the vaccine is pain at the injection site. To date, the HPV vaccine has not been shown to have any direct adverse effects. Newer vaccines like the nonavalent (9 HPV types) HPV vaccine are also being developed.

TABLE 6.5   Types and Characteristics of Currently Available HPV Vaccines

	Quadrivalent Vaccine	Bivalent Vaccine
Protect against the following HPV sub-types	6, 11, 16, 18	16, 18
Vaccination schedule	0, 2 and 6 months	0, 1 and 6 months, or as advised by your doctor
Approved indications	Prevention of cervical cancer, vulvar cancer, vaginal cancer and genital warts	Prevention of cervical cancer
Approved age for use	Girls and women aged 9 to 26 years, or as advised by your doctor	Girls and women aged 9 to 25 years, or as advised by your doctor

Secondary Prevention of Cervical Cancer

Cervical cancer screening

The purpose of screening is to identify asymptomatic individuals who have a higher risk of developing cervical cancer. Numerous studies have shown that an organised cervical cancer screening programme has led to significant reduction in the incidence and mortality of women due to cervical cancer.

Since the introduction of an organised cervical screening programme in the United Kingdom in 1988, the incidence and mortality rate from cervical cancer has been reduced by more than 50%.[4]

Screening methods

There are currently 3 main types of screening methods for cervical cancer used clinically worldwide. These include:

(1) Cytology-based
(2) HPV testing
(3) Visual inspection

(1) Cytology-based screening

Cytology-based screening is a method initially introduced by Dr. George Papanicolaou (hence the Pap smear) in the 1940s. Since its introduction more than 50 years ago, it is currently the most common method used for cervical cancer screening worldwide.

A Pap smear involves gentle brushing of the cervix using a device to exfoliate cervical cells, to allow for microscopic inspection for specific nucleic changes in the cell that may indicate the presence of cervical intraepithelial neoplasia, that may lead to cervical cancer if not treated.

One single Pap smear has a low sensitivity of about 50% in detecting high grade CIN. However, due to the long natural history of development of cervical cancer from high grade CIN, regular attendance for cervical cancer screening has been shown to increase its sensitivity to up to more than 80%.

The Pap smear, however, has a high specificity for detecting high grade abnormalities and invasive cervical cancer. It is less specific for low grade lesion.

Conventional method. This is the original sampling method using a wooden spatula. The Ayre's spatula is a wooden spatula that was introduced in 1847. It is still currently used by doctors to take a Pap smear.

The disadvantage of this method is the high incidence of unsatisfactory Pap smears. This may be due to operator-dependent factors, poor slide preparation, laboratory interpretation error or the presence of other materials on the slide, such as blood.

The use of liquid-based cytology has been shown to reduce the number of unsatisfactory Pap smears that are seen in the conventional method.

Liquid-based cytology (LBC). In LBC the sampling method is the same as the conventional method. However, instead of smearing the sample onto a slide, the sample is washed into a liquid medium. The liquid medium is then sent to the laboratory where it is processed to produce a monolayer of cells on the slide. This results in a 'cleaner' slide for clearer assessment by the cytologist, hence reducing the number of unsatisfactory slides.[5]

Another advantage of the LBC is that the sample medium can be kept and used for HPV DNA testing.

(2) HPV testing

ASCUS triage. The most common abnormal Pap smear result obtained is ASCUS. The majority of ASCUS are due to low risk HPV infection which does not lead to cervical cancer.[6]

In ASCUS triage, women who have had an ASCUS Pap smear are offered an HPV test. The HPV test will differentiate those women who had ASCUS Pap smears due to a low risk HPV from those with an oncogenic HPV infection. This will allow more efficient referral of women who are at higher risk of cervical cancer to further assessment by colposcopy.[6]

Test of cure. In test of cure, women who have had treatment for proven preinvasive cervical disease i.e. CIN3 will be offered an HPV test at a 6–12 month interval to prove that the disease has been eradicated. Those women who have a negative HPV test have been shown to have a lower risk of recurring high grade CIN or cervical cancer, and it is safe for them to resume routine three yearly cervical cancer screening.[7]

Primary HPV screening. Primary HPV screening will involve exchanging the method of cervical cancer screening from cytology-based (Pap smear) to HPV test. There is currently increasing evidence that primary HPV testing is a more sensitive and efficient way to screen for cervical cancer compared to cytology-based screening. Australia, for example, has already incorporated HPV primary screening into their cervical cancer screening programme. With increasing evidence for primary HPV testing for cervical cancer screening, it is anticipated that more and more countries will adopt this method of screening in future.[8]

(3) Visual inspection

Screening by visual inspection involves applying 3–5% acetic acid or Lugol's iodine onto the cervix, with direct observation of specific changes. These changes are seen immediately and allow treatment to be done at the same time.[9]

This method is used widely in countries with low resource settings.

Cervical screen Singapore

Singapore introduced its national cytology based cervical screening program in 2004. Sexually active women between the ages of 25 to 69 years old are invited for a Pap smear test every three years.

Pap smear reporting

Reporting of Pap smear results is a very important part of cervical cancer prevention. It is currently the main drive in the management of preinvasive disease and cervical cancer prevention.[10]

Essentially, Pap smear results can be placed into three main categories:

(1) Unsatisfactory
(2) Negative for malignancy
(3) Abnormal smears

Unsatisfactory smears are usually due to either not enough cells for adequate assessment, or the cells being obscured (by blood for example), preventing a definitive Pap smear result.

Negative for malignancy is the most common Pap smear result. It shows no evidence of dyskaryotic or malignant cells i.e. no cytological evidence of CIN, glandular dysplasia or malignancy. This category includes those in which cells can show reactive changes. Micro-organisms such as *Candida* or *Chlamydia* can also be identified in a negative Pap smear.

Abnormal Pap smear results can be categorised further into squamous abnormality, glandular abnormality, invasive cancer or others (Table 6.6).

ASCUS smears are the most common abnormal Pap smear result obtained.

There are various terminologies used worldwide for reporting Pap smear results.

Two of the most common Pap smear reporting systems are:

(1) 1973 WHO system: Borderline, mild, moderate and severe dyskaryosis. Invasive cancer and adenocarcinoma.
(2) 2001 Bethesda system (see Table 6.6).

TABLE 6.6 Summary of the Bethesda Reporting System 2001[10]

Pap smear results

(1) Unsatisfactory smear

(2) Negative for malignant cells

(3) Abnormal smears

Squamous abnormality		Glandular abnormality	
High grade	Low grade	High grade	Low grade
ASC-H:	ASCUS	AGC — favour neoplastic	AGUS
HSIL	LSIL	AIS	

Invasive cancer	
Squamous cell carcinoma (SCC)	Adenocarcinoma

Definition:	Definition:
ASCUS: Atypical squamous cell of undetermined significance	AGUS: Atypical glandular cells of undetermined significance
ASC-H: Atypical squamous cell, cannot exclude HSIL	AGC — favour neoplastic: Atypical glandular cells that favour neoplastic
LSIL: Low squamous intraepithelial lesion	AIS: Adenocarcinoma *in situ*
HSIL: High squamous intraepithelial lesion	

Colposcopy

Principles of colposcopy

Colposcopy is a procedure where the cervix is visualised using a colposcope to identify the presence of preinvasive cervical disease.

It is important to appreciate that Pap smear is a screening test and is performed in asymptomatic women. Pap smear is not able to identify the lesion or the degree of abnormality. This is why colposcopy examination also plays an important role in cervical cancer screening and prevention.

The first ever colposcope was invented by Hinselmann in 1925. Colposcopy allows the cervix to be examined by low power microscopy with bright illumination, aided by 3–5% acetic acid and Lugol's iodine.

Colposcopy allows the identification different specific cervical topography and vascular patterns that may indicate the presence of preinvasive cervical disease (Tables 6.7 and 6.8).

TABLE 6.7 Importance of Colposcopy in Management of Abnormal Pap Smears

(1) Locates the lesion on the cervix
(2) Indicates severity of intraepithelial neoplasia
(3) Its most important function is to exclude invasive cervical cancer
(4) Allows selection of sites on the lesion to biopsy to confirm suspicions
(5) Facilitates local ablative and excisional treatment

TABLE 6.8 Summary of the Common Indications for Referral to Colposcopy Clinic

Common Indication	Action
ASCUS	Repeat Pap smear in six months and refer for colposcopy if persistently abnormal
ASC-H LSIL HSIL All glandular abnormalities	Colposcopy
Malignancy	Urgent referral to gynaecologist/gynaeoncologist
Other referrals to colposcopy	Suspicious looking cervix Suspicious symptoms that may indicate the presence of cervical cancer i.e. post coital bleeding *Important: Preinvasive disease DOES NOT cause unscheduled bleeding*

Cervical intraepithelial neoplasia (CIN)

CIN is a histological diagnosis (compared to Pap smear result which is a cytological reporting). It is diagnosed following a cervical punch biopsy or excisional biopsy, usually during a colposcopy examination.

Tertiary Prevention of Cervical Cancer

Tertiary prevention of cervical cancer is out of the scope of this chapter. For further details regarding tertiary cervical cancer prevention, please refer to chapter on Carcinoma of Cervix.

Treatment of Preinvasive Cervical Disease

The aim of treatment for cervical preinvasive disease is to locally remove the abnormal epithelial lining of the cervix using ablation or excisional technique (Table 6.9).

TABLE 6.9   Types of Treatment for Cervical Preinvasive Disease

Treatment Option for Preinvasive Cervical Disease	Types of Treatment
Ablative techniques	Cold coagulation Laser ablation/vaporisation Cryotherapy Electrocoagulation diathermy Radical diathermy
Excisional techniques	LEEP/LLETZ Cone biopsy: – Laser – Needle – Cold knife Trachelectomy Hysterectomy

Conclusion

Cervical cancer is still one of the biggest causes of death in women worldwide but it is the only cancer at the moment that can be effectively prevented and screened. Health providers have an important responsibility to increase awareness of cervical cancer screening and prevention, which can potentially lead to total eradication of cervical cancer in the future.

TABLE 6.10 Glossary of Terms

Term	Explanation
HPV	Human papillomavirus
Squamocolumnar junction (SCJ)	Where the squamous and columnar epithelium meet. This is not fixed and depends on the degree of metaplasia
Transformation zone (TZ)	A zone formed by squamous metaplasia and bound by the original and new squamocolumnar junctions
Squamous metaplasia	Squamous metaplasia is a permanent change of columnar epithelium to squamous epithelium
Dysplasia	A histological term describing the architectural abnormality within tissue
Dyskaryosis	A cytological term describing nuclear abnormalities in a cell
CIN	Cervical intraepithelial neoplasia. Usually it is graded from CIN 1–3
AIS	Adenocarcinoma *in situ*. A precursor for adenocarcinoma of cervix.
LEEP	Loop electrosurgical excision procedure

References

1. Ferlay J, Steliarova-Foucher E, Lortet-Tieulent J, *et al.* (2013) Cancer incidence and mortality patterns in Europe: estimates for 40 countries in 2012. *Eur J Cancer* **49**: 1374–1403.
2. Annual Registry Report. (2014) Trends in Cancer Incidence in Singapore 2009–2013. Singapore Cancer Registry. *Singapore Cancer Registry.*
3. Zur HH. (2002) Papillomaviruses and cancer: from basic studies to clinical application. *Nat Rev Cancer* **2**:342–350.
4. Canfell K, Barnabas R, Patnick J, Beral V. (2004) The predicted effect of changes in cervical screening practice in the UK: results from a modelling study. *Br J Cancer* **91**:530–536.
5. Cox JT. (2004) Liquid-based cytology: evaluation of effectiveness, cost-effectiveness, and application to present practice. *J Natl Compr Canc Netw* **2**:597–611.
6. Arbyn M, Martin-Hirsch P, Buntinx F, *et al.* (2009) Triage of women with equivocal or low-grade cervical cytology results: a meta-analysis of the HPV test positivity rate. *J Cell Mol Med* **13**:648–659.
7. Kitchener HC, Almonte M, Thomson C, *et al.* (2009) HPV testing in combination with liquid-based cytology in primary cervical screening (ARTISTIC): a randomised controlled trial. *Lancet Oncol* **10**:672–682.
8. Wright TC, Jr, Stoler MH, Behrens CM, *et al.* (2012) The ATHENA human papillomavirus study: design, methods, and baseline results. *Am J Obstet Gynecol* **206**:46.

9. Almonte M, Ferreccio C, Winkler JL, *et al.* (2007) Cervical screening by visual inspection, HPV testing, liquid-based and conventional cytology in Amazonian Peru. *Int J Cancer* **121**:796–802.
10. Solomon D, Davey D, Kurman R, *et al.* (2002) The 2001 Bethesda System: terminology for reporting results of cervical cytology. *JAMA* **287**:2114–2119.

7

ABNORMAL VAGINAL DISCHARGE AND PRURITUS VULVAE

Shakina Rauff

Introduction

Abnormal vaginal discharge is one of the commonest complaints that gynaecologists encounter and is often a source of worry among women. In order to understand what constitutes an "abnormal vaginal discharge", it is first necessary to comprehend what is "normal vaginal discharge".

A clear or white discharge resulting from cervical and vaginal secretions is normal in women who are of the reproductive age group. The consistency and amount of discharge may vary throughout the menstrual cycle as well — it becomes more stretchy (akin to egg-white) peri-ovulation and may be thicker and slightly yellow during the luteal phase of the menstrual cycle. Normal healthy discharge usually does not have a strong odour and does not cause itchiness, although some women may experience more wetness from the discharge than others.

Pruritis vulvae refers to itch of the vulva. Although most women will experience some vulval itch occasionally, pruritis vulvae refers to the pathological condition which occurs when the itch is persistent and causes distress. It is a symptom and not a diagnosis and may be caused by excessive vaginal discharge, infections, urinary incontinence, malignancy or other non-neoplastic vulval epithelial disorders.

Physiology of Normal Vaginal Discharge

In young girls, the vagina is lined by a simple cuboidal epithelium with a neutral pH. After puberty and the rise in oestrogen, the vaginal mucosa of a woman in her reproductive years is lined by stratified squamous epithelium about 10–30 cells thick. The vaginal pH is maintained between 3.5–4.5 by the lactobacilli (Doderlein's bacilli) found in the vagina. The lactobacilli act on the glycogen released by the shedding vaginal cells to produce lactic acid and hydrogen peroxide. The acidic environment prevents multiplication of pathogenic organisms. After menopause, atrophic changes occur due to the loss of oestrogen, and the bacterial flora is similar to that of the skin, with the pH rising once again to a neutral level.

There are a large number of bacteria found in the vagina which constitute the normal flora — the main group are lactobacilli, which form 80–90%. Others include *Staphylococci, Ureaplasma, Streptococci, Gardnerella, E. coli, Candida* spp. and some anaerobes. However, some of these are potential pathogens that can cause symptoms as well.[1-3]

Thus, normal vaginal secretions consist of a transudate containing desquamated vaginal epithelial cells and mucous secreted by the cervical glands, which are mixed with the normal flora found in the vagina. Normal vaginal discharge is white and becomes yellowish on contact with air due to oxidation.

Physiological discharge can be increased in pregnancy and discharge may be more excessive in women with a large cervical ectropion.

Abnormal Vaginal Discharge

It is often difficult for the woman to differentiate between normal and abnormal vaginal discharge and she may give a very nebulous history without any specific causative factor identifiable. One of the best ways to discriminate the abnormal from normal vaginal discharge is to ask whether the amount or character of the discharge has altered significantly from the woman's usual pattern.

Most women will be aware of what their normal pattern is like and they do realise there is some variation throughout the menstrual cycle. They often seek help and reassurance when there is a change in consistency or colour, an unusually large amount of discharge, if there is associated itchiness or a bad smell, or if the discharge is associated with other symptoms like abdominal-pelvic pain or abnormal vaginal bleeding e.g. inter-menstrual or post-coital bleeding.

TABLE 7.1   Causes of Abnormal Vaginal Discharge

Causes of Abnormal Vaginal Discharge	
Physiological	Pregnancy
	Oral contraceptive pill users
	Cervical ectropion
	Emotional stress

(Continued)

TABLE 7.1 *(Continued)*

Causes of Abnormal Vaginal Discharge

Infective	Bacterial vaginosis
	Monilial vaginosis (*Candida* infection)
	Trichomonal vaginosis (*Trichomonas*)
	Sexually transmitted infections e.g. *Neisseria gonorrhoea*, *Chlamydia*, genital herpes
Malignancy	Vaginal cancer
	Cervical cancer
	Endometrial cancer
	Fallopian tube cancer
Miscellaneous	Foreign body e.g. retained tampon or incarcerated ring pessary
	Fistula e.g. vesico-vaginal or recto-vaginal fistula
	Bartholin's abscess
	Infestations e.g. pubic lice or scabies

About 90% suffer from infections caused by bacterial vaginosis, *Candida* or *Trichomonas*, and each of these conditions will be described in more detail below.[4]

Candida Vulvovaginosis

More than 75% of women will experience at least one episode of vaginal candidiasis or thrush infection at some point in their lives. A minority (~5%) will have recurrent infections (four or more infections per year). Most women have *Candida* as a commensal in the vagina and are asymptomatic, as the normal vaginal secretions and flora prevent it from becoming pathogenic. Symptoms arise when the natural environment is upset and *Candida* multiplies. Vaginal thrush is not a sexually transmitted infection but it can be passed on during intercourse.

Aetiology and Predisposing Factors

Most episodes occur without an obvious cause, although there is a strong association with sexual activity and the physical trauma of intercourse. Over 90% of cases of vaginal thrush are caused by *Candida albicans*. The rest are due to other *Candida* species e.g. *Candida glabrata* or *Candida krusei*.

In some women, there are recognisable risk factors which make them more prone to vaginal candidiasis:

- Broad-spectrum antibiotics, especially if chronic use
- Immunosuppression and immunosuppressive therapy e.g. steroids
- Human immunodeficiency virus (HIV) infection
- Diabetes mellitus
- Pregnancy
- Vaginal douching, bubble baths, shower gel, tight-fitting undergarments
- Underlying dermatosis e.g. eczema

Uncomplicated thrush refers to mild thrush that occurs sporadically or infrequently, for the first time or with mild to moderate symptoms or findings. Complicated thrush is characterised by recurrent episodes, severe symptoms or clinical appearance or infection with *Candida* species other than *Candida albicans*.

Clinical Features

The features of infections caused by the different types of *Candida* species i.e. *Candida albicans* versus non-*Candida albicans* cannot be differentiated clinically.

The woman will usually present with:

(1) Discharge that is curdy, thick and white (like cottage cheese) with a yeast odour, but may be thin and watery or odourless as well.
(2) Vulvo-vaginal itching.
(3) Dyspareunia due to soreness or a burning sensation at the introitus.
(4) There may be a stinging sensation on micturition due to abrasions caused by scratching.

In severe cases:

(1) The whole vulva area is red, swollen and fissured.
(2) The woman's partner may complain of itching of the glans penis and foreskin.
(3) Speculum examination may reveal a white, curdy discharge that is adherent to the vaginal walls and cervix.

Diagnosis and Investigations

A vaginal swab should be taken during examination and sent for microscopy and culture, as this is the most sensitive test. The presence of more than 10 yeast colonies confirms the diagnosis. The pH of the vaginal fluid is usually normal.

If there is a predisposing condition(s) suspected, additional tests can be carried out to confirm them. For example, a random glucose level or an oral glucose tolerance test can be performed to check if the patient is diabetic, or an HIV test can be done.

Management

Asymptomatic women who have thrush incidentally diagnosed do not require treatment. General rules are that

- Patients should avoid local irritant, douching, perfumed soaps and bath gels and tightly fitting garments
- Avoidance of intercourse is necessary until the infection has cleared
- Local treatment is generally preferred over systemic treatment to minimise the risk of systemic side effects
- Topically applied anti-fungals like azoles (clotrimazole, econazole, miconazole, itraconazole) should be used with vaginal pessaries for a one-week duration. There is no evidence that any one imidazole is more effective than another
- If vaginal treatment fails or oral treatment is preferred, a single dose of fluconazole 150 mg is effective
- Complementary therapies like bathing the area with plain bio-live yoghurt have not been proven to be effective, though it does not cause harm

*In patients with recurrent symptoms (~5–10%), it is important to exclude diabetes and assess for underlying risk factors e.g. immunodeficiency, steroid use or frequent antibiotic use, although up to half will not have any identifiable risk factors. In these patients, longer courses of treatment and subsequent maintenance therapy may be required. An induction regime of oral fluconazole 150 mg repeated every three days for a total of three doses to induce clinical remission, followed by maintenance suppressive fluconazole prophylaxis of 150 mg weekly for six months will prevent symptomatic episodes in more than 90% of patients within the six months. Ketoconazole may also be used, but liver function tests should be done at the beginning of treatment and again after three months, as it can rarely cause liver damage. The optimal treatment for non-albicans vulvo-vaginal candidiasis not well-established, but boric acid capsules or non-fluconazole azole therapy may be attempted.

Pregnant women represent a special group of patients in which oral treatment should not be used. They also require a longer duration of treatment compared to non-pregnant women.

Bacterial Vaginosis (BV)

BV is the commonest cause of abnormal vaginal discharge in women of childbearing age and affects 10–20% of women. Normally, about 60% of the lactobacilli in the vagina produce hydrogen peroxidase but in BV, only 6% do. This results in an increase in the vaginal pH which can then range from 4.5–7.0. The rise in vaginal pH causes an overgrowth of predominantly anaerobic organisms like *Gardnerella vaginalis*, *Mycoplasma hominis*, *Bacteroides*, *Prevotella* spp. and *Mobiluncus* spp.

BV can arise and recur spontaneously in both sexually active and non-sexually active women. It is also associated with an increased risk of preterm labour in pregnancy, late miscarriage, preterm pre-labour rupture of membranes and post-partum endometritis.

Predisposing Factors

BV is more common in:

- Black women compared to white women
- Smokers
- Those with use of an intrauterine contraceptive device
- Women undergoing elective termination of pregnancy
- Women using scented soaps and bubble baths
- Those who perform douching and the use of vaginal deodorants
- Those with multiple sexual partners, although it can occur in virgins

Clinical Features

About half of women with BV infection are asymptomatic. In those who have symptoms, the commonest symptoms are:

- An offensive, fishy discharge, particularly after sexual intercourse
- Does not usually cause vaginal itching or soreness
- The discharge may be white or grey and its consistency is thin and watery

On examination, there is usually a thin, homogenous discharge coating the walls of the vagina and vestibule. The discharge may be white or yellow.

Diagnosis

The Ansel's criteria are used for diagnosing BV and three out of four of the following should be present to make a diagnosis:

- Characteristic thin, white homogenous discharge on examination
- Vaginal pH > 4.5

- Presence of "clue cells" on microscopy: "Clue cells" are vaginal epithelial cells so heavily coated with bacteria that their borders are obscured
- Release of a fishy smell on adding an alkali — usually 10% potassium hydroxide

A vaginal swab that has been taken for Gram-stain can also be used to diagnose BV. In this situation, a reduced number or absent lactobacilli (large Gram-positive bacilli) are noted but there are increased numbers or Gram-positive and Gram-negative cocci. Culture is not so useful as *Gardnerella vaginalis* can be grown in more than half of women with normal vaginal discharge and, thus, is not diagnostic of BV.

Management

Simple measures can be taken to reduce the chance of BV infection and this includes avoidance of vaginal douching, the use of shower gels and antiseptic bath agents. There is no evidence to prove that probiotics such as those found in yoghurts can prevent or treat BV.

In women who are asymptomatic, no treatment is needed. In those with symptoms, the simplest and most cost-effective treatment would be the antibiotic Metronidazole. Oral Metronidazole can be given as a single 2 g dose or the alternative of 400 mg twice daily for 5–7 days. There are topical intravaginal preparations available in the form of Metronidazole gel in some countries. Vaginal pessaries with a combination of Metronidazole and Nystatin (Flagystatin) are available locally, and one pessary can be used nightly for 5–7 nights. An alternative antibiotic cream — 2% Clindamycin cream — can also be employed once daily for a week. The initial cure rates are as high as 80% but relapse rate is also high.

The commonest side effects of Metronidazole are nausea and vomiting. The drug may also leave a slight metallic taste in the mouth so it is best taken after meals. Alcohol should also be avoided while on Metronidazole treatment and for 48 hours after finishing the last dose. Metronidazole can also be taken in pregnancy. However, intravaginal treatment is recommended during breastfeeding as it can affect the taste of breast milk.

Male partners of women who have BV infection need not be treated as this has not shown to reduce the recurrence rates. There is no consensus on the optimal treatment of women with recurrent BV infections, although regular treatment may be helpful in those with frequent episodes.

There are no firm recommendations about screening women with a history of preterm labour or routine screening of pregnant women for BV. However, women undergoing elective termination of pregnancy should be treated for BV if this is found, as this may reduce the subsequent risk of endometritis and pelvic inflammatory disease.

Trichomoniasis

This is a sexually transmitted infection caused by the flagellated protozoon, *Trichomonas vaginalis*. This tiny single-celled parasite can be found in the vagina, urethra and paraurethral glands in women. In men, the infection most commonly affects the urethra. *Trichomonas* infection in pregnancy is associated with an increased risk of preterm labour and low birth weight infants.

Predisposing Factors

Transmission is almost always:

- By unprotected sexual intercourse in adults
- Having multiple sexual partners is not a significant risk factor as anyone who is sexually active can acquire the infection and pass it on. Trichomoniasis cannot be transmitted by oral or anal sex, kissing or sharing cutlery and toilets

Clinical Features

Up to 50% of women are asymptomatic and the infection can be carried for several months before becoming symptomatic. As it mainly affects the vagina and urethra, symptoms of Trichomoniasis include:

- Yellowish-green vaginal discharge which may be thick, thin or frothy
- The discharge can be quite profuse and is sometimes associated with an unpleasant smell
- Soreness, itching and inflammation around the vagina
- Dyspareunia and dysuria are also presenting complaints
- Lower abdominal discomfort and pain may be present as well
- On clinical examination, there is evidence of vulvitis, vaginitis and cervicitis
- The classical appearance of a "strawberry cervix" due to punctate haemorrhages is found in 2% of cases

Diagnosis

Culture is able to confirm the diagnosis in 95% of cases, compared to microscopy and direct observations which detect only about 60–80% of cases. When reported as an incidental finding on cervical cytology, a vaginal swab should be sent off for culture to confirm the presence of *Trichomonas*, as the sensitivity of cytology-detected infection is lower.

Management

- Systemic therapy is preferable and more effective than local intravaginal therapy as the urethral and paraurethral glands are often affected as well
- Metronidazole is the standard treatment used and can be given as single oral dose of 2 g or 400 mg twice daily for 5–7 days
- Alcohol should be avoided during the duration of treatment and for 48 hours after completion due to the disulfiram-like effect
- This regimen results in a cure rate of more than 90%
- Important to treat the current sexual partner as well. Ideally, recent partners should be traced, tested and treated accordingly
- Intercourse should be avoided until the treatment is over, or there is a risk of re-infection

Cervicitis

Cervicitis refers to inflammation of the cervix and is diagnosed clinically by the finding of mucopurulent discharge at the cervical os and endocervical canal. There may be contact bleeding on examination.

Aetiology

Cervicitis is usually caused by a sexually transmitted infection and the male partner may have accompanying features of urethritis. The commoner pathogens involved are *Chlamydia* and gonorrhoea and, less frequently, trichomoniasis and herpes. It can also be caused by non-infective sources such as an intrauterine contraceptive device or an allergic reaction to condoms.

Clinical Features

- Majority are asymptomatic
- May present with post-coital bleeding
- Complain of purulent vaginal discharge
- Pain during intercourse

Diagnosis and Investigations

- Purulent discharge can be seen at the cervical os, and
- There may be redness and erythema of the cervix

- Vaginal walls can appear inflamed and swollen as well
- A cervical smear should be taken for cytology
- Swabs for sexually transmitted infections like *Trichomonas*, *Chlamydia* and gonorrhoea
- A bimanual examination is mandatory to ensure there are no uterine or adnexal abnormalities e.g. pelvic inflammatory disease
- Rarely, colposcopy and a cervical biopsy are required, and these are indicated if an underlying malignancy or preinvasive lesion is suspected

Treatment

Treatment is tailored according to the causative factor:

- Anti-microbials for bacterial infections
- Chronic cervicitis can lead to scarring of the cervix. If symptoms persist after completion of medical therapy and no further causative organism is isolated, the inflamed area on the cervix can be cauterised by cold coagulation or laser ablation

Genital Herpes

A diagnosis of herpes can be distressing for a number of women, as not only do they feel pain from the symptoms, but they also feel there is a stigma attached to having herpes. Genital herpes is a sexually acquired infection and is caused by the herpes simplex virus which exists in two types — herpes simplex type 1 virus (HSV-1) and herpes simplex type 2 virus (HSV-2). HSV-1 is the usual cause of orolabial herpes or oral cold sores but can also cause genital herpes in up to 40% of cases. The remainder of cases of genital herpes is caused by HSV-2.

After the primary infection, the virus lies dormant in the dorsal root ganglia and may be re-activated periodically to cause recurrent outbreaks.

Clinical Features

The first clinical attack of genital herpes is usually the most severe in terms of symptoms and duration, and recurrent episodes are usually less painful and shorter.

Primary Infection

- Presents most commonly with painful vulval ulcers or blisters which are found mainly on the inner surfaces of the labia majora
- Abnormal discharge
- Dysuria
- In severe cases, urinary retention can occur
- Genital infection may be preceded by, or coexist with, a low-grade fever and myalgia or flu-like symptoms
- Can also experience vulval itch or a burning sensation

Recurrent Attacks

- Are usually less severe in terms of pain and are self-limiting
- The virus, which has established a latent infection in the sensory ganglia, is re-activated and travels down the neural axons to the skin
- Symptoms include a tingling, burning or itching sensation around the genital area and sometimes around the inner thighs
- Followed by small crops of painful blisters appearing around the genital region
- Possible triggers of HSV re-activation include stress, having flu or being unwell or immunocompromise

Diagnosis

In primary herpes, there is usually:

- Widespread involvement of the vulva with blistering and multiple, shallow, painful ulcers
- The vagina and cervix can also be affected making a pelvic examination quite difficult at times
- The whole vulva may be swollen, oedematous and there may be vesicles present on the vaginal walls and cervix as well
- A secondary bacterial infection can occur, exacerbating the swelling and pain
- The inguinal lymph nodes may be palpable and tender. Peri-urethral lesions can be present which lead to severe dysuria and in some cases, acute urinary retention

Investigations

- Swabs must be taken from the base of the fresh lesions and transported directly to the microbiology laboratory in a special viral culture medium

- Polymerase chain reaction (PCR) which tests for HSV DNA is available locally for diagnosis and is more accurate than culture. However, this method of analysis is not ubiquitous
- Serology is not commonly required to reach a diagnosis but can be used to diagnose an acute infection versus a recurrent attack by measuring serum IgG and IgM levels

Over 5–7 days, the fresh lesions will crust over, dry up and heal slowly, although in first attacks, this make take place over two weeks. Recurrent episodes heal faster. Swabs taken from lesions that are healed or dried up may not yield a diagnosis.

It is worthwhile offering patients with herpes a full STI screening evaluation which includes testing for *Chlamydia*, gonorrhoea, hepatitis B, hepatitis C, HIV, syphilis and *Trichomonas* infections. This should be done at the appropriate time and suggested with sensitivity.

- A urine culture can also be sent off if a concurrent urinary tract infection is suspected

Treatment

- Bathing the area with a warm saline bath to reduce the oedema and soothe the vulval area
- Patient should keep herself well-hydrated so that her urine is not concentrated as this will reduce the pain on micturition
- Sexual intercourse should, of course, be avoided until the patient is completely healed
- Tight clothing is not advised as this may irritate the blisters and ulcers
- Suprapubic catheterisation may be necessary in patients with retention of urine who cannot void
- If there is a superimposed bacterial infection, broad-spectrum antibiotics can be prescribed as well
- Analgesia in the form on non-steroidal anti-inflammatory drugs (NSAIDs)
- Topical anaesthetic gels like lignocaine gel. This can be applied for pain relief a few minutes before the patient micturates
- Anti-viral drugs like acyclovir (200 mg five times a day), valaciclovir (500 mg twice daily) or famciclovir (250 mg thrice a day) are useful in reducing the duration and severity of the attack
- However, they are usually effective only when the lesions are still fresh and developing i.e. within five days of the start of the episode
- Topical agents like acyclovir cream are less effective, and are not helpful once the lesions have crusted over

- Intravenous therapy is indicated if oral treatment cannot be tolerated, if complications like meningitis occur or if the patient is immunocompromised
- Valaciclovir and famciclovir are more expensive than acyclovir but have greater bioavailability

Clinical Course and Sequelae

Women who have faced this infection may encounter significant psychological distress and the relationship with her partner can be affected. She may be afraid of recurrent attacks or dyspareunia and want to avoid intercourse. In these situations, counselling and psychological support are useful.

In about 30% of women, a single recurrent episode occurs and in about 2–5%, multiple recurrent attacks may happen. If a patient has more than recurrent outbreaks in a year, she will warrant suppressive treatment with acyclovir twice daily for 6–12 months.

Neurological sequelae are unusual, and patients who are immunocompromised are at higher risk for complications of the central nervous system (CNS). CNS involvement can present as aseptic meningitis, transverse myelitis or autonomic neuropathy.

Herpetic infections can also involve the eye and herpes keratitis that can result in corneal scarring and blindness.

Pruritis Vulvae

Vulval itch is a common presenting complaint among women and can be non-specific. One must remember that, in this situation, the cause of vulval itch may not be purely gynaecological in origin. The vulva may be affected by other systemic diseases like dermatological disorders, emotional problems or urinary incontinence.

About 1 in 10 women consult a doctor about persistent vulval itch at some stage of her life and it can be upsetting, troublesome and distressing for the woman. Thus the history should be taken with a sensitive and non-judgemental approach and patient confidentiality should be maintained.

Regardless of the cause of pruritis vulvae, the itch is generally caused by a histamine release. The itch leads to scratching which further aggravates the itch. This itch-scratch cycle results in a variety of histological changes in the vulval skin. It is essential to break the cycle in order to allow the healing process to take place.[5]

Classification of Vulval Skin Disorders

Classification of vulval epithelial disorders by the International Society for the Study of Vulval Disease has led to less confusion over some of the terminology used in categorising vulval skin diseases (see Table 7.2).

TABLE 7.2 Classification of Epithelial Vulval Disorders (ISSVD)
Non-neoplastic epithelial disorders of skin and mucosa
Lichen sclerosus
Squamous hyperplasia
Allergic dermatitis
Lichen planus
Other dermatoses e.g. psoriasis
Intraepithelial neoplasia
Squamous intraepithelial neoplasia:
VIN, usual type (a. VIN, warty type b. VIN, basaloid type c. VIN, mixed type)
VIN, differentiated type
Non-squamous intraepithelial neoplasia:
Paget's disease
Tumours of melanocytes, non-invasive (melanoma *in situ*)
Mixed non-neoplastic and neoplastic epithelial disorders
Invasive tumours

General skin diseases or medical conditions that can manifest as pruritis vulvae include: psoriasis, intertrigo, scabies, contact or allergic dermatitis, abnormal vaginal discharge or vaginal infections (thrush, BV), nutritional deficiency problems or even psychosomatic disorders. Even common products like deodorants, perfumes, scented shower gels or soaps may cause sensitisation in some patients. The menopause, an inevitable process in aging, results in the vulval epithelium becoming thin, with a loss of elasticity and collagen. The absence of oestrogen causes atrophy and dryness of the vulvo-vaginal epithelium, which in turn may lead to vulval irritation.

History-Taking

The history is very important in establishing predisposing factors and eliciting a cause and one must realise that the history extends beyond a standard gynaecological history. It has to include the medical, drug and family history, as well as symptoms at other skin sites, and establish the patient's personal habits. Psychological problems and sexual relationships are sensitive topics that have to be addressed.

Besides the standard gynaecological history, the following details should be established:

- Drug history — self-medication or previous treatment and duration of treatment, use of hormone replacement therapy in those who are menopausal; drug allergies or contact dermatitis
- Medical history — any immunosuppressive illness; personal history of atopic conditions e.g. hay fever, eczema, asthma; personal history of autoimmune conditions (the most common autoimmune conditions in women with lichen sclerosus are thyroid disorders, alopecia areata, pernicious anaemia, type I diabetes and vitiligo)
- Psychiatric history — emotional problems
- Sexual history — number of partners, any previous STIs, sexual abuse (if appropriate)
- Previous abnormal cervical cytology/HPV infection
- Family history of atopic conditions or autoimmune diseases
- History of urinary or faecal incontinence
- Personal habits and hygiene of the patient — bathing versus showering, douching, type of shower gel used and if antiseptic bath wash used, type and material of underwear used; use of pantyliners, tampons, sanitary pads; if any emollient, powder or moisturiser is used on the area

Physical Examination

Good lighting and adequate exposure are necessary to examine the patient and this should ideally be done in the lithotomy position with a bright white light. Colposcopy may or may not be required depending on the clinical findings and suspicion.

It is important to:

- Ask the woman to indicate where the itchy area is and to observe the general skin condition of the vulva
- If a lesion(s) is seen, the size, shape, colour, location, texture, margins and involvement of any surrounding organs should be noted
- If there is a suspicion of VIN or malignancy, application of 5% acetic acid may help and a biopsy must be taken
- The other lower genital tract sites like the vagina, cervix and perianal skin should be inspected in cases where VIN or a malignancy is a possibility

- The rest of the body should be examined for evidence of dermatosis as well, and this includes the mouth for signs of lichen planus and the scalp, elbows, knees and nails for psoriasis. Eczema can affect any area on the skin and this should be recorded too

Investigations

- If the patient complains of abnormal vaginal discharge, a swab of the discharge should be taken for culture.
- A cervical cytology can be taken opportunistically if this has not been updated.
- In high risk patients, testing for *Chlamydia* can be done concurrently.
- In patients who have failed to respond to treatment, a skin scraping can be taken.
- If, on inspection and examination, there is a suspicion of VIN or malignancy, a biopsy should be taken.
- Testing for other causes, especially autoimmune or medical conditions, can be performed.
- If lichen sclerosus or lichen planus is diagnosed, serum autoantibodies can be screened for.
- In women with vulval dermatitis, skin patch testing and serum ferritin levels should be checked as correction of iron-deficiency anaemia can relieve vulval symptoms. Skin patch testing can identify specific allergens.
- Other general medical conditions like diabetes should be considered and either a random glucose level or checking for glycosuria should be performed.

Management

Treating the cause (when a cause can be found) will naturally improve the pruritis vulvae. Some aetiologies need more prolonged and complex treatment. In some cases, the treatment may just involve avoiding an allergen that may be sensitising to the vulval skin, or local hormone therapy for menopausal women with atrophic vaginitis.

General Measures

There are some measures most women can take to help with the vulval itch regardless of the cause:

- Using a bland moisturiser, or an emollient like aqueous cream, protects the skin and restores skin barrier function. They can be used liberally and as a soap substitute. Soap substitutes with water should be used for washing the area,

instead of water alone or water with soap. Taking a shower instead of a bath is better as it is easier to ensure that all soap is washed off
- Avoidance of potential irritants that may aggravate vulval symptoms is key to allow healing of the vulval skin. Irritants and allergens commonly found are perfumed products, soaps, detergents, textile dyes, tight underwear and sanitary protection. Wearing loose-fitting silk or cotton underwear and trousers is better than leggings or tight jeans. When at home, or sleeping at night, consider not wearing any underwear to avoid contact with potential irritants and to allow the vulval area to remain cool and dry. Synthetic undergarments should be avoided
- The itch-scratch cycle should be broken if possible, and:
  — The woman should try not to scratch at all.
  — Her nails should be kept short and nail varnish removed. Excessive scratching can cause thickening of the vulval skin which then becomes even itchier, exacerbating the cycle. Furthermore, scratching can damage the vulval skin and predispose one to infections.
  — Shaving should be avoided, as this can cause micro-abrasions, which can lead to folliculitis and a superimposed bacterial infection.

Specific Measures

Treating the underlying cause or aetiological factor is the best method of curing pruritis vulvae.

- Medical therapy is the mainstay of treatment for lichen sclerosus and squamous cell hyperplasia
- Those with VIN or malignancy should be referred to a gynaecologic oncologist for surgical management

  In some cases, where no cause can be found, the above general measures should help ease some symptoms.

- Sometimes, a mild steroid ointment or cream can be used for a short course to alleviate the itch and break the itch-scratch cycle
- Long durations of topical steroid treatment and frequent regular use are not encouraged as this may cause vulval skin thinning
- High-potency steroid creams like Dermovate (clobetasol) are usually reserved for women with lichen sclerosus and lichen planus
- If the itch is severe and interferes with the woman's sleep, anti-histamines can be prescribed nightly. Although the anti-histamine may not cure the problem or have a significant impact on the itch, it can cause drowsiness and help her to sleep

- The impact of the vulval disorder on the woman's sexual relationship should not be neglected, and the disorder may have a profound effect on her body image and sexual function. Advice on sexual behaviour, the use of lubricants and the availability of psychosexual counselling are essential

Lichen Sclerosus (LS)

This is one of the commoner causes of vulval itch in older women but can also be found in younger women. It is associated with an increased risk of personal, or family history of, autoimmune disorders e.g. alopecia areata, vitiligo, thyroid disease. LS is a chronic lymphocytic mediated dermatosis and is characterised by epithelial thinning, inflammation and distinct histological changes in the dermis.

Clinical Features

The woman usually:

- Presents with chronic pruritis
- Pain, soreness and dyspareunia, especially if there are fissures and ulcerations present on the vulval area. If the woman has been scratching the area, it may become thickened (lichenified)
- On examination, the anogenital area is most affected, with typical lesions of atrophic shiny white plaques
- The skin can be reddish or normal coloured and may be crinkled or parchment-like in appearance
- The changes usually extend to the anal area in a figure-of-eight pattern. The normal anatomy of the vulva may have changed such that:
  - Labial adhesions may have formed
  - Labia minora may be atrophied
  - There is loss of the clitoral hood with narrowing of the vaginal orifice
- Unlike lichen planus, LS does not involve the vagina and cervix

Diagnosis

Although the diagnosis may be clinically obvious, a vulval biopsy will show epidermal thinning, the horny layer will be unchanged or hyperkeratinised with disappearance of the rete pegs. The dermis is oedematous with some degree of hyalinisation and collections of round cells.

Management

The aim is symptom-control and to detect any malignant changes with regular follow-up. Women with LS have a lifetime risk of developing invasive vulval cancer of about 4–9% and should be reviewed regularly.

- General measures as outlined above, like wearing cotton underwear, avoidance of pantyliners, perfumed soaps, bubble baths etc., should be followed
- The patient may require a lubricant to enable intercourse to be more comfortable
- Bland emollients can be used liberally
- Ultrapotent topical corticosteroids are used as the initial medical treatment for LS and clobetasol propionate (Dermovate) is the most potent one available

Most patients will respond to this and go into complete remission, requiring no further treatment, whereas others will continue to have flares and remissions and require long-term maintenance treatment.

References

1. Monga A, Dobbs S. (2011) *Gynaecology by Ten Teachers*, 19th edn.
2. Edmond K. (2012) *Dewhurst's Textbook of Obstetrics and Gynaecology*, 8th edn.
3. Hacker NF, Gambore JC, Hobil CJ. (2010) *Essentials of Obstetrics and Gynaecology*, 5th edn.
4. Mann M, editors: Luesly Dm, Baker PN. (2004) *An Evidence-based Text for MRCOG*. Chapter 64.1, Infection and sexual health. Edward Arnold Ltd., London, pp. 735–752.
5. Tzakas E, Redman C, editors: Luesly Dm, Baker PN. (2004) *Obstetrics and gynaecology: An Evidence-based Text for MRCOG*. Chapter 65, Benign vulval problems. Edward Arnold Ltd., London, pp. 771–780.

8

SEXUALLY TRANSMITTED DISEASES AND PELVIC INFLAMMATORY DISEASES

Lim Min Yu

Introduction

There are more than 30 different pathogens that cause sexually transmitted infections (STIs). They are mainly spread by sexual contact, but some may also be spread through non-sexual means such as blood products and tissue transfer. They may also be transmitted from mother to child during pregnancy and childbirth.

Eight of the more than 30 known pathogens have been linked to the greatest incidence of illness. Four are currently curable:

- Syphilis
- Gonorrhoea
- Chlamydia
- Trichomoniasis

The other four are viral infections. They are incurable, but there is treatment available to reduce symptoms and the chance of transmission:

- Hepatitis B
- *Herpes simplex*
- Human immunodeficiency virus (HIV)
- Human papillomavirus (HPV)

The World Health Organisation estimates that, globally, more than one million people acquire an STI every day. Each year, 500 million people acquire one of the four curable STIs listed above. STIs rank among the top five reasons for adults to seek healthcare. Therefore, there is a very significant impact on health resources.

Long Term Sequelae

Beyond the immediate impact of infection, STIs can also have other far-reaching consequences. Some STIs increase the risk of acquiring HIV. Mother-to-child transmission can result in congenital abnormalities, stillbirth or neonatal death, premature birth and sepsis. HPV infection causes cervical cancer (530,000 cases; 275,000 deaths each year). STIs are associated with pelvic inflammatory disease, infertility and ectopic pregnancy.

Prevention of STIs

One of the most important methods of reducing the health burden of STIs is through education. Programs should be put in place to inform the public about the method of transmission of STIs, i.e. through unprotected sexual intercourse, especially if people have more than one sexual partner.

There are key populations that are at high risk of catching an STI, such as adolescents and sex workers. Intensive efforts should be made to reach out to these groups and give them safe sex counselling, particularly on the importance of using barrier contraception.

Education may enable recognition of symptoms and seeking medical help. However, barriers include social stigma around STIs, lack of public awareness and limited resources.

Seven out of the eight infections listed above will be discussed in turn, with the exception of HPV, as this will be covered in the chapter on cervical screening.

Syphilis

Organism

Treponema pallidum

Classification

Congenital
- Early (diagnosed within 2 years of life)
- Late (presenting after 2 years)

Acquired
- Early
  - Primary
  - Secondary
  - Early latent (< 2 years of infection)

- Late
  - Late latent (> 2 years of infection)
  - Tertiary

Clinical Features

Primary
Painless ulcer (chancre), typically in the anogenital region. Indurated with a clean base discharging clear serum. Usually single, but may be multiple. Average 21 days from infection to appearance. Lasts three to six weeks, and heals without treatment.

Secondary
Multisystem involvement within the first two years of infection. There is often a rash involving the palms and soles (macular, papular or maculo-papular), condylomata lata, mucocutaneous lesions and generalised lymphadenopathy. Less commonly there may be patchy alopecia, anterior uveitis, meningitis, cranial nerve palsies, hepatitis, splenomegaly, periosteitis and glomerulonephritis. Usually the rash is not itchy.

Latent
The latent stage begins when primary and secondary symptoms disappear. It is diagnosed on serological testing in the absence of symptoms or signs. Latent

syphilis can last for years. Early latent syphilis is the first year of infection and beyond that, it is defined as late latent syphilis.

Symptomatic late syphilis (may develop in one third of untreated individuals)
Neurosyphilis
Cardiovascular syphilis
Gummatous syphilis

Congenital syphilis
Early; includes a rash, condylomata lata, vesiculobullous lesions, snuffles, haemorrhagic rhinitis, osteochondritis, periosteitis, pseudoparalysis, mucous patches, perioral fissures, hepatosplenomegaly, generalised lymphadenopathy, non-immune hydrops, glomerulonephritis, neurological or ocular involvement, haemolysis and thrombocytopenia.

Late; including stigmata: Interstitial keratitis, Clutton's joints, Hutchinson's incisors, mulberry molars, high palatal arch, rhagades, deafness, frontal bossing, short maxilla, protuberance of mandible, saddlenose deformity, sterno-clavicular thickening, paroxysmal cold haemoglobinuria, neurological or gummatous involvement.

Diagnosis

Dark field microscopy
PCR
Serological tests:
Treponemal

- Treponemal EIA
- TPPA (Treponema Pallidum Particle Agglutination)
- TPHA (Treponema Pallidum Haemagglutination Assay)

Confirm a positive screening test with a different treponemal test
Non-treponemal

- VDRL (Venereal Disease Research Laboratory)
- RPR (Rapid Plasma Reagin)

If positive, needs to be confirmed by a treponemal test.

Quantitative VRDL/RPR should be performed when treponemal tests indicate syphilis. This helps stage the disease and indicates the need for treatment. VDRL/RPR titre > 16 and/or positive IgM test indicates active disease and need for treatment. They are also performed serially to monitor serological response to treatment.

Management

Notifiable disease
Offer screening for other STIs, including HIV
Refrain from sexual activity until lesions healed or first follow-up serology known.

Early syphilis
(1) Benzathine penicillin G 2.4 MU i.m. single dose
(2) Procaine penicillin G 600,000 units i.m. daily × 10 days.

Late latent, cardiovascular and gummatous syphilis
(1) Benzathine penicillin 2.4 MU i.m. weekly for two weeks (three doses)
(2) Procaine penicillin 600,000 units i.m. o.d. for 17 days.

Follow-up

For early syphilis, minimum clinical and serological (VDRL or RPR) follow-up should be at months 1, 2, 3, 6 and 12, then six monthly until VDRL/RPR negative or serofast.

For late syphilis, minimum serological follow-up is three monthly until serofast.

Partners

Partner notification should be discussed. For primary cases, partners in the past three months should be notified. Partner notification may have to extend to two years for patients in secondary syphilis, with clinical relapse or in early latent syphilis.[1]

Pregnancy

All pregnant women should be screened for syphilis at the initial antenatal visit. Syphilis may be transmitted transplacentally at any stage of pregnancy and may result in polyhydramnios, miscarriage, preterm labour, stillbirth, hydrops and congenital syphilis.

If treatment is required, a single dose of benzathine penicillin G 2.4 MU is effective in most cases. When maternal treatment is initiated in the third trimester, a second dose of benzathine penicillin is recommended to be given one week after the first, because of altered drug pharmacokinetics in pregnancy.

Gonorrhoea

Organism

Neisseria gonorrhoeae

Clinical Features

Up to 50% will be asymptomatic
- Increased or altered vaginal discharge is the most common symptom (up to 50%)
- Lower abdominal pain
- Urethral infection may cause dysuria but not frequency
- Intermenstrual bleeding
- Menorrhagia

Diagnosis

Nucleic Acid Amplification Test (more sensitive), or culture from endocervical swab or vaginal swab.

Commercial NAAT tests offer dual capability to also test for *Chlamydia* in the same sample. Dual test for both pathogens maximises sensitivity and operational ease of specimen collection, transport and processing.

N. gonorrhoeae may coexist with other genital mucosal pathogens, notably *Chlamydia trachomatis*, *Trichomonas vaginalis* and *Candida albicans*. If symptoms are present, they may be attributable to the co-infecting pathogen.

Management

Notifiable disease
Offer screening for other STIs. About 40% of women are co-infected with *Chlamydia*.

Patients should be advised to abstain from sexual intercourse until they and their partner(s) have completed treatment.

Uncomplicated anogenital infection:
Ceftriaxone 500 mg intramuscularly as a single dose, with azithromycin 1 g oral as a single dose.

Azithromycin is recommended as co-treatment irrespective of the results of *Chlamydia* testing to delay the onset of widespread cephalosporin resistance. There is some *in vitro* evidence of synergy between azithromycin and cephalosporins.[2]

Follow-up

Test of cure two weeks after completion of antibiotics.

Partners

Partner notification should be performed for all partners within the last three months.

Pregnancy

Same treatment regimen as non-pregnant.

Chlamydia

Organism

Chlamydia trachomatis

Clinical Features

More than 70% of women are asymptomatic. However, possible symptoms include:
- vaginal discharge
- post-coital/intermenstrual/breakthrough bleeding
- inflamed/friable cervix (which may bleed on contact)
- urethritis
- lower abdominal pain
- reactive arthritis

In a local paper, 8% of women requesting termination of pregnancy were found to have *C. trachomatis* infection. However, the prevalence is age related: 16.2% of women aged under 25 were infected, compared to 3.1% of those 25 and older.[3]

Diagnosis

Endocervical swab or vaginal swab or urine
NAAT
Dual testing with gonorrhoea

Management

Notifiable disease
Azithromycin 1 g single dose (preferred because of compliance)
Doxycycline 100 mg BD for 7 days
Chlamydial salpingitis (PID) should be treated with doxycycline 100 mg twice daily for 14 days, plus metronidazole 400 mg twice daily for 14 days.[4]

Follow-up

Test of cure need not be performed in patients who have adhered to therapy and in whom there is no risk of re-infection. However, as re-infection rates are high, consider tests for re-infection in the 12 months following a positive diagnosis.

Partners

Partner notification should be performed in all partners within the last six months, or the most recent sexual partner if outwith that time period.

Pregnancy

Azithromycin 1 g single dose (preferred because of compliance)
Erythromycin 500 mg QDS for 7 days
Amoxicillin 500 mg TDS for 7 days
Test of cure should be routine during pregnancy. (Higher chance of positive test after treatment than in non-pregnant).
Risk of neonatal conjunctivitis if infected.

Trichomoniasis

Organism

Trichomonas vaginalis, a flagellated protozoon

Clinical Features

Up to 50% asymptomatic[5]
Vaginal discharge. Classically frothy yellow in up to 30%.
Vulval itching
Dysuria
Offensive odour
Low abdominal pain
2% have strawberry cervix

Diagnosis

Direct microscopy of vaginal secretions
Vaginal swab for
- culture; or
- NAAT (also tests for *Candida albicans* and *Gardnerella vaginalis* simultaneously)

Management

Offer screening for coexistent STIs
Metronidazole 2 g orally single dose or
Metronidazole 400–500 mg BD for 5–7 days
Intravaginal treatment showed cure rates around 50%, unacceptably low, and
   therefore not recommended.

Follow-up

Test of cure only recommended if patient remains symptomatic following treatment, or if symptoms recur.

Partners

Any partners within the last four weeks should be notified and screened for STIs. Should be treated for trichomonas irrespective of investigation results. Avoid intercourse for one week after treatment and follow-up.

Pregnancy

Metronidazole safe to use in pregnancy. No difference from non-pregnant.

Herpes Simplex

Organism

HSV-1 (orolabial)
HSV-2 (genital)

Classification

Initial and recurrent[6]

Clinical Features

Initial
May be asymptomatic
Papular lesions progressing to vesicles then ulcers with local lymphadenitis.
Virus then becomes latent in the sensory root ganglion.
Recurrent
May be asymptomatic
Prodromal symptoms then lesions develop
Features highly variable
Recurrences usually self-limiting, generally minor symptoms. May be managed supportively, with episodic antivirals or suppressive antivirals.
Risk of transmission highest during lesional recurrences or prodrome: should abstain from intercourse
Subclinical viral shedding can cause transmission in absence of lesions
HSV-2 seropositivity increases the risk of HIV transmission.

Diagnosis

Take swab from base of lesion (vesicles should be unroofed first)
HSV DNA detection by PCR
Viral isolation in cell culture (slow)

Serology is recommended for:
- History of recurrent or atypical genital disease when direct virus detection methods have been negative. HSV-2 antibodies are supportive of a diagnosis of genital herpes; HSV-1 antibodies do not differentiate between genital and oropharyngeal infection.
- First-episode genital herpes, where differentiating between primary and established infection, guides counselling and management. At the onset of symptoms, the absence of HSV IgG against the virus type detected in the genital lesion is consistent with a primary infection. Seroconversion should be demonstrated at follow-up.
- Sexual partners of patients with genital herpes, where concerns are raised about transmission. Serodiscordant couples can be counselled about strategies to reduce the risk of infection and disease.

Management

Genital herpes is a notifiable disease
Offer screening for other STIs
Saline baths and appropriate analgesia
Lignocaine gel
Treat any secondary bacterial infection

First episode genital herpes
Patients presenting within five days of the start of the episode, or while new lesions are still forming, should be given oral antiviral drugs. Optimal benefit if started within 72 hours of onset. Treat for 7–10 days.

Acyclovir 400 mg three times a day, or
Famciclovir 250 mg three times a day, or
Valaciclovir 1 g two times a day
Complications: urinary retention, meningism, severe constitutional symptoms. May require admission.

Recurrent genital herpes
Patient initiated treatment within 24 hours of lesion onset or during prodrome is most effective.
Episodic antivirals

Short course therapy
  Acyclovir 800 mg three times daily for 2 days, or
  Famciclovir 1 g twice daily for one day, or
  Valaciclovir 500 mg twice daily for 3 days
Suppression if high recurrence rate (>6/year)
  Acyclovir 400 mg BD or
  Valaciclovir 250 mg BD
  Review therapy after 9–12 months to see if recurrence rate warrants continued suppressive treatment.

Follow-up

Offer follow-up until the episode has resolved.

Partners

High population prevalence. Low physical morbidity. Disclosure should be tailored to patient.

Pregnancy

1st episode genital herpes
  1st or 2nd trimester infection: manage in line with clinical condition. Manage pregnancy expectantly and anticipate vaginal delivery.
  Daily suppressive acyclovir 400 mg three times daily from 36 weeks of gestation reduces HSV lesions at term and hence the need for delivery by caesarean section.[7]
  3rd trimester infection: recommended to deliver by CS. Risk of neonatal transmission by vaginal birth is > 40%. If serology shows HSV IgG, then the episode is recurrent and CS is not required to prevent neonatal transmission.

Recurrent genital herpes
Risk of neonatal transmission is low (0–3%), even if genital lesions are present at time of delivery, therefore CS not required to prevent neonatal transmission. Daily suppressive acyclovir 400 mg three times daily should be considered from 36 weeks of gestation.

Human immunodeficiency virus (HIV)

Organism

HIV-1 and HIV-2. Most infections in Singapore are caused by HIV-1.

Classification

Retrovirus

Clinical Features

Clinical HIV infection undergoes 3 distinct phases:
(1) Acute seroconversion
    Infection becomes established. Lasts from a few weeks to several months. Symptoms include fever, flu like illness, lymphadenopathy and rash.
(2) Asymptomatic infection
    Exhibit no or few signs and symptoms for up to a decade or more.
(3) AIDS
    Significant opportunistic infections, or CD4 count less than 200/microlitre.

Diagnosis

Antibodies are identified by the use of a screening test, usually an enzyme-linked immunosorbent assay (ELISA), followed by definitive diagnosis using a Western Blot assay.

A positive ELISA test is usually observed within 3–6 weeks following infection.

The Western Blot is the definitive diagnostic test for HIV infection. The Western Blot (WB) assay detects antibodies in patient sera that react with a number of different viral proteins.

It is possible that an indeterminate result is due to early HIV infection and incomplete evolution of the anti-HIV immune response. An indeterminate test result should be repeated at 1, 2 and 3 months to exclude an evolving pattern.

PCR for HIV DNA is available in special circumstances e.g. for infants of mothers with HIV infection to distinguish active infection of the infant from passive transfer of maternal antibodies, and in cases where the WB test is indeterminate in a patient with high-risk behaviour.

Management

HIV infection and AIDS are notifiable conditions.

Each HIV-infected patient entering into care should have a complete medical history, physical examination, and laboratory evaluation and should be counselled regarding the implications of HIV infection. Newly diagnosed HIV-infected persons should receive psychosocial evaluation including ascertainment of behavioural factors indicating risk for transmitting HIV. Women should be counselled or appropriately referred regarding reproductive choices and contraceptive options.

Patients need to be started on antiretroviral therapy (ART). There are more than 20 approved antiretroviral drugs, and they fall into six different classes.

Listing all treatment regimes is beyond the scope of this summary, but selection of a regimen should be individualised based on virologic efficacy, toxicity, pill burden, dosing frequency, drug–drug interaction potential, resistance testing results, and the patient's comorbid conditions.

Patients with HIV are managed by an infectious diseases specialist.

Partners

HIV-infected patients should be encouraged to notify their partners and to refer them for counselling and testing. If the patient is unwilling to notify his/her partner, the first step should be for the doctor to make the notification. The doctor is empowered to do so under the Infectious Diseases Act.

Pregnancy

Aim is to prevent mother to child transmission (MTCT).

The prevalence of HIV in Singapore resident women is about 0.2 per 1000. Women from sub-Saharan Africa approximately 2–3%, UK born women 0.5 per 1000.

(There were a total of 417 women aged 20–49 newly diagnosed with HIV in Singapore between 1985 and 2013. 1.9 million women in that age group in 2013.)

MTCT about 25% without intervention, below 1% with antiretroviral therapy.

Routine antenatal screening in Singapore.

Newly diagnosed HIV-positive pregnant women do not require any additional baseline investigations compared with non-pregnant HIV-positive women other than those routinely performed in the general antenatal clinic.

In women who either conceive on combination antiretroviral therapy (cART) or who do not require cART for their own health there should be a minimum of one CD4 cell count at baseline and one at delivery.

In women who commence cART in pregnancy a viral load should be performed 2–4 weeks after commencing cART, at least once every trimester, at 36 weeks and at delivery.

In women commencing cART in pregnancy, liver function tests should be performed as per routine initiation of cART and then at each antenatal visit.

It is recommended that women conceiving on an effective cART regimen should continue this even if it contains efavirenz or does not contain zidovudine.

Women requiring ART for their own health should commence treatment as soon as possible as per Singapore Communicable Disease Centre guidelines.

All women should have commenced ART by week 24 of pregnancy.

There is most evidence and experience in pregnancy with zidovudine plus lamivudine.

A woman who presents after 28 weeks should commence cART without delay.

For women taking cART, a decision regarding recommended mode of delivery should be made after review of plasma viral load results at 36 weeks:[8]

< 50 HIV RNA copies/mL: in the absence of obstetric contraindications, a planned vaginal delivery is recommended.

50–399 HIV RNA copies/mL: pre-labour Caesarean Section (PLCS) should be considered, taking into account the actual viral load, the trajectory of the viral load, length of time on treatment, adherence issues, obstetric factors and the woman's views.

≥ 400 HIV RNA copies/mL: PLCS is recommended.

Vaginal birth after Caesarean section (VBAC) should be offered to women with a viral load < 50 HIV RNA copies/mL.

Hepatitis B

Organism

Hepatitis B virus

Classification

DNA Hepadna virus

Clinical Features

Incubation period 40–160 days

Up to 50% of adults in the acute phase of infection may have no symptoms (especially likely in those with HIV coinfection).

Two phases of acute illness:

(1) Prodromal illness: flu-like symptoms (malaise, myalgia, fatigue), often with right upper quadrant pain. This phase usually lasts between 3 and 10 days.

(2) Icteric illness: jaundice (hepatic and cholestatic) associated with anorexia, nausea, fatigue, liver enlargement and tenderness. This usually lasts for 1–3 weeks, but can persist for 12 or more weeks in a minority of patients who have symptoms of cholestasis such as itching and/or deep jaundice.

Chronic carriers are usually asymptomatic but may have fatigue or loss of appetite.

Often, there are no physical signs of chronic infection. After many years of infection, depending on the severity and duration, there may be signs of chronic liver disease.

Chronic infection (> 6 months) occurs in 5–10% of symptomatic cases.

Diagnosis

In acute Hepatitis B infections, the order of appearance of markers, and their clinical significance is

- HBsAg (Hepatitis B surface antigen) — presence of HBV
- HBeAg (Hepatitis B envelope antigen) — viral replication: high infectivity
- antiHBc IgM, (IgM antibody to Hepatitis B core antigen) — acute infection
- antiHBe (Hepatitis B envelope antibody) — loss of viral replication: low infectivity
- antiHBc IgG (IgG antibody to Hepatitis B core antigen) — late acute or chronic infection
- antiHBs (Hepatitis B surface antibody) — protective antibody.

There are 4 phases of chronic carriage:

- Immune Tolerant (HBe Ag +ve, normal ALT levels, little or no necroinflammation on liver biopsy)
- Immune Active, HBe Ag +ve phase (HBe Ag +ve, raised ALT, progressive necroinflammation and fibrosis)
- Inactive hepatitis B carrier (HBsAg+ve, HBeAg -ve, low levels of HBV DNA and normal ALT)
- HBeAg -ve chronic active hepatitis (precore, core promotor mutations, HBeAg -ve, detectable HBV DNA, progressive inflammation and fibrosis).

Types 2 and 4 may progress to cirrhosis and liver cancer, with type 4 generally progressing fastest.

Management

Acute viral hepatitis is notifiable.

Patients should be advised to avoid unprotected sexual intercourse until they have become non-infectious or their partners have been successfully vaccinated.

Management of patients with chronic hepatitis B should be tailored according to the clinical state of liver disease (compensated versus decompensated liver disease) as well as virologic and biochemical status (i.e. the liver function test, in particular the serum transaminase levels).

Treatment of chronic infection is usually managed by a gastroenterologist or hepatologist. Antiviral treatments include lamivudine, adefovir, tenofovir, telbivudine and entecavir. Interferon treatment is another option.

Partners

Should be vaccinated.

Pregnancy and breastfeeding

Routine screening is performed antenatally.

Vertical transmission of infection occurs in 90% of pregnancies where the mother is HBeAg +ve and in about 10% of HBsAg +ve, HBeAg -ve mothers. More than 90% of infected infants become chronic carriers.

Infants born to infectious mothers are vaccinated from birth, usually in combination with Hepatitis B specific Immunoglobulin 200 i.u. i.m. This reduces vertical transmission by 90%.

There is some evidence that treating the mother in the last month of pregnancy with lamivudine may further reduce the transmission rate if she is highly infectious, but this needs to be further substantiated.

Infected mothers should continue to breastfeed as there is no additional risk of transmission.

Reporting of Notifiable Diseases

In Singapore, HIV/AIDS, gonorrhoea, syphilis, chlamydia, herpes and viral hepatitis have to be notified under the Infectious Diseases Act.

However, other than HIV/AIDS, notification is for epidemiological analysis, not for case detection or contact tracing.

Acute Pelvic Inflammatory Disease

Overview

Acute pelvic inflammatory disease (PID) is usually an ascending infection from the endocervix, leading to endometritis, salpingitis, parametritis, oophoritis, tubo-ovarian abscess and pelvic peritonitis.

The original infection may be sexually transmitted (e.g. *Chlamydia* or gonorrhoea) or a vaginal infection.

PID is a common cause of morbidity and accounts for 1 in 60 GP consultations by women under 45 years of age. If PID is not treated promptly it can cause long-term problems such as infertility, chronic pelvic pain and ectopic pregnancy.

Acute PID is not easy to diagnose since many of the symptoms can be caused by other conditions. However, since a delay of only a few days can have long-term sequelae, acute PID should be treated before a positive diagnosis is made.[9]

Aetiology

PID is often polymicrobial. There are both sexually transmitted and non-sexually transmitted pathogens.

Sexually-transmitted pathogens
> *N. gonorrhoeae*
> *C. trachomatis*
> *Mycoplasma genitalium*
> *Mycoplasma hominis*
> *Ureaplasma urealyticum*

Non-sexually transmitted pathogens
> Anaerobic bacteria (e.g. *Prevotella*, *Atopobium* and *Leptotrichia*)
> *Gardnerella vaginalis*
> Gram-negative rods
> Streptococci

Presenting Symptoms and Signs

Women with acute PID commonly present with bilateral lower abdominal tenderness, which may also radiate to the legs. They often have an abnormal vaginal or cervical discharge. They may also be pyrexial, with a temperature greater than 38°C.

Another associated feature of acute PID is abnormal vaginal bleeding. This bleeding may be intermenstrual, post-coital or breakthrough bleeding.

Because of the inflammation of the cervix, uterus and surrounding tissues, women may complain of dyspareunia, especially on deep penetration.

When a woman with acute PID is examined, this will be expressed as cervical motion tenderness on bimanual vaginal examination. The adnexae are also likely to be tender. Further, there may or may not be a palpable adnexal mass.

Differential Diagnosis

There are several different reasons for abdominal pain in young women. Important conditions to exclude are:

Ectopic pregnancy
Acute appendicitis
Endometriosis
Irritable bowel syndrome
Complications of an ovarian cyst
Urinary tract infection
Functional pain

Management

It is important to ascertain that the patient is stable. Unstable patients require prompt resuscitation.

History including full sexual history

- Recent sexual exposures — usually the last and second last partner, spouse, casual or regular partner, whether local or overseas
- Type of sexual exposure — vaginal, anal or oral
- Use of condoms — for vaginal, anal, oral sex
- Use of other contraceptives
- Previous STI

Physical Examination

Abdominal palpation
Pelvic Examination

Investigations

Pregnancy test
Full Blood Count, C-Reactive Protein
Screening for STIs including HIV
Ultrasound scan

Treatment

It is likely that delaying treatment increases the risk of long-term sequelae such as ectopic pregnancy, infertility and pelvic pain. Because of this, and the lack of definitive diagnostic criteria, a low threshold for empirical treatment of PID is recommended. Broad spectrum antibiotic therapy is required to cover *N. gonorrhoeae*, *C. trachomatis* and a variety of aerobic and anaerobic bacteria commonly isolated from the upper genital tract in women with PID.

Outpatient versus Inpatient Treatment

While many patients may be treated as outpatients, admission for parenteral therapy, observation, further investigation and/or possible surgical intervention should be considered in the following situations:

- A surgical emergency cannot be excluded
- Lack of response to oral therapy
- Clinically severe disease
- Presence of a tubo-ovarian abscess
- Intolerance to oral therapy
- Pregnancy

Parenteral therapy is recommended for patients with more severe clinical disease e.g. pyrexia > 38°C, clinical signs of tubo-ovarian abscess, signs of pelvic peritonitis.

Recommended Regimens

Outpatient

Ceftriaxone 500 mg i.m. single injection with Doxycycline 100 mg orally twice daily for 14 days and Metronidazole 400 mg orally twice daily for 14 days.

Inpatient

Ceftriaxone 2 g i.v. daily, plus i.v./oral Doxycycline 100 mg twice daily, plus oral Metronidazole 400 mg twice daily for a total of 14 days.

Patients should be advised to avoid unprotected intercourse until they, and their partner(s), have completed treatment and follow-up.

PID in Pregnancy

This is rare, but if it does occur, there is an increase in both maternal and fetal morbidity. However, none of the above evidence-based regimens are of proven safety in this situation. Coverage of gonorrhoea, *Chlamydia* and anaerobic infections may be achieved with I.M. ceftriaxone, I.V. or oral erythromycin, plus I.V. or oral metronidazole.

Role of Laparoscopy

Laparoscopy enables specimens to be taken from the tubes and Pouch of Douglas. The procedure can provide information on the severity of PID as well as exclude alternative pathology. As such, laparoscopy is considered the gold standard in making the diagnosis of PID. This conclusion is based on a Swedish study published by Jacobson et al from the 1960s. However, laparoscopy is not without risks and is not commonly used for primary diagnosis. Furthermore, in 15–30% of cases there is no evidence of acute infection despite organisms being isolated.[10]

However, surgical treatment may at times be appropriate. For example, surgical treatment should be considered in severe cases, or where there is clear evidence of a pelvic abscess, drainage can lead to earlier resolution of PID and decrease the likelihood of long-term sequelae.

Ultrasound guided aspiration of pelvic fluid collection is less invasive and may be equally effective.

Complications

Fitz-Hugh-Curtis syndrome
This refers to perihepatic adhesions that are secondary to pelvic infection, most commonly with *C. trachomatis*. This is usually only diagnosed at laparoscopy. Some women may have right upper quadrant pain.

IUCD
Removal of an IUCD may result in better short term clinical outcome, however the decision whether to remove an IUCD or leave it *in situ* should be made on a case by case basis, as it needs to be balanced against the risk of pregnancy.

Patient Counselling

When counselling patients, the following should be considered:

- The treatment being given and its possible adverse effects
- Fertility is usually maintained but there remains a risk of future infertility, chronic pelvic pain or ectopic pregnancy
- Clinically more severe disease is associated with a greater risk of sequelae
- Repeat episodes of PID are associated with an exponential increase in the risk of infertility
- The earlier treatment is given the lower the risk of future fertility problems
- Future use of barrier contraception will significantly reduce the risk of PID
- The need to screen her sexual contacts for infection to prevent her becoming re-infected.

References

1. UK Guidelines on the Management of Syphilis 2008 DOI: 10.1258/ijsa.2008.008279.
2. UK national guideline for the management of gonorrhoea in adults, 2011 DOI: 10.1258/ijsa.2011.011267.
3. Gopalakrishnakone D, Appan DP, Singh K. (2009) Prevalence of Chlamydia trachomatis in Singaporean women undergoing termination of pregnancy. *Ann Acad Med Singapore* **125**(38):457–460.
4. SIGN 109: Management of genital Chlamydia Trachomatis infection. http://www.sign.ac.uk/pdf/sign109.pdf.
5. United Kingdom National Guideline on the Management of Trichomonas vaginalis 2014. http://www.bashh.org/documents/UK%20national%20guideline%20on%20the%20management%20of%20TV%20%202014.pdf.
6. European guideline on management of genital herpes.
7. RCOG BASHH joint guideline on management of genital herpes in pregnancy.
8. British HIV Association guidelines for the management of HIV infection in pregnant women 2012.
9. UK National guideline on PID 2011. http://www.bashh.org/documents/3572.pdf.
10. Jacobson L, Weström L. (1969) Objectivized diagnosis of acute pelvic inflammatory disease. Diagnostic and prognostic value of routine laparoscopy. *Am J Obstet Gynecol.* **1**;105(7):1088–1098.

9

PELVI-ABDOMINAL MASS AND BENIGN OVARIAN TUMOURS

Ida Ismail-Pratt and Jeffrey Low

Introduction

Pelvi-abdominal mass is not an uncommon finding in gynaecology. It can present at any age. A woman with a pelvi-abdominal mass can present with various symptoms that can be menstrual, urological, bowel or pressure related symptoms. In a good majority of women, the mass can be asymptomatic and discovered incidentally.

Differential Diagnosis of Pelvi-Abdominal Mass

When a woman presents with a pelvi-abdominal mass, the two key issues are:

(1) Where does the mass come from?
(2) Is it benign or malignant?

The most common mass in a woman of reproductive age is pregnancy. As such a high index of suspicion is necessary. The most common non-pregnancy related benign gynaecological mass is a fibroid uterus. Enlargement or pathology in other pelvic organs such as the bladder and colon may also give rise to pelvi-abdominal masses.

TABLE 9.1 Differential Diagnosis of a Pelvi-Abdominal Mass

	Gynaecological	
	Benign	**Malignant**
Uterus	• Gravid uterus	
	Non -pregnancy related • Fibroid • Adenomyosis • Pyometra	Carcinoma Sarcoma
Fallopian tubes	Tubo-ovarian abscess Hydro-salpinx	Tubal cancer
Ovaries	Physiological cyst • Follicular • Haemorrhagic Benign tumour • Dermoid • Cystadenoma • Fibroma Endometrioma	Malignant tumour Borderline tumour
	Non-gynaecological	
Bladder	Distended bladder	Bladder carcinoma
Bowel	Faecal loading in the colon	
	Diverticular abscess	Colorectal carcinoma
	Appendiceal abscess	
Rertroperitoneal	Pelvic kidney	Renal carcinoma

History

Take a good and thorough general history including age, obstetric and menstrual history, surgical, medical and drug history, family and social history.

Obtain information specifically pertaining to her key symptoms, as well as other symptoms that will narrow down the differential diagnoses.

TABLE 9.2   Symptoms in Presenting Complaints and Associated History

Presenting Complaint	Specific Symptoms
Abdominal swelling/distension	*Most common abdominal swelling in a reproductive age woman is pregnancy. Rule this out.* *Persistent abdominal distension/swelling of more than two weeks in a non-pregnant woman is usually associated with a pelvic tumour, such as ovarian malignancy.*
Acute or chronic pain *Mnemonic (**SOCRATES**)* • *Site* • *Onset* • *Character* • *Radiation* • *Alleviating factors/Associated symptoms* • *Timing* • *Exacerbating factors* • *Severity*	*Acute pain* • *If pregnant, an ectopic pregnancy must be ruled out.* • *If associated with fever and foul smelling vaginal discharge, the diagnosis of pelvic inflammatory disease (PID) with tubo-ovarian abscess is most likely.* • *Cyclical acute pain may be due to endometriosis and the presence of an endometrioma or adenomyosis.* *Chronic pain* • *Cyclical pain may be due to longstanding endometriosis and endometrioma.* • *A tubo-ovarian abscess and previous history of PID may cause chronic pelvic pain*
Pressure symptoms *The mass may be pressing on other organs, thus causing pressure symptoms*	• *Urological: Frequency of micturition or voiding difficulties.* • *Bowel: Constipation or bloatedness.* • *General heaviness in the abdomen or pelvis.*
Menstrual dysfunction • *Heavy menstrual bleeding* • *Postmenopausal bleeding* • *Intermenstrual bleeding* • *Post-coital bleeding*	• *Fibroids are usually associated with heavy menstrual bleeding.* • *Irregular menses in a premenopausal woman, or postmenopausal bleeding, may be due to uterine malignancy.* • *The most common reason for intermenstrual or postcoital bleeding is pelvic/vaginal infection, and if associated with a pelviabdominal mass, a tubo-ovarian abscess or hydrosalpinx is more likely.* • *Cervical cancer may also present with postcoital bleeding.*

Physical Examination

General Examination

This is important, in particular looking for pallor, breast lumps, any palpable lymphadenopathy or lower limb oedema.

Abdominal Examination

Refer to Table 9.3 and Table 9.4.

TABLE 9.3   Components of Abdominal Examination in a Woman with Pelvi-Abdominal Mass

Abdominal examination	
Inspection	• *Presence of any scars* — help in predicting the difficulties of future abdominal surgery, if required • *Abdominal distension* — can be due to the 7F's: *Fat, Fluid, Fetus, Flatus, Faeces, Filthy big tumours or False pregnancy* • *Local (e.g. surgical hernia) or general abdominal swelling* • *Other findings*: prominent veins, pulsations, skin lesions
Abdominal palpation	(1) Presence of an acute abdomen: Guarding, rigidity, rebound tenderness (2) Intra-abdominal mass (see Table 9.4 below) (3) Other organs: hepatosplenomegaly, inguinal lymph node enlargement
Specific test	• Ascites; shifting dullness or fluid thrill • Palpation for supraclavicular node enlargement

TABLE 9.4   Descriptive Features of a Pelvi-Abdominal Mass

For any abdominal mass, the following should be determined:

(1) Site: Region involved
(2) Tenderness
(3) Size (must be measured) and shape
(4) Surface: Regular or irregular
(5) Edge: Regular or irregular
(6) Consistency: Hard or soft
(7) Mobility and movement with inspiration
(8) Pulsatile or not
(9) Whether or not can get below the mass — which indicates this is most likely a pelvic mass

The Pelvic Examination

The components of a pelvic examination are inspection, speculum examination and digital vaginal examination.[1]

Inspection

Inspection of the external female genitalia is important prior to proceeding to speculum and vaginal examination.

- Skin discoloration or pigmentation: leukoplakia, lichen sclerosis
- Signs of infection: redness, swelling, excoriation
- Lumps or bumps: ulceration, warts, vulval abscess
- Vaginal discharge: purulent, clear, bloodstained
- Check for stress incontinence
- Check for ureovaginal prolapse

Speculum examination

Assessment made during speculum examination includes:

- Presence and nature of vaginal discharge
- Appearance of the cervix: cervical atrophy/cervicitis, cervical polyp, nabothian follicle, cervical ectropion, cervical cancer
- Appearance of the vaginal walls: atrophy/vaginitis, vaginal lumps/lesions

Digital bimanual vaginal examination

Vaginal examination involves assessment of:

- Uterus: bimanual palpation of the uterus allows for assessment of its size, shape, mobility, ante/retroversion position, tenderness and consistency
- The cervix: normally points towards the posterior vaginal wall. Note the position, size, shape, consistency, tenderness including cervical excitation and mobility
- Vaginal fornices: There are four fornices. Anterior, posterior left and right fornices. This allows assessment of the adnexa and parametrial area. This will also allow further assessment of a pelvic mass

Rectal examination

A rectal examination is an important part of a physical examination, especially if malignancy is suspected. The rectal exam will allow for the assessment of the Pouch of Douglas.

Investigations

Urine Pregnancy Test

- Should be performed in all women of reproductive age

Diagnostic Imaging

Pelvic ultrasound scan

- Pelvic ultrasound scan is the most sensitive radiological investigation in the assessment of a pelvic mass.[2] Specific features on a pelvic ultrasound scan suggestive of malignancy are:
  - Solid cystic appearance
  - Septations
  - Bilaterality
  - Intra-abdominal nodules
  - Presence of ascites/free fluid

CT scan

- If malignancy is strongly suspected
- Can help to assess for the presence of metastases or lymph node involvement

Blood Investigations

If a malignant ovarian mass is suspected, serum tumour markers may be of some value in the initial assessment.[2,3] However, these are neither very sensitive nor specific and should only be used as a guide to management.

- Ca-125 — Elevation could be due to physiological, benign or malignant causes
- CEA — GI tract tumours
- CA 19-9 — Mucinous tumours
- LDH — Dysgerminoma
- AFP — Yolk sac tumour
- bHCG — Ovarian choriocarcinoma (extremely rare)

Management of Ovarian Tumours

Ovarian tumours or neoplasms may be broadly classified as:

- Benign
- Malignant

Benign Ovarian Tumours

These can be further classified as:

- Physiological e.g. follicular cysts, corpus luteum cysts
- Pathological e.g. endometriotic cysts, benign cystadenoma

Benign ovarian cysts are far more common than ovarian malignancies. Their size can vary tremendously, from a few cm to sizes large enough to fill the entire abdominal cavity. They may be unilateral or bilateral and the majority are cystic tumours.[4]

Management principles

- Observation

Especially when the cysts are smaller than 5 cm in diameter, physiological cysts will tend to resolve spontaneously

- Surgical options[4] include:
  - Cystectomy — preservation of the normal ovarian tissue and uterus
  - Salpingo-oophorectomy — preservation of the uterus and contralateral tube and ovary
  - Total hysterectomy and bilateral salpingo-oophorectomy — especially in postmenopausal women

Malignant Ovarian Tumours

Ovarian malignancies form the 5th most frequent cancers of females in Singapore.[5] They constitute 5.4% of all the cancers in females in Singapore and have an age-specific rate of 12.5 per 100,000. This is discussed in the chapter on Ovarian Cancer.

References

1. RCOG Greentop Guideline No. 62: (2011) *Management of Suspected Ovarian Masses in Premenopausal Women.*
2. Sari R, Buyukberber S, Sevinc A, *et al.* (2000) The effects of abdominal and bimanual pelvic examination and transvaginal ultrasonography on serum CA-125 levels. *Clin Exp Obstet Gynecol* **27**:69–71.
3. Aggarwal P, Kehoe S. (2010) Serum tumour markers in gynaecological cancers. *Maturitas,* **67**:46–53.
4. Curtin JP. (1994) Management of the adnexal mass. *Gynecol Oncol* **55**:S42–S46.
5. Annual Registry Report. (2014) Trends in Cancer Incidence in Singapore 2009–2013. Singapore Cancer Registry.

10

UTERINE FIBROIDS AND ADENOMYOSIS

Ng Ying Woo

Fibroids and Adenomyosis are two common conditions that a gynaecologist will encounter in his/her daily work. When one mentions fibroids, most women seem to know a fair bit about the condition and its management. But surprisingly, far fewer women are aware of adenomyosis and its sequelae. Nevertheless, both conditions have a great impact on a woman's quality of life, as they often present with menstrual disorders or fertility issues.

Fibroids

Introduction

The incidence of uterine fibroid tumours increases with age, and they may occur in more than 30% of women after the age of 40.[1] Uterine fibroid tumours tend to arise during the reproductive years, enlarge during pregnancy and regress after menopause. Their growth rate is influenced by oestrogen. Risk factors include nulliparity, obesity, family history, black race, and hypertension.

Pathology and Terminology/Location

Fibroids (Leiomyomata) grossly appear as round, well circumscribed (but not encapsulated), solid nodules that are white or tan, and show whorled appearance on histological section. Microscopically, tumour cells resemble normal cells (elongated, spindle-shaped, with a cigar-shaped nucleus) and form bundles with different directions (whorled).

An International Federation of Gynecology and Obstetrics (FIGO) staging scheme for fibroid location has recently been proposed to describe fibroids.[2] The new FIGO classification gives eight positions: submucous (0, 1, 2), interstitial (3, 4, 5), subserous (6, 7), others e.g. cervical or parasitic (8) (Fig. 10.1).

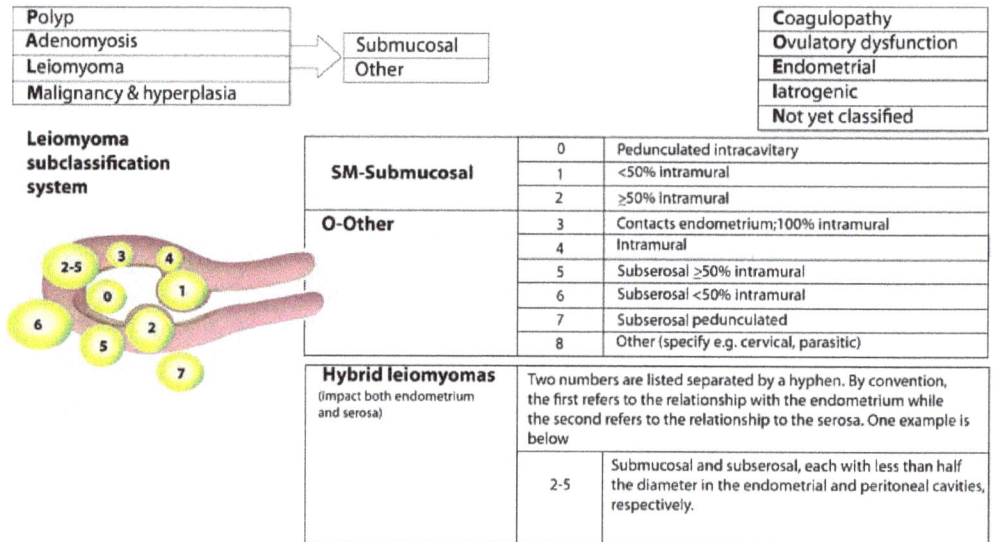

Polyp		
Adenomyosis	→	Submucosal
Leiomyoma		Other
Malignancy & hyperplasia		

| | |
| Coagulopathy |
| Ovulatory dysfunction |
| Endometrial |
| Iatrogenic |
| Not yet classified |

Leiomyoma subclassification system

SM-Submucosal		0	Pedunculated intracavitary
		1	<50% intramural
		2	≥50% intramural
O-Other		3	Contacts endometrium;100% intramural
		4	Intramural
		5	Subserosal ≥50% intramural
		6	Subserosal <50% intramural
		7	Subserosal pedunculated
		8	Other (specify e.g. cervical, parasitic)

Hybrid leiomyomas (impact both endometrium and serosa)	Two numbers are listed separated by a hyphen. By convention, the first refers to the relationship with the endometrium while the second refers to the relationship to the serosa. One example is below
2-5	Submucosal and subserosal, each with less than half the diameter in the endometrial and peritoneal cavities, respectively.

FIGURE 10.1 ■ Staging of fibroids and location.

Clinical Features

Fibroids, particularly when small, may be entirely asymptomatic. Symptoms also depend on the location, size and number of the lesions. Symptoms can be broadly categorised into three entities: menstrual abnormalities, pelvic discomfort/pain and fertility problems.

Menstrual Abnormalities

Menorrhagia (regular heavy menstrual flow) is the most common symptom associated with uterine fibroid tumours.[3] Other menstrual patterns, such as intermenstrual bleeding or postmenopausal bleeding, are **NOT** characteristic of myomas and should be investigated to rule out endometrial pathology, especially malignancy.

Often the location of the fibroid contributes to the presence and degree of uterine bleeding, with size of secondary importance. For example, submucosal myomas that protrude into the uterine cavity (e.g. types 0 and 1) are most frequently related to significant menorrhagia. Women with intramural myomas, especially those that distort the uterine cavity, may also experience heavy or prolonged menstrual bleeding. The mechanism(s) of profuse menses are unclear, but may include dysregulation of local growth factors, vascular abnormalities, impaired endometrial haemostasis, or molecular dysregulation of angiogenic factors.[4]

Pelvic Discomfort/Pain

Fibroids may cause specific symptoms due to direct pressure at particular locations, such as urinary frequency or urgency when pressing on the bladder. Rarely, urinary obstruction can occur with a posterior fibroid pushing the entire uterus forward and pressing on the mid-urethral. Direct compression on the ureters due to large fibroid leading to renal hydronephrosis is rare.[5]

Back pain may, on occasion, be related to the presence of myomas. Very large uterine fibroids may compress the vena cava and lead to increase in thromboembolic risk.[6] Infrequently, fibroids can cause acute pain due to degeneration (e.g. red degeneration during pregnancy) or torsion of a pedunculated tumour.

Infertility

The role of fibroid tumours in infertility is controversial. Fibroids that distort the uterine cavity (submucosal or intramural with an intra-cavitary component) may result in difficulty conceiving a pregnancy and an increased risk of miscarriage.[7] In addition, fibroids can be associated with adverse pregnancy outcomes (e.g. placental abruption, foetal growth restriction, malpresentation, and preterm labour and birth).

Diagnosis — The presumptive diagnosis of uterine myoma is usually based upon the clinical finding of an irregularly enlarged uterus on bimanual pelvic examination. Typically, an ultrasound is used to confirm the diagnosis and exclude the possibility of other pathology or an adnexal mass.

Pelvic examination — A thorough pelvic examination should be performed. On bimanual pelvic examination, an irregularly enlarged uterus is consistent with a leiomyomatous uterus. The size, contour, and mobility of the uterus should be noted, along with any other findings (e.g. adnexal mass, cervical mass). Infrequently, on speculum exam, a prolapsed submucosal fibroid may be visible at the external cervical os.

When a myoma is suspected based upon symptoms or pelvic examination findings, ultrasound imaging or hysteroscopy are useful to affirm the diagnosis.

Ultrasound — Transvaginal ultrasound has high sensitivity (95% to 100%) for detecting myomas in the uterus. In addition, it is also useful to determine the size, number and location of these myomas. This is the most widely used modality, due to its easy availability and cost-effectiveness. Besides confirming the diagnosis, it can exclude the possibility of other pathology or an adnexal mass.

Differential Diagnosis — The differential diagnosis of an enlarged uterus includes both benign and malignant conditions:

Differential diagnosis

- Leiomyoma
- Uterine adenomyosis or adenomyoma
- Leiomyoma variant
- Adenomatoid tumours
- Pregnancy

- Haematometra
- Uterine sarcoma
- Uterine carcinosarcoma
- Endometrial carcinoma
- Metastatic disease (typically from another reproductive tract primary)

Treatment Options

Relieving the symptoms (e.g. abnormal uterine bleeding, pain, pressure) is the major goal in management of women with uterine fibroids. Treatment plan should be customised and individualised to the patient, based upon factors such as:

Factors to consider when customising treatment plan:

- Type and severity of symptoms
- Size of the myoma(s)
- Location of the myoma(s)
- Age of the patient
- Reproductive plans and obstetrical history

Expectant Management

Expectant management with observation is increasingly recognised as a reasonable course for women with asymptomatic fibroids, especially if they are near to their presumed menopause. The risk of a malignant leiomyosarcoma is small (0.23%).[8]

Levonorgestrel-releasing intrauterine system (Mirena®)

Studies have shown a reduction in uterine volume and bleeding, and an increase in hematocrit after placement of Mirena for treatment of menorrhagia related to uterine fibroids. The device is widely used for control of heavy menstrual bleeding and is now approved by the US Food and Drug Administration (FDA) for this indication. An addition advantage of this treatment is its contraceptive effect for women who do not desire pregnancy.

Surgery

Surgery is the mainstay of therapy for fibroids. Hysterectomy is the definitive procedure; myomectomy by various techniques, endometrial ablation, uterine artery embolisation, magnetic resonance-guided focused-ultrasound surgery, and myolysis are alternative procedures. Indications for surgery include abnormal menstrual bleeding or bulk-related symptoms, and /or infertility or recurrent pregnancy loss.

Hysterectomy. Leiomyomas are one of the most common indications for hysterectomy. The main advantage is that it eliminates both current symptoms and the chance of recurrent problems from leiomyomas. For many women who have completed childbearing, this freedom from future problems makes hysterectomy an attractive option. Nevertheless, we have to bear in mind the operative risks associated with this option.

Myomectomy. Myomectomy is an alternative for women who have not completed childbearing or otherwise wish to retain their uterus. Although myomectomy is an effective therapy for menorrhagia and pelvic pressure, the disadvantage of this procedure is the risk of recurrences, intra-operative bleeding and fertility issues.

Over the years, the traditional laparotomy approach has been replaced by laparoscopic and robotic-assisted procedures in removing subserosal or intramural myomas. Intra-cavitary myomas (submucosal and intramural myomas that protrude into the uterine cavity) can be effectively removed via hysteroscopic approach.

Adenomyosis

Introduction

Adenomyosis refers to a disorder in which there is presence of ectopic endometrial glands within the uterine musculature (uterine adenomyomatosis). These ectopic endometrial tissues appear to induce hypertrophy and hyperplasia of the surrounding myometrium, which results in a diffusely enlarged uterus.

Pathology

The pathogenesis of adenomyosis is not known. The two major theories are that it either develops from endomyometrial invagination of the endometrium or de novo from mullerian rests.[9]

Microscopic Appearance — The pathognomonic feature of adenomyosis is the presence of endometrial tissue within the myometrium at a distance of at least one low power field from the endomyometrial junction. A zone of myometrial hypertrophy and hyperplasia surrounds the adenomatous tissue. The ectopic endometrium may show a functional response to oestrogen and progesterone, but usually has an immature proliferative pattern.

Clinical Manifestations — Heavy and painful menstruation are the major symptoms of adenomyosis, occurring in approximately 60% of affected women.[10] The heavy menstrual flow is possibly related to the increased endometrial surface of the enlarged uterus, while pain may be due to bleeding and swelling of endometrial islands confined by myometrium.

As discussed above, physical examination usually reveals diffuse uterine enlargement (often termed "globular" enlargement). The uterus may be tender on palpation.

Diagnosis — A definitive diagnosis of adenomyosis can only be made from histological examination of a hysterectomy specimen. The pre-operative diagnosis is suggested by characteristic clinical manifestations i.e. heavy menstrual bleeding and dysmenorrhea with a uniformly enlarged uterus.

Transvaginal ultrasound — Ultrasound evidences for adenomyosis include (1) asymmetric thickening of the myometrium (with the posterior myometrial typically thicker), (2) myometrial cysts, (3) linear striations radiating out from the endometrium, (4) loss of a clear endomyometrial border, and (5) increased myometrial heterogeneity.

Treatment — The definitive treatment for adenomyosis is hysterectomy. Since disease is confined to the uterus, ovarian conservation can be employed unless there are other contraindications.

Hormonal manipulation with progestins (including the levonorgestrel-releasing intrauterine contraception, gonadotropin-releasing hormone analogs, or aromatase inhibitors may be effective for reducing the menstrual flow and dysmenorrhea, as in endometriosis.

With these findings in mind, hysterectomy appears to be the treatment of choice for women with significant symptoms who have completed childbearing. Nevertheless, for younger women with extensive adenomyosis, exploration of alternative treatments for symptomatic relief is warranted.

References

1. Lurie S, Piper I, Woliovitch I, Glezerman M. (2005) Age-related prevalence of sonographically confirmed uterine myomas. *J Obstet Gynaecol* **25**: 42–44.
2. Munro MG, Critchley HO, Fraser IS. (2011) FIGO Menstrual Disorders Working Group. The FIGO classification of causes of abnormal uterine bleeding in the reproductive years. *Fertil Steril* **95**: 2204.
3. Fraser IS, Critchley HO, Munro MG, *et al.* (2007) A process designed to lead to international agreement on terminologies and definitions used to describe abnormalities of menstrual bleeding. *Fertil Steril* **87**: 466.
4. Stewart EA, Nowak RA. (1996) Leiomyoma-related bleeding: a classic hypothesis updated for the molecular era. *Hum Reprod Update* **2**: 295.
5. Bansal T, Mehrotra P, Jayasena D, *et al.* (2009) Obstructive nephropathy and chronic kidney disease secondary to uterine leiomyomas. *Arch Gynecol Obstet* **279**: 785.
6. Fletcher H, Wharfe G, Williams NP, *et al.* (2009) Venous thromboembolism as a complication of uterine fibroids: a retrospective descriptive study. *J Obstet Gynaecol* **29**: 732.
7. Pritts EA, Parker WH, Olive DL. (2009) Fibroids and infertility: an updated systematic review of the evidence. *Fertil Steril* **91**: 1215.

8. Parker WH, Fu YS, Berek JS (1994) Uterine sarcoma in patients operated on for presumed leiomyoma and rapidly growing leiomyoma. *Obstet Gynecol* **83**: 414–418.
9. Ferenczy A. (1998) Pathophysiology of adenomyosis. *Hum Reprod Update* **4**: 312.
10. McElin TW, Bird CC. (1974) Adenomyosis of the uterus. *Obstet Gynecol Annu* **3**: 425.

11

UNPLANNED PREGNANCY

Lim Li Min and Kuldip Singh

Introduction

Abortion refers to the termination of a pregnancy before the birth of the child. This is usually performed before the limit of fetal viability. In Singapore, abortion is allowed up to 24 weeks of gestation.

According to the World Health Organisation (WHO), the estimated worldwide rate for induced abortion in 2008 was 28 per 1,000 in women aged from 15 to 44. In Asia, abortion rates across subregions held steady between 2003 and 2008, with 36 per 1,000 in Southeast Asia. 21.6 million women experience an unsafe abortion worldwide each year; 18.5 million of these occur in developing countries. 47,000 women die from complications of unsafe abortion each year. Deaths due to unsafe abortion remain close to 13% of all maternal deaths.[1]

Indications for Abortion

Maternal Reasons

- Cardiac disease
- Malignancy
- Renal disease
- Acute psychosis

Fetal Reasons

- Chromosomal and structural anomalies of the fetus

Social Reasons

- Financial costs of raising a child
- Need to defer starting a family

History of Abortion Legislature in Singapore

Before 1967: Legal abortion was restricted only to cases where maternal life was endangered

1967: *Abortion Authorisation Board set up*

Abortion extended to those with fetal malformations, where the mother was a victim of sex crime, or sexual intercourse with a mentally insane person

1968: *First Abortion Bill*

Law liberalised to allow abortion for family, social and economic reasons

1974: *New Abortion Act*

Abortion could be performed at the request of any female up to 24 weeks of pregnancy, by a registered doctor with prescribed qualification, in an approved institution. This resulted in a dramatic increase in the number of abortions performed, beginning in 1974. The rate peaked at 23,512 abortions in 1985. There were 42,484 live births in that year, indicating 35% of all pregnancies were terminated in 1985 (Figs. 11.1 and 11.2).

1987: *Mandatory pre-abortion counselling was introduced*

Consent for procedure could only be given 48 hours after counselling. This led to a decline in the number of abortions.

In Singapore, the number of abortions fell to a 30-year low in 2013 when 9,282 abortions were performed. During that same period, there were 39,720 births, indicating about 19% of pregnancies were terminated. The number of abortions has been falling steadily in the last five years[2] (Figs. 11.1 and 11.2).

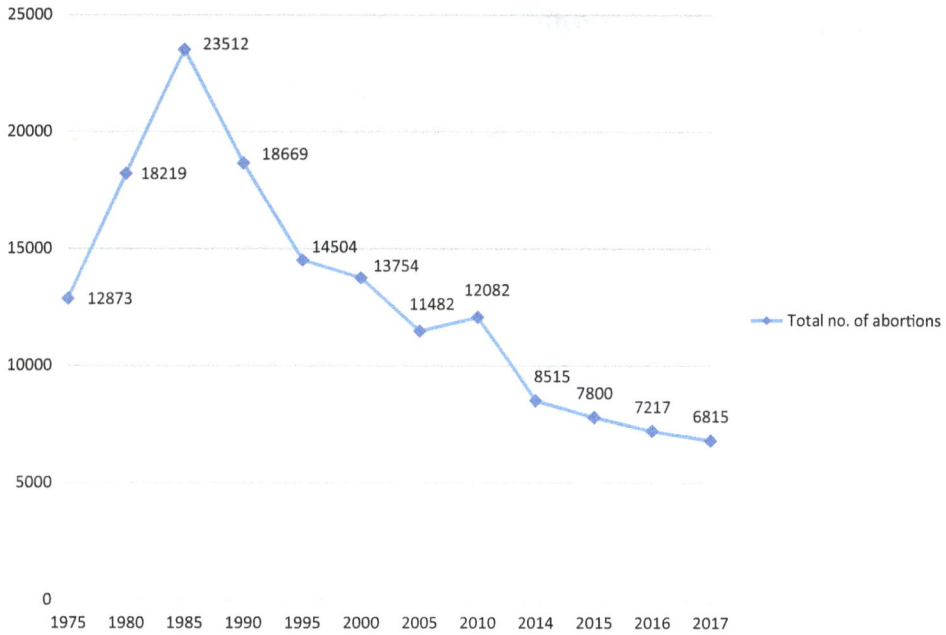

FIGURE 11.1 ■ Abortion trends in Singapore from 1975 to 2017 (total number of abortions).

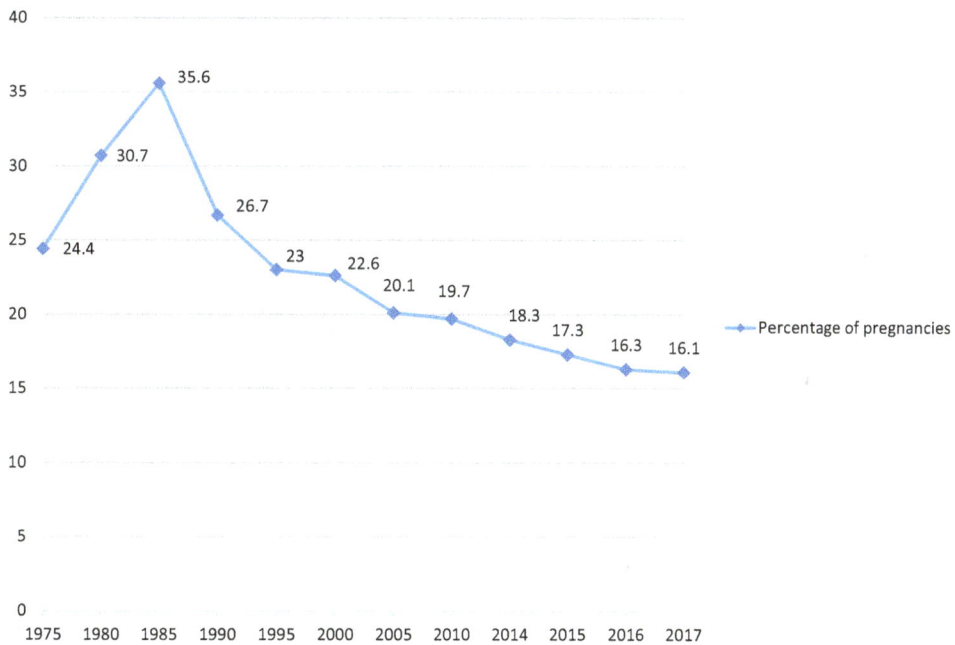

FIGURE 11.2 ■ Abortion trends in Singapore from 1975 to 2017 (percentage of pregnancies).

Abortion Laws in Singapore

Singapore's laws on abortion are encapsulated in the Termination of Pregnancy Act.[2]

Termination of pregnancy act

This act states that every treatment for terminating pregnancy shall be carried out by an authorised medical practitioner in an approved institution. An authorised medical practitioner shall not carry out treatment for the termination of pregnancy on any pregnant woman other than:

(a) A citizen of Singapore or the wife of a citizen of Singapore.
(b) A holder, or the wife of a holder, of a work permit pass or employment pass.
(c) A person who has been resident in Singapore for at least four months.

Unless it is immediately necessary to save the life of the pregnant woman.

No treatment for terminating a pregnancy of more than 24 weeks can be carried out unless the treatment is immediately necessary to save the life, or to prevent grave permanent injury to the physical or mental health, of the pregnant woman.

Pre-abortion counselling must be provided for a pregnant woman, regardless of her marital status. The Act requires the pregnant woman to sign a declaration that she has been counselled, and there is a mandatory waiting period of 48 hours after the counselling is conducted before the procedure can be done.

Special groups
(a) *Girls below 16 years of age (except for rape victims)*
It is mandatory to refer an unmarried girl below 16 years of age for pre-abortion counselling at the Health Promotion Board Counselling Centre when she seeks treatment to terminate pregnancy. A Certificate of Attendance (COA) will be issued to her by the Health Promotion Board Counselling Centre. No termination of pregnancy can be performed unless the COA is produced by the girl.
(b) *Mentally disabled women* require certification by a psychiatrist that continuation of the pregnancy will be harmful to the mother before medical procedures can be done.

Pre-Abortion Considerations

History and Examination

Firstly, the woman's reasons for terminating the pregnancy must be explored and any misconceptions should be clarified.

A full medical history should be obtained including parity, previous surgeries and abortions, any complications during previous abortion. A thorough examination should be performed, in particular to assess uterine size (to correlate to gestation) and any adnexal tenderness or masses.

Gestational dating: The use of the woman's last menstrual period (if she is sure of the dates and her periods are regular) should be confirmed by pelvic examination of the uterine size. Pregnancy location, viability and gestation must be confirmed by a pelvic ultrasound examination.

Investigations

- Full blood count: to assess haemoglobin
- Rhesus status
- *Chlamydia* screening:

Chlamydia is a common infection. According to the WHO 2008 report, there was a 4.1% increase in new cases worldwide compared to 2005, with an estimated incidence of 29.7/1,000 women. In Southeast Asia, incidence of *Chlamydia* was 9.2/1,000 women.[3] In Singapore, the incidence of *Chlamydia* among females decreased from 62 per 100,000 in 2008 to 32 per 100,000 in 2013.[4]

The U.S. Preventive Services Task Force recommends screening of asymptomatic women for *Chlamydia trachomatis* infection in the following high risk groups: all sexually active women age 25 years or younger, sexually active women older than 25 years with risk factors (e.g. a new sex partner in prior 60 days, more than one sex partner, inconsistent condom use, unmarried, or history of STI).[5]

In Singapore, the estimated prevalence of *Chlamydia trachomatis* in Singaporean women undergoing termination of pregnancy was 8%, similar to the prevalence rates among women requesting an abortion in the United Kingdom.[6] Thus, opportunistic screening for *Chlamydia* would be justified in our local context.

Infective prophylaxis

Universal antibiotic prophylaxis at the time of abortion is associated with a reduction in the risk of subsequent infective morbidity of around 50%. Antibiotic prophylaxis has been shown to decrease the incidence of post-abortal infection in surgical abortions, thus routine antibiotic prophylaxis should be given. In areas where universal antibiotic prophylaxis is not practised, *Chlamydia* screening should be considered.

Antibiotic prophylaxis effective against both *Chlamydia trachomatis* and anaerobes should be considered.

The following regimens may be considered for surgical abortions[7]:

- Azithromycin 1 g orally on the day of the abortion, plus metronidazole 1 g rectally or 800 mg orally prior to, or at the time of, the abortion
  OR
- Doxycycline 100 mg orally twice daily for seven days, starting on the day of the abortion, plus metronidazole 1 g rectally or 800 mg orally prior to, or at the time of, the abortion
  OR
- Metronidazole 1 g rectally or 800 mg orally prior to, or at the time of, abortion for women who have tested negative for *C. trachomatis* infection.

Counselling

Pre-operative counselling includes a thorough discussion of the various types of pregnancy termination procedures (medical or surgical): the risks, benefits, and expected outcome of each procedure. Alternatives must be discussed (e.g. continuing pregnancy and adoption) as well. A signed informed consent should be obtained from all women.

Contraceptive options should be discussed and should cover both reversible methods as well as irreversible methods, where appropriate. The woman may choose to start long acting reversible contraception on the same day after the abortion, or even choose to have methods such as the intrauterine contraceptive device (IUCD) or implant inserted after a surgical abortion under anaesthesia.

Options for Termination

Options for termination of pregnancy can be broadly divided into: **medical** or **surgical** abortion.

The type of abortion chosen depends on gestation, operator experience or preference, availability of resources, the woman's fitness for surgery and her preference. Surgical abortion has the attendant risks of anaesthesia and surgery but can be completed in one visit. Medical abortion avoids the risks of surgery and anaesthesia, but the woman may experience prolonged bleeding as well as side effects of the medication as detailed below.

First Trimester Termination of Pregnancy

Medical

- Mifepristone-misoprostol combined regimen, or
- Misoprostol (prostaglandin E1) only

A combined regimen of mifepristone and misoprostol is universally recommended as it is more effective than misoprostol alone (96–97% versus 88%).[8,9] A misoprostol-only regimen can be considered when mifepristone is not available.

Mifepristone (RU-486)

Mifepristone (RU-486) is an anti-progesterone and is contraindicated in women with porphyria, chronic adrenal failure, on concurrent long-term corticosteroid therapy or who are at risk of haemorrhage. Mifepristone administered alone results in complete termination of pregnancy in 64–85%. Mifepristone elicits an increase in sensitivity to prostaglandin 24–48 hours after its administration. Thus the rational for a combined effect of mifepristone and misoprostol (prostaglandin E1). This permits greater efficacy of prostaglandin at lower doses, thus minimising potential side effects.[8-10]

Misoprostol

This is a synthetic prostaglandin E1 analogue. It is prescribed for the treatment of gastric ulcers but is commonly used in abortions. It is generally well tolerated, inexpensive, can be stored at room temperature, and is widely available. Common side effects are nausea, diarrhoea and fever which are self-limiting. These side effects are reported more frequently in women taking oral rather than vaginal misoprostol. Asthma is not a contraindication to use of misoprostol. Misoprostol can be administered via vaginal, oral, sublingual, buccal, or rectal routes. At less than eight weeks' gestation, vaginal misoprostol (initial dose of 800 mcg then 400 mcg every three hours up to three doses) has been shown to approach the efficacy of surgical abortion, with 96% success rate.[9]

Currently research has shown that the best method of terminating a first trimester unwanted pregnancy up to 10 weeks gestation is a dose of 200 mg of mifepristone followed 24 hours by an oral/buccal dose of 800 µg of misoprostol. This result has a success rate of 97% medical abortion.[9]

In the first trimester medical abortion the woman must be assessed

- Clinically to have an intrauterine pregnancy by ultrasound.
- Beta HCG, a human chorionic gonadotopin is determined
- The date of 200 mg of mifepristone is given followed by 800 μg of misoprostol buccally/orally 24 hours later
- The woman is reviewed at 7 to 10 days with a repeat beta HCG. In a successful abortion, there will be a fall in the beta HCG level close to 80 to 90%. In general ultrasound assessment is limited as often some blood clots/echogenic areas would be seen, whereas a specific drop in beta HCG is more assuring
- If there is a suboptimal drop of beta HCG, a second dose of 800 μg of misoprostol may be given and the beta HCG evaluated a week later
- With an optimal drop of beta HCG, the woman can be reviewed in 6 to 8 weeks to assess return of menses. The woman needs to be assured that until the beta HCG becomes negative, she can be expected to have some spotting or bleeding.

Surgical

Vacuum aspiration

This is an appropriate method at this early gestation only when there are safeguards to ensure complete abortion. There is a higher risk of retained products of conception or continuing pregnancy at this gestation. These safeguards include confirmation of products of conception (POC) at aspiration (by placing POC in sterile water or saline to wash away the blood and look for fetal membranes or fronds of chorionic villi) or ultrasound confirmation of a complete evacuation after the procedure (by assessing the endometrial cavity and endometrial thickness). Surgical vacuum aspiration performed at less than 7 weeks gestation are 3 times more likely to fail than those performed between 7 and 12 weeks.[7]

Pre-cervical priming before surgical abortion

Cervical priming is beneficial where difficulty in cervical dilatation is expected, especially in nulliparous women.

Methods include:

- Osmotic dilators (e.g. natural: Laminaria tents; synthetic: Dilapan-S)
- Rigid dilators (e.g. Hegar dilators)
- Pharmacological agents (e.g. misoprostol)

A combination of methods may be needed. Adequate cervical preparation can help minimise the occurrence of procedure-related complications, such as cervical laceration and uterine perforation.

Misoprostol is 97% effective in cervical dilation in the first trimester.[21] This method is less uncomfortable for the woman and more convenient. Both oral and vaginal misoprostol given at dosages of 400 mcg are effective for cervical priming when administered three hours prior to surgical vacuum aspiration.[11,12]

Second Trimester Termination of Pregnancy

Medical

- Medical abortion: mifepristone–misoprostol combined regimen or misoprostol only regimen
- Intra-amniotic instillation of abortifacients e.g. prostaglandin F2-alpga, hypertonic saline

Combined mifepristone–misoprostol regimens have been consistently found to be safe and effective in the second trimester. This combined regimen has been shown to be associated with a shorter induction-to-abortion interval and lower analgesic requirements compared to misoprostol only regimens.[13,14] Mifepristone and misoprostol regimens, alone or in combination, result in fetal expulsion in >90% of abortions within 24 hours. Surgical evacuation is not required routinely after mid-trimester medical abortion.

The recommended mifepristone–misoprostol regimen[15]:

- Mifepristone 200 mg orally, followed 36–48 hours later by misoprostol 80 mcg vaginally, then misoprostol 400 mcg orally or vaginally, 3-hourly, to a maximum of four further doses. If abortion does not occur, mifepristone can be repeated three hours after the last dose of misoprostol, and 12 hours later misoprostol may be recommenced.

The recommended prostaglandin only regimen:

- Prostaglandin E1 analogues e.g. misoprostol

A recommended regimen is misoprostol 400 mcg vaginally 3-hourly for up to five doses. Women who fail to expel the foetus after five doses may wait up to 12 hours before starting another cycle of misoprostol up to five doses.[16] Vaginal administration was shown to be more effective and associated with a shorter induction-to-delivery interval compared with oral administration.[17,18]

- Prostaglandin E2 analogues e.g. dinoprostone (Prostin): 3 mg intravaginal pessary every 3–4 hours, with a maximal exposure of 24 hours. The mean time to abortion is 13–14 hours, and 90% of women abort by 24 hours.[19]

Successful abortion rates are similar between vaginal misoprostol (400 mcg every 3 hours) or intra-amniotic PGF2alpha (carboprost 1.5 mg), but vaginal misoprostol is associated with a shorter mean induction-to-abortion interval. Fever and shivering are more common with vaginal misoprostol compared with intra-amniotic PGF2alpha.[16]

Oxytocin fails to effectively induce labour compared to the above agents because the uterus has less oxytocin receptors at less than 20 weeks of gestation. Oxytocin is associated with side effects such as postpartum haemorrhage and water intoxication.

Hysterotomy or hysterectomy may be considered after failed medical abortion when dilatation and evacuation cannot be safely performed, such as in situations where multiple obstructing myomas are present, with pelvis peritoneal malignancy or after an abdominal cerclage.[20]

Table 11.1 Summary of Methods of Induced Abortion

First Trimester Methods of Abortion		Second Trimester Methods of Abortion	
Efficacy		**Efficacy**	
Medical abortion	96–97% with combined mifepristone–misoprostol regime up to 7 weeks;[8,9] 88–96% with misoprostol only regime (up to 8 weeks)[9,10]	**Systemic abortifacients**	97% successful abortion rates with combined mifepristone–misoprostol regime.[15] 95.1% successful abortion rates (at 48 hours) with misoprostol only regime[16]
Surgical abortion	98–99% with vacuum aspiration[9]	**Intra-amniotic instillation of abortifacients**	93% successful abortion rates with combined mifepristone–misoprostol regime[16]
		Dilation and evacuation	93% successful abortion rates[20]

Surgical

- Dilatation and evacuation (D&E)

The procedure must only be performed by an experienced operator with adequate cervical preparation (e.g. osmotic dilators or prostaglandins). For gynaecologists lacking the necessary expertise and case-load, medical abortion may be appropriate. Anaesthetic options include conscious sedation, regional block, and general anaesthesia. A vacuum cannula can be used, although forceps may be required after 16–17 weeks.[20]

Postoperative Care

Women should be observed for vaginal haemorrhage or changes in vital signs for at least four hours before discharge. Women may be told to expect mild lower abdominal cramps 2–4 days after the procedure, which can be treated with non-steroidal anti-inflammatory drugs. They should also expect some light vaginal bleeding up to a week after the procedure.

Women who are Rh(D)-negative and unsensitised should receive Anti-D IgG within 72 hours following abortion (surgical or medical).

All women should receive a 24-hour contact number in case of emergency. The woman should be advised to seek medical consult immediately if she experiences heavy bleeding, fever, or abdominal pain. She should be advised to refrain from vaginal intercourse or tampon use for two weeks post procedure to reduce the risk of infection.

The woman's chosen contraceptive should be started immediately. Intrauterine contraceptives/implants can be inserted immediately following medical and surgical abortion at all gestations, so long as it is reasonably certain that the woman is not still pregnant. Women who have yet to decide on contraception should be offered information on contraceptive options.

Complications of Pregnancy Termination

- Mortality — <0.1 per 1,000
- Complication rate -1–2 per 1,000
- Complications of abortions increase
  - With gestational age
  - In teenage pregnancies

Immediate Complications of Induced Abortion[20]

Trauma (surgery-related)

This includes: cervical tears (<1% risk) , uterine perforation (<0.1–0.4% risk), uterine rupture during medical abortions (0.1%), bowel or blood vessel injury. Further treatment e.g. laparoscopy or laparotomy may be required for repair. The risk is lower for early abortions and with more experienced operators.

Major haemorrhage (< 0.1–0.4% risk)

Blood transfusion may be required in the event of acute heavy bleeding, or rarely, hysterectomy. This risk increases beyond 20 weeks.

Infection (< 0.1–1% risk)

This includes endometritis and urinary tract infection which may require additional treatment with antibiotics, and sometimes prolonged hospital stay for intravenous antibiotics. The risk is higher in the presence of chlamydial or gonorrhoeal infections.

Retained products of conception (< 5% risk)

Further intervention may be required e.g. surgical evacuation of uterus after medical abortion or re-evacuation following surgical abortion.

Venous thromboembolism

Women at risk of thromboembolism include those with known thrombophilia or family history of thrombophilias, obese, smoker and age more than 35 years old.

Failed abortion (< 1%)

The risk to an ongoing pregnancy after medical termination cannot be quantified, but the woman must be warned of this risk if she chooses to continue with the pregnancy. Misoprostol has been associated with the development of congenital abnormalities including scalp or skull defects, cranial nerve palsies (Mobius syndrome), and limb deficiencies (e.g. equinovarus). This may be related to vascular disruption.[21]

Late Complications of Induced Abortion

Uterine rupture during subsequent pregnancy <0.1%

Cervical incompetence

Some studies have found an increased risk of cervical insufficiency with rapid mechanical dilation or an increasing number of abortion procedures. Cervical priming before surgical evacuation must be considered in order to reduce this risk.

Infection — pelvic inflammatory disease

Additional treatment of antibiotics and sometimes prolonged hospital stay for intravenous antibiotics may be required.

Intrauterine adhesions (Asherman's syndrome)

Asherman's syndrome may present with secondary amenorrhoea and may require hysteroscopic adhesiolysis.

Psychological sequelae

Women are no more or less likely to suffer adverse psychological sequelae whether they have an abortion or continue with the pregnancy and have the baby. However, those women who have existing mental health problems should be closely monitored.

Impact on subsequent pregnancy

There is evidence that women with a previous termination have a slightly higher rate of retained placenta but no difference in the risk of placenta praevia.[22] There is insufficient evidence regarding the risk of preterm birth or preterm pre-labour rupture of membranes.[23]

Follow-Up after Pregnancy Termination

Immediate Follow-Up (1–2 Weeks)

The woman should be assessed to rule out a possibility of retained products of conception (prolonged or heavy bleeding, fever, abdominal pain) or endometritis (foul-smelling discharge, fever, uterine tenderness). Psychological support should be offered as needed. Contraceptive advice should be given if she has not started on any method.

Delayed Follow-Up (6–8 Weeks)

The return of her menstruation should be checked.

If the woman has prolonged bleeding after two weeks: the possibility of retained products of conception (POC) or endometritis should be ruled out. Signs indicating retained POC: cervical os is open, POC seen at cervical os or in the vaginal canal, thickened endometrial lining on US pelvis. If endometrium is thin, then may consider treating with antibiotics for endometritis.

If there is no return of menstruation, a urine pregnancy test should be checked. If not pregnant, the woman should be reviewed again in one month. If she still has no menses one month later, combined contraceptive pills should be started for one cycle. If there is no response, then Asherman's syndrome must be excluded.

Duties of Doctor to Patient

(1) Ensure proper indication for any abortion
(2) Abortion counselling, emphasising dangers
(3) Obtain informed consent
(4) Post abortion counselling and advice on family planning to prevent recurrence
(5) Patient confidentiality should be respected. Issues of child protection or under-age sexual intercourse should adhere to local policy

References

1. Department of Reproductive Health and Research, WHO. (2011) *Unsafe abortion: global and regional estimates of incidence of unsafe abortion and associated mortality in 2008*. WHO, 6th edn.

2. Ministry of Health (Singapore) guidelines and statistics (accessed 30/12/14).

3. Department of Reproductive Health and Research, WHO. (2012) *Global incidence and prevalence of selected curable sexually transmitted infections — 2008.*

4. MOH. (Singapore) Report (2013) Communicable Diseases Surveillance in Singapore 2013.

5. LeFevre ML. (2014) Screening for Chlamydia and gonorrhea: US Preventive services task force recommendation statement. *Ann Intern Med* **161**(12): 902.

6. Gopalakrishnakone D, Appan DP, Singh K. (2009) Prevalence of Chlamydia trachomatis in Singaporean women undergoing termination of pregnancy. *Ann Acad Med Singapore* **38**(5):457–460.

7. Royal College of Obstetricians and Gynaecologists. (2011) The Care of Women Requesting Induced Abortion: Evidence-based Clinical Guideline Number 7.

8. Spitz IM, Bardin CW, Benton L, *et al.* (1998) Early Pregnancy Termination with Mifepristone and Misoprostol in the United States. *N Engl J Med* **338**(18): 1241–1247.

9. Yi-Ling Tan, Kuldip Singh. Kok Hian Tan, *et al.* (2018) Acceptability and feasibility of outpatient medical abortion with mifepristone and misoprostol up to 70 days gestation in Singapore. *Eur J Obstet Gynecol Reprod Biol* **229**:144–147.

10. Singh K, Fong YF, Dong F. (2003) A viable alternative to surgical vacuum apiration: Repeated doses of intravaginal misoprostol over 9 hours for medical termination of pregnancies up to eight weeks. *BJOG* **110**(2):175–80.

11. Singh K, Fong YF, Prasad RN, *et al.* (1998) Randomized trial to determine optimal dose of vaginal misoprostol for preabortion cervical priming. *Obstet Gynecol* **92**(5):795–798.

12. Singh K, Fong YF. (2000) Preparation of the cervix for surgical termination of pregnancy in the first trimester. *Hum Reprod Update* **6**(5):442–448.

13. Rodger MW, Baird DT. (1990) Pretreatment with mifepristone (RU 486) reduces interval between prostaglandin administration and expulsion in second trimester abortion. *Br J Obstet Gynaecol* **97**:141e5.

14. Webster D, Penney GC, Templeton A. (1996) A comparison of 600 and 200 mg mifepristone prior to second trimester abortion with the prostaglandin misoprostol. *Br J Obstet Gynaecol* **103**:706e9.

15. Ashok PW, Templeton A, Wagaarachchi PT, Flett GM. (2004) Midtrimester Medical Termination of Pregnancy: A Review of 1002 Consecutive Cases. *Contraception* **69**(1):51–58.

16. Su LL, Biswas A, Choolani M, *et al.* (2005) A prospective, randomized comparison of vaginal misoprostol versus intra-amniotic prostaglandins for midtrimester termination of pregnancy. *Am J Obstet Gynecol* **193**(4):1410–1414.

17. Bebbington MW, Kent N, Lim K, *et al.* (2002) A randomized controlled trial comparing two protocols for the use of misoprostol in midtrimester pregnancy termination. *Am J Obstet Gynecol* **187**:853.

18. Dickinson JE, Evans SF. (2003) A comparison of oral misoprostol with vaginal misoprostol administration in second-trimester pregnancy termination for fetal abnormality. *Obstet Gynecol* **101**:1294.

19. Surrago EJ, Robins J. (1982) Midtrimester pregnancy termination by intravaginal administration of prostaglandin E2. *Contraception* **26**:285e94.

20. Lim LM, Singh K. (2014) Termination of pregnancy and unsafe abortion. *Best Pract Res Clin Obstet Gynaecol* **28**(6):859–869. DOI:10.1016/j.bpobgyn.2014.05.005. Epub 2014 Jun 4.

21. Gonzalez CH, Marques-Dias MJ, Kim CA, *et al.* (1998) Congenital abnormalities in Brazilian children associated with misoprostol misuse in first trimester of pregnancy. *Lancet* **351**(9116):1624.

22. Zhou W, Nielsen GL, Larsen H, *et al.* (2001) Induced abortion and placenta complications in the subsequent pregnancy. *Acta Obstet Gynecol Scand* **80**(12):1115.

23. Akhlouf MA, Clifton RG, Roberts JM, *et al.* (2014) Adverse pregnancy outcomes among women with prior spontaneous or induced abortions. *Am J Perinatol* **31**(9): 765–772. DOI:10.1055/s-0033-1358771. Epub 2013 Dec.

12

FAMILY PLANNING

Arundhati Gosavi and Kuldip Singh

Introduction

Birth control, also known as **contraception** and fertility control, involves methods or devices used to prevent unplanned or unwanted pregnancy.

Contraception is essential for physical, mental and social well-being of a woman of reproductive age. It empowers woman to decide when and how often to reproduce.

An ideal contraceptive method should be 100% effective, acceptable, safe, free from any side effects, economic, simple to use, readily available, requiring minimal motivation and supervision, with immediate return to fertility and conferring as many health benefits as possible.

TABLE 12.1   Factors that May Influence the Choice of Contraception

Extrinsic Factors	Intrinsic Factors (Related to Method)
Age, parity, coital history	Efficacy of method
Future fertility intention	Mode of action
Medical condition	Duration of action
Family history	Return to fertility
Social history — e.g. smoking	Side effects of a method
Sexual history — e.g. number of partners	Advantages
Socioeconomic factors	Disadvantages
Education	Non-contraceptive benefits
Motivation	
Influence of peers, partner or culture	
Availability of a method	
Government policies	

The efficacy of a contraceptive method is calculated as follows using the Pearl Index.[1]

$$\frac{\text{Number of accidental pregnancies} \times 1200}{\text{Number of patients observed} \times \text{months of use}} = \text{Pregnancy failure rate/HWY (hundred woman years)}$$

TABLE 12.2   Efficacy of Various Contraceptive Methods

Method	Typical Use (%)	Perfect Use (%)
No method	85	85
Withdrawal	22	4
Male condom	18	2
Diaphragm	12	6
Combined oral contraceptive pills	9	0.3
Progestogen only pill	9	0.3
EVRA patch	9	0.3
Nuva ring	9	0.3
Depo provera	6	0.2
Intrauterine contraceptive device	0.8	0.6
Levonorgestrel intrauterine system — Mirena	0.2	0.2
Implant	0.05	0.05
Female sterilisation	0.5	0.5
Male sterilisation	0.15	0.10

Comparison of the percentage of women experiencing an unintended pregnancy during the first year of contraceptive method use.[2]

Typical use: refers to failure rates for women and men whose use is not consistent or always correct.

Correct use: refers to failure rates for those whose use is consistent and always correct.

Methods of Contraception

The term contraception includes all temporary and permanent methods of prevention of pregnancy.

TABLE 12.3   Contraceptive Methods

Contraceptive Methods	
REVERSIBLE	**IRREVERSIBLE**

NATURAL
Safe period method
Abstinence
Withdrawal method
	Sterilisations
	Male (vasectomy)
	Female
	Minilaparotomy e.g.
	  • Modified Pomeroy's technique
	  • Uchida's method

BARRIER METHODS
Mechanical
  • Male — condom
  • Female — condom, diaphragm, cervical cap
Chemical e.g.
  • Nonoxynol-9 cream
  • Sponge foam tablets
	Laparoscopy
	  • Silastic band/ring application
	  • Hulka clips
	  • Filshie clips
	
	Hysteroscopy
	Essure

HORMONAL METHODS
Combined Oestrogen + Progestogen methods
  • Combined oral contraceptive pills
  • Vaginal ring
  • Transdermal patch
Progestogen only methods
  • Progesterone Only Pills
  • Injection
  • Subdermal Implant
  • Intra-Uterine System (LNG-IUS)	

NON-HORMONAL METHODS
Intra-Uterine Contraceptive Devices (IUCD)
  • Inert
  • Copper containing	

Reversible Methods

Natural methods

Rhythm method — It is based on identification of the fertile period of a cycle. Various methods can be used to determine timing of ovulation, like recording the menstrual cycles (Calendar method), noting the basal body temperature (BBT method), noting the excessive mucus in the vaginal discharge etc. The method used may be abstinence or withdrawal method.

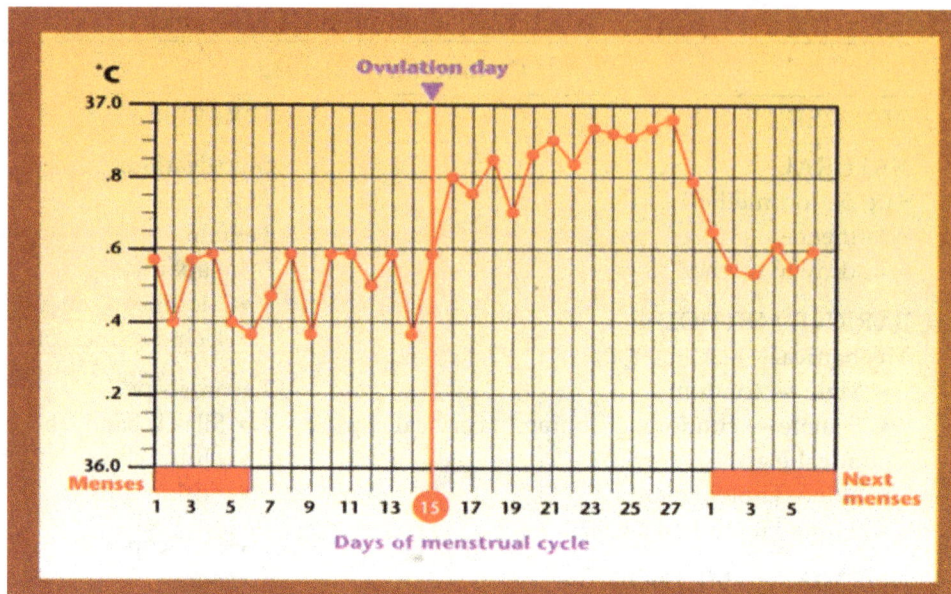

FIGURE 12.1 ■ Basal body temperature chart.

Mechanism of action — Prevent fertilisation
Efficacy — Has a high failure rate of 6% with perfect use
Advantages — No cost, no side effect.
Disadvantages

- The calculation may be inaccurate, hence high failure rate.
- Not applicable in women with irregular menstrual cycles.

Reversibility — Immediate

Barrier contraceptives

These methods use a barrier to prevent sperm deposition in the vagina. This can be achieved with:

- Physical barriers, like condoms in males and females, OR diaphragm or cervical cap in females.
- Chemical methods like Nonoxynol-9 (spermicidal cream) or aerosol foam tablets.

Male condom

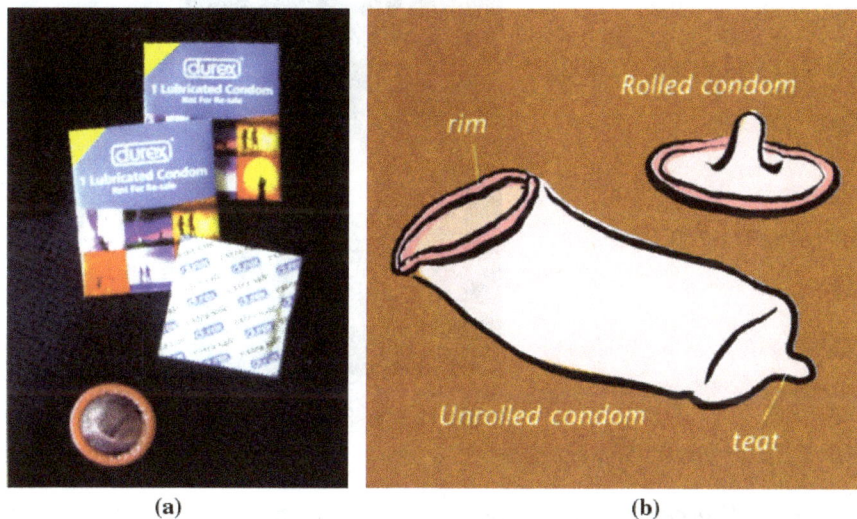

FIGURE 12.2a, b ■ Male condoms.

The most widely used method is the male condom. They are made of latex.

Mechanism of action — physical barrier for the union of sperm and ovum

Efficacy — The failure rate is 18% with typical use and 2% with perfect use after one year of usage. The efficacy can be increased with concurrent use of spermicidal creams.

Advantages

- It is cheap, simple to use and dispose and easily available without prescription
- It is coitus dependent, hence couples with infrequent coital frequency are spared from consumption of pills/hormones throughout the month.
- It protects against sexually transmitted infections (STI), pelvic inflammatory diseases (PID), Human Papilloma Virus (HPV) and cervical cell abnormalities.

Disadvantages

- The failure rate is high and varies widely amongst users.
- It may accidentally slip/break off.
- It interferes with sexual pleasure.

Side effects — some users may experience latex allergy.

Reversibility — immediate

Female condom — e.g. Femidom

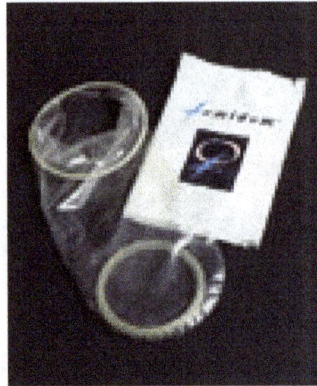

FIGURE 12.3 ■ Female condom.

It covers the cervix, lines the vagina and shields the introitus, thus providing a physical barrier between male and female genitalia and secretions during sexual intercourse. It has an anchor (like a ring/frame) outside the vagina to prevent the condom from being pushed inside the vagina during use and to aid removal.

Mechanism of action — Physical barrier for the union of sperm and ovum

Efficacy — Failure rate is 21% with typical use and 5% with perfect use

Advantages

- Protects against STIs and PID
- No delay in return of fertility following discontinuation of the method
- Can be placed before intercourse, as compared to the male condom

Disadvantages

- Some women find it difficult to insert and remove
- Higher failure rates in preventing pregnancy compared to the male condom.
- Not widely available worldwide
- It may not be appropriate for women who are not comfortable touching their genitals, or who may have other problems with insertion

Reversibility — Immediate

Hormonal methods

They can be either:

- Combined Oestrogen and Progestogen (E + P) methods, or
- Progestogen only methods.

Combined Oestrogen + Progestogene (E + P) methods

They can be used by various routes:

- Daily Combined Oral Contraceptive pills (COC pills)
- Weekly trans-dermal patch
- Monthly vaginal ring
- Monthly injections.

Combined Oral Contraceptive pills (COC pills)

It is a combination pill that contains Oestrogen and Progestogen. Low dose oral contraceptives are referred to the products containing less than 50 mcg of Ethinyl Estradiol.

The following oestrogens and progestogens may be used in various formulations.[3]

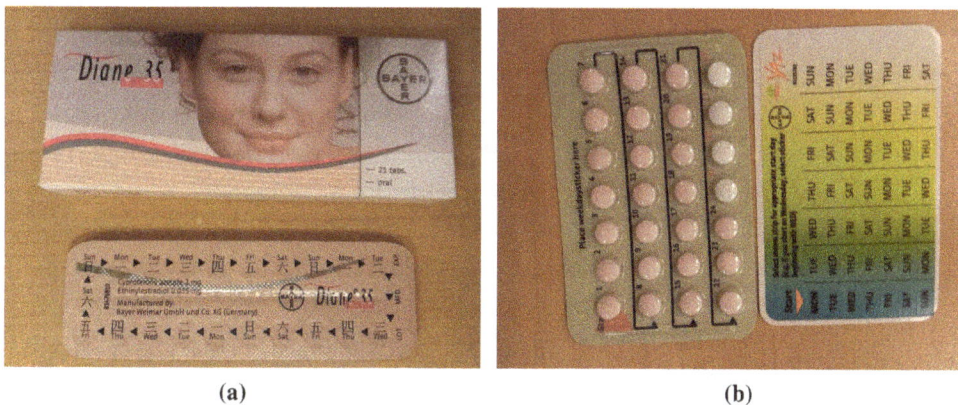

(a)   (b)

FIGURE 12.4 ■ (a) Pill pack 21 pills. Rear side with instructions. (b) Pill packet of 28 pills.

TABLE 12.4   Oestrogens and Progestogens in Contraceptive Formulas

Oestrogens	Progestogens	
Ethinyl oestradiol, Mestranol or Estradiol valerate	**17-Alfa hydroxyl-progesterone derivatives**	**19-Nortestosterone derivatives**
	Medroxyprogesterone acetate	Norethisterone (1st generation)
	Chlormadione	Norethynodrel
	Megestrol	Levonorgestrel (2nd generation)
		Desogestrel (3rd generation)
		Gestodene (3rd generation)
		Norgestimate (3rd generation)

Examples of some commonly prescribed COC pills are: Mercilon, Microgynon, Marvellon, Diane 35, Yasmin etc.

Mechanism of action — Progestin primarily suppresses LH secretion and thus prevents ovulation, while the oestrogenic agent suppresses FSH secretion and prevents the emergence of a dominant follicle.[3]

Administration — Some pill packets have 21 pills and others have 28 pills. The 21 day pill packets are to be taken for 21 days, with one week of pill-free period. The 28 day pill packets have seven placebo pills at the end of 21 active pills, hence the woman continues to take pills daily.

Efficacy — Highly effective, with failure rates of 0.3% with perfect use and 9% in typical use. Non-compliance is responsible for the majority of failures.

Missed pills

- If one pill is missed — take that pill as soon as remembered. Continue remaining pills at usual time. Emergency Contraception (EC) is not needed.
- If two pills are missed — take most recent pills as soon as remembered and continue remaining pills at usual time. Use condoms for the next seven days, until seven active pills have been taken. Consider EC if these two pills are missed in the first week, and omit pill free interval if in the last week.[4]

Advantages

- Highly effective, non-invasive, convenient method that gives regular menses
- **Confer the following non-contraceptive benefits:**[3]
  - Regulates cycles, relieves dysmenorrhoea and reduces menstrual loss.
  - Protects against epithelial ovarian cancer and endometrial cancers — use of COC pills protects against endometrial (by 50%) and ovarian cancers (by 40%) even after 12 months of usage. This protective effect increases with duration of use, continues for 20 years after stopping the pill and is seen with all low dose COC pills.
  - Protection against colorectal cancer — there is a 40% reduction in the risk of colorectal cancers with eight years of COC pill usage
  - Reduce benign breast disease and possibly benign ovarian cysts
  - Suppresses endometriosis
  - Reduces mid-cycle ovulation pain and pre-menstrual syndrome
  - Useful for the treatment of women with hyperandrogenism (most often due to polycystic ovary syndrome)
  - Withdrawal bleeding is predictable and adjustable

Disadvantages

- Need to take pill daily
- Not ideal for women who forget to take daily medications, or less motivated women.

TABLE 12.5   Side Effects/Risks of COC Pills

Minor Side Effects/Risks	Serious Risks
Nausea, vomiting	Cardiovascular disease
Breast fullness, tenderness	Venous thromboembolic disease
Headache/giddiness	Liver disease
Acne, facial pigmentation	Cancers
Breakthrough bleed	
Post pill amenorrhoea	
Decreased libido, mood	

Cardiovascular — There is a very small increase of risk of myocardial infarction (MI) and stroke with low dose pills. MI is an extremely rare event in these women, increased in users over age 35 years who smoke, most likely due to thrombotic mechanism.[5]

Venous thromboembolism (VTE) — The risk of VTE in women with low dose COC pills is three times higher than in healthy non-pregnant women. However, the absolute risk is small and less than the risk conferred by pregnancy. The factors influencing VTE are obesity, age and type of progestin used.[6]

Liver disease — Oestrogens affect the synthesis of hepatic cell enzymes and transport of biliary components. Long-term COC users are at risk of having benign hepatocellular adenomas. This risk is related to duration of COC use and to the dose of steroid.[7]

Cancers — Breast cancer — Available data on breast cancer risk with COC use are conflicting. Hence, a woman should be told that current and recent use of COC pills may be possibly associated with a slightly increased risk of pre-menopausal breast cancer. There is no effect of past use or duration of contraceptive use on risk of breast cancer.[8–10]

Cervical cancer — Studies have reported a small increase in the incidence of cervical cancer with use of COC pills. However, it may be related to confounding factors like age of first sexual intercourse, number of partners and HPV infection. Recent studies have shown that the relative risk of cervical cancer increases two fold with 10 years of use and are mostly confined to HPV positive cases.[3]

Pregnancy outcome — Women who become pregnant while taking COC pills should be advised that the risk of miscarriage is not increased, and that of significant congenital anomalies is not greater than the incidence in general population.[3]

Drug interactions — Drugs that reduce contraception efficacy of COC pills are: Anticonvulsants e.g. phenytoin, phenobarbitone; Antibiotics e.g. rifampicin, griseofulvin, broad spectrum antibiotics; and Sedatives, like chlordiazepoxide.

Some drugs may require dosage adjustment when taken concurrently with COC pills e.g. doses of anticoagulants, tricyclic antidepressants, insulin/oral hypo-glycaemics may need to be increased due to increased metabolism.[1]

TABLE 12.6   Contraindications to use of COC Pills

Absolute Contraindications	Relative Contraindications
Thromboembolic disorders	21–42 days postpartum
Cerebrovascular accidents	Obesity
Cardiovascular — coronary artery disease, IHD, complicated valvular heart disease	Adequately controlled hypertension
	Known hyperlipedemias
SLE with positive (or unknown) antiphospholipid antibodies	Uncomplicated valvular heart diseases
Impaired liver function	Diabetes
Hepatocellular adenoma, hepatoma	Migraine without aura
Migraine headaches with aura	Gall bladder disease
Vascular disease	Epilepsy on anticonvulsants
Current oestrogen dependent malignancy: breast, endometrium	Sickle cell disease
	Gall bladder disease
Pregnancy and postpartum < 21 days	SLE
Uncontrolled severe hypertension	Mitral valve prolapse
Age > 35 years and heavy smokers (15 sticks/day)	Elective surgery and immobilisation

Return to fertility — No significant delay with current low dose pills.[3]

Trans-dermal combined E + P patch (EVRA patch)

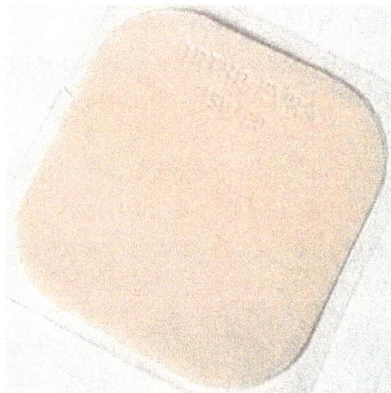

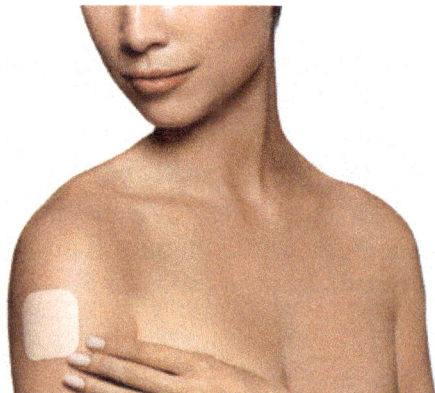

FIGURE 12.5 ■ Combined E + P patch (EVRA patch).

The 20 cm² patch contains 600 µg Ethinyl Estradiol and 6,000 µg Norelgestromin. It is a trans-dermal patch applied to clean, intact and dry skin on the upper outer arm, buttocks, abdomen or thigh.

Mechanism of action — The same as COC pills

Administration — A woman applies her first patch on the first day of her menstrual cycle, changes it weekly, and must remember the "patch change day"

Efficacy — Failure of 0.3% with perfect use and 9% with typical use

Advantages

• The patch is a simple and convenient form of birth control.
• Only requires weekly attention, giving better continuation rates.
• Avoids gastrointestinal malabsorption and hepatic first pass effect.
• Non-contraceptive benefits are the same as COC pills.

Disadvantages

• Women may forget the patch change day.
• Patch may fall off due to sweat/scratching.

Side effects

• Breast discomfort, engorgement or pain
• Headache, nausea
• Application site reaction and lint ring formation around the edge of the patch
• Menstrual cramps and rarely breakthrough bleeding.

Most of these side effects tend to go away after two or three months.

Contraindications — The same as COC pills.

Combined E + P injection

These are monthly injections, preferred by women who are satisfied by COC pills and who are keen for regular withdrawals but do not want daily oral dosing, or in women with gastrointestinal malabsorption.

A few examples of preparations are: Cyclofem, Lunelle and Cyclo-Provera (not available in Singapore).

Efficacy — Failure rate is 0.3% with perfect use.

Mechanism of action, contraindications and drug interactions are the same as COC pills.

Administration — Once a month intramuscular injection into the deltoid, gluteus maximus or anterior thigh.

Advantages and non-contraceptive benefits — Same as COC pills.

Disadvantages and side effects — Same as COC pills.

E + P vaginal ring

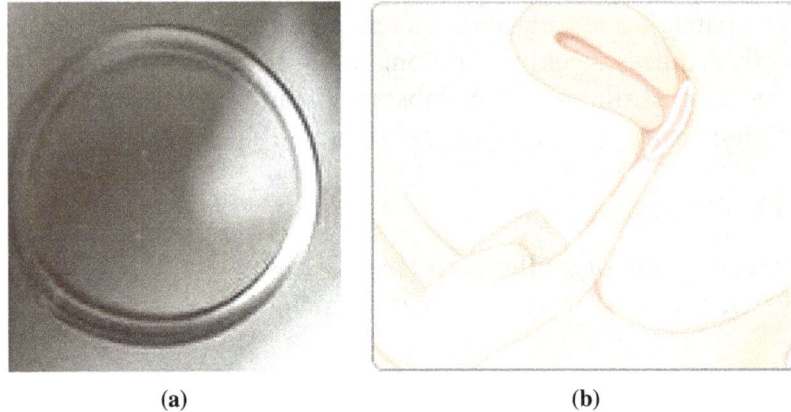

(a)   (b)

FIGURE 12.6 ■ Nuva Ring.

A combined hormonal contraceptive vaginal ring, available in pharmacies, is NuvaRing. It is a flexible plastic (ethylene-vinyl acetate copolymer) ring, two inches in diameter, which releases a low dose of a progestin and estrogen over three weeks. NuvaRing delivers 120 µg of etonogestrel and 15 µg of ethinyl estradiol each day of use.

Mechanism of action — It works primarily by preventing ovulation.

Administration — The ring should be inserted into the vagina for a three-week period and then removed for one week, during which the user will experience a menstrual period. It usually stays securely in place, even during exercise or sex. Women can check the contraceptive ring periodically with their finger.

Efficacy — Failure rate is 0.3% with perfect use.

Advantages

- Once-a-month self-administered, increasing compliance
- Convenience
- Ease of use and privacy
- Maintains regular menstrual cycles
- Avoids gastrointestinal absorption problems and renders lower systemic oestrogen exposure
- Avoids hepatic first pass effect

- Lower estrogen exposure than with COC pills
- Lower oestrogenic side effects, like nausea and breast tenderness

Disadvantages

- Rarely may fall out during sexual intercourse, while straining before or during a bowel movement, or while removing a tampon.
- Contraceptive efficacy is reduced if the ring is removed, accidentally expelled, or left outside of the vagina for more than three hours, and a backup method of contraception must be used until the ring has been used continuously for a subsequent seven days.
- Not appropriate for women who do not like touching their genitals

Side effects

- Breakthrough bleeding occurs in 2.0 to 6.4% of users
- Vaginitis, vaginal discharge

Risks and contraindications — Same as COC pills.

Progestogen only methods

These include:

- The oral pills
- Injections
- Subdermal implant
- Intrauterine system

Progesterone only pills (POPs)

Pills contain very low doses of a progestin and need to be taken at the same time of the day each day, without a gap between packets. They are also called "minipills". They do not affect milk production.

There are various POPs available — e.g. Micronor and Cerazette.
Mechanism of action

— Thickening cervical mucus, thereby reducing sperm viability and penetration.
— Prevents ovulation in 40–50% of women.

Administration — Orally, daily at the same time, continuously.
Efficacy — Failure rate 0.3% with perfect use and 9% with typical use in the first year of use.
Advantages

- Can be taken safely during breastfeeding.
- Can be taken by women who cannot use methods with oestrogen.

- Safe in women with varicose veins or in smokers.
- Suitable for women of any age; and can be started immediately after abortion, miscarriage or ectopic pregnancy.
- No significant metabolic effects (lipid levels, carbohydrate metabolism and coagulation factors remain unchanged).

Disadvantages

- It needs motivation to be taken at the same time of day. If taken more than three hours late, generally a backup method is necessary for 48 hours.
- It does not protect against STIs.
- Patients using medications that increase liver metabolism (Carbamazepine, Lamotrigine, Nevirapine, Phenobarbital or Phenytoin) should avoid this method of contraception due to the risk of failure.

Side effects

- Changes in bleeding pattern including:
  — Frequent or prolonged irregular bleeding.
  — In breastfeeding women, periods of amenorrhoea may be lengthened.

- Headache, mood changes and occasionally acne
- Nausea and breast tenderness occur that are reduced after 3–4 months.

Return to fertility — No delay.

TABLE 12.7 **Contraindications for all Progestogen only Methods**

Absolute Contraindications	Relative Contraindications
Active thromboembolic disease	Uncontrolled diabetes mellitus
Acute liver disease	Previous thromboembolic event
Undiagnosed genital bleeding	Cardiovascular disease
Benign or malignant liver tumours	Past history of breast cancer with no evidence of disease for 5 years
Current breast cancer	HIV infected women on antiretroviral agents (depending on drug interactions)
	Hepatocellular adenomas or hepatomas
	SLE with antiphospholipid antibodies
	Patients on certain anticonvulsant agents — rifampicin or rifabutin

Injectable progestogens

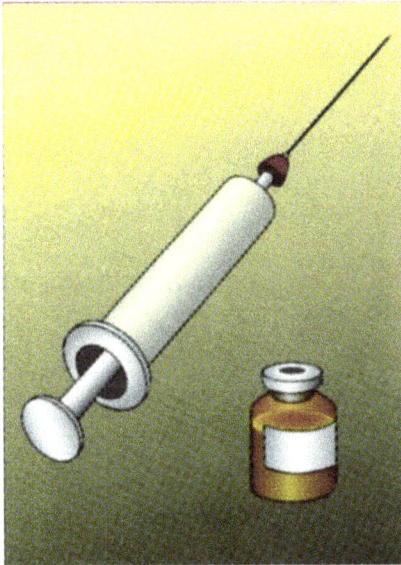

The preparations available are depot injection of:

• Medroxyprogesterone acetate (DMPA)
• Norethisterone enanthate (NET-EN).

FIGURE 12.7 ■ Injectable progestogens.

Mechanism of action — Inhibition of ovulation by suppressing the LH surge and thickening of cervical mucus, preventing sperm penetration.

Administration — Both are administered as deep intramuscular injection in the deltoid or gluteus muscle. DMPA in a dose of 150 mg every 12 weeks and NET-EN in dose of 200 mg 8 weekly.

Efficacy — The pregnancy rate associated with injectable DMPA is very low: 0.2% with perfect use and 6% with typical use.

Advantages

• 3 monthly dosing schedules, convenient.
• Safe during lactation.
• No oestrogen related side effects.
• Menstrual symptoms of dysmenorrhoea and menorrhagia are reduced.
• Can be administered immediately after first- or second-trimester abortion and postpartum.
• In women who are mentally challenged due to ease of administration.

Disadvantages

• Unpredictable and irregular menstrual bleeding can be annoying and lead to discontinuation of method and failure in early months.

- Reversible loss of bone mineral density is observed, particularly with use for more than a year. However, there is no evidence that DMPA use increases risk of fracture. Hence, care should be taken in recommending DMPA to adolescents and women older than 40 years.

Side effects

- IM injection can be painful and cause bruising
- Need to come every three months

Contraindications — Same as POP and in women with high risk factors for osteoporosis.

Return to fertility — Can be delayed by 9–12 months from the last injection.

Progestogen implant

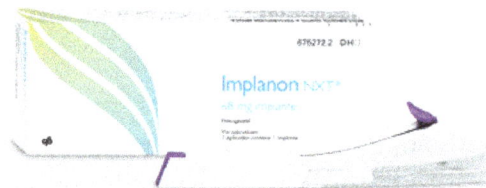 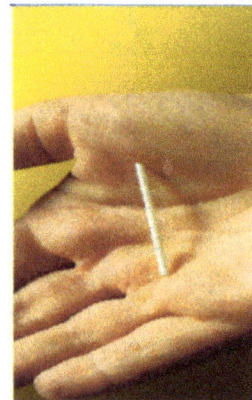

(a)   (b)

FIGURE 12.8a, b ■

Early first generation implants were Norplant check 6 rod system followed by the 2 rod system e.g. Norplant2 and Jadelle. They have now been replaced by the current device Implanon NXT.

Implanon NXT

It is a soft, flexible, non-biodegradable, single-rod, sub-dermal contraceptive implant that contains Etonogestrel 68 mg on an ethylene vinyl acetate (EVA) copolymer core. It is 4 cm long and 2 mm thick. It comes in a pre-loaded applicator for easy and accurate sub-dermal insertion. It confers protection for three years.

Mechanism of action — Acts primarily by maintaining ovulation suppression and increasing cervical mucus viscosity.

Administration — Insertion and removal are done under local anaesthesia by a trained professional.

Efficacy — The failure rate of the implant is 0.05% for both perfect use and typical use because the method requires no user action after insertion.

Advantages

- Long-term contraception
- Very high efficacy
- Quick insertion and removal, easy technique
- Quick return to fertility
- Women can breastfeed when using the implant
- Reduces menstrual blood flow and dysmenorrhoea

Disadvantages

- Irregular, unpredictable, prolonged, frequent or infrequent bleeding or even experience amenorrhea. Hence, proper counselling prior to insertion is important.
- Implant migration
- Needs removal as it is non-biodegradable

Side effects

- Headache, breast tenderness or changes in mood can occur.

Complications

- Bruising and mild discomfort are common after insertion
- Rarely, serious infection
- The small risk of neurovascular damage or misplacement
- Deep insertion
- Non-insertion of device may occur.

Return to fertility — There is no delay in return to fertility.

Intrauterine contraceptive devices (IUCD)

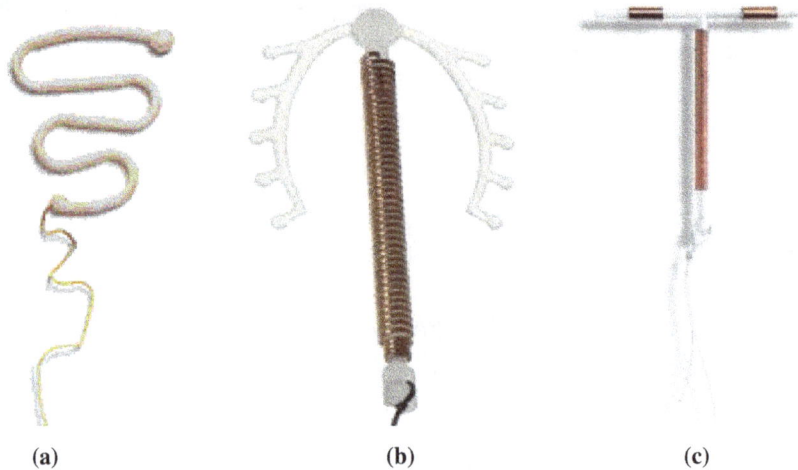

(a)   (b)   (c)

FIGURE 12.9 ∎ (a) Lippes loop. (b) Multiload 375. (c) Copper T 380 A.

IUCDs can be:

- First generation — Inert (e.g. lippes loop) — not currently used
- Second generation — Copper containing e.g. Multiload-375, Copper T-380A (ParaGard)
- Third generation — Hormone containing (LNG IUS or Mirena).

The stem has threads at the lower tip that hang below the cervix that aid in removal of the device.

Copper IUCD

Mechanism of action — It acts by creating a non-specific inflammatory response that renders the endometrium unimplantable. Macrophages cause phagocytosis of the spermatozoa, decrease sperm transport and impede the ability of sperm to fertilise the ovum.

Administration — It is inserted under aseptic precautions using non-touch technique. Confers protection for five years.

Efficacy — Failure rate is 0.6% with perfect use and 0.8 % with typical use.

Advantages

- Highly effective, reversible, long term contraceptive
- Most cost-effective even after one year of use

Disadvantages

- Needs to be inserted and removed by a trained person

- No protection against STIs
- Insertion can be painful.

Side effects

- Syncopal episode at the time of insertion
- Abdominal cramps, per vaginal spotting can occur for a short duration
- Infection — There may be an increased risk of pelvic infection in the 20 days following insertion of intrauterine contraception, but the risk is the same as the non-IUD-using population thereafter.
- Menstrual irregularity in some women.

Complications

- Uterine perforation
- Expulsion, leading to failure
- **Missing IUCD thread** — If history confirms that it is not expelled, then ultrasound scan can help to locate it. If in the uterus, then can remove it with artery forceps/IUCD hook/Novak's curette or by hysteroscopy. If it is translocated into the abdominal cavity, refer to a specialist to discuss laparoscopic removal.
- **Pregnancy with IUCD** — Ectopic pregnancy should be excluded. In case of intra-uterine pregnancy, and if the woman wishes to continue pregnancy, the IUCD should be removed if strings are seen. There is a small risk of miscarriage after this procedure. If strings are not seen and the IUCD is seen in the uterine cavity on ultrasound, she can continue the pregnancy with an understanding that she is at increased risk of a miscarriage, premature labour or uterine infection, and should be followed up closely and checked for IUCD at time of delivery.
- **Risk of ectopic pregnancy** — There is a small increase in the risk of ectopic pregnancy, if pregnancy occurs with IUCD. However, since IUCDs are such effective contraceptives, the absolute risk of pregnancy (intra-uterine and ectopic) while using these methods is very low.

TABLE 12.8. Contraindications to use of IUCD

Absolute Contraindications	Relative Contraindications
Pregnancy, puerperal sepsis, septic abortion	Between 48 hours and < 4 weeks postpartum
Unexplained vaginal bleeding	
Gestational trophoblastic neoplasia when serum hCG concentrations are abnormal	Current VTE (on anticoagulants)
	Women with ovarian cancer
Cervical or endometrial cancer	
Uterine fibroids or uterine anatomical Abnormalities distorting the uterine cavity	
Current PID or purulent cervicitis	
Known pelvic tuberculosis	

Return to fertility — Immediate.

Levonorgestrel Intrauterine Device (LNG-IUD or the IUS or hormone IUD-MIRENA)

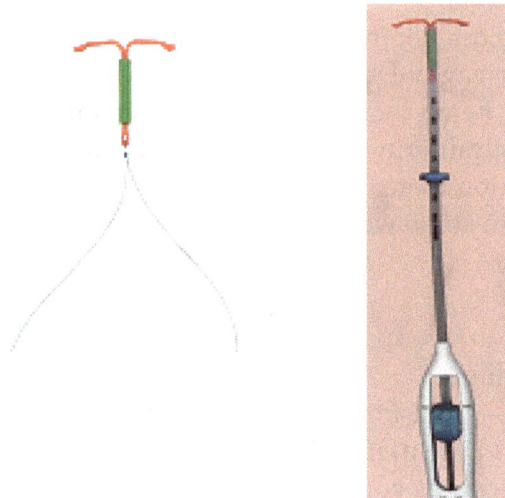

- T-shaped polyethylene frame with a collar
- Steadily releases small amounts of levonorgestrel daily
- MIRENA contains 52 mg of levonorgestrel
- Release rate of 20 mcg/day
- Efficacy lasts for five years

FIGURE 12.10 ■ Levonorgestrel intrauterine device.

Mechanism of action — The progestin effect is primarily local but suppresses ovulation in many women.

Administration — Same as copper IUCD

Efficacy — The failure rate is 0.2% with typical and perfect use.

Advantages

- It is a hormonal method with minimal systemic hormonal effects
- It is an effective treatment of idiopathic menorrhagia, iron deficiency anaemia and dysmenorrhoea[11]
- Suppresses symptoms of endometriosis[11]
- It is an effective option in the treatment of non-atypical endometrial hyperplasia[12]
- Protects endometrium in women using oestrogen replacement therapy[3]
- It may decrease the risk of PID, as observed with other progestin-containing contraceptives by thickening the cervical mucus, possibly reducing the ascending infection
- It can be used safely and effectively in adolescents, nulliparous and older women[13]

Disadvantages: The same as IUCD.

Side effects

- Irregular bleeding pattern — Prolonged spotting, bleeding or amenorrhoea
- Breast tenderness, mood changes and acne
- Insertion can be painful due to the thick vertical arm, particularly in nulliparous women

Complications: The same as IUCD.
Return to fertility — Immediate

TABLE 12.9. Contraindications to Use of Hormonal IUCDs

Absolute Contraindications	Relative Contraindications
Current breast cancer Others: Same as IUCD	Between 48 hours and < 4 weeks postpartum Current VTE (on anticoagulants) Ischaemic heart disease Past history of breast cancer with no recurrence in last five years Active viral hepatitis, severe decompensated cirrhosis Liver tumours (benign or malignant)

Long-acting reversible contraceptive (LARC) methods

LARC, a commonly used terminology, is defined as contraceptive methods that require administration less than once per cycle or month. They are currently recommended as first-line methods[14] because medical professionals place them and ensure compliance, so they are the most effective form of reversible contraceptives available. They include:

- Copper intra-uterine devices
- Progestogen-only intra-uterine systems
- Progestogen-only injectable contraceptives
- Progestogen-only sub-dermal implants.

All currently available LARC methods are more cost-effective than the combined oral contraceptive pill, even at one year of use.[14] The intra-uterine devices, intrauterine system and implants are more cost-effective than injectable contraceptives.

Permanent/Irreversible Methods — Sterilisation

The permanent surgical methods of contraception include male sterilisation by vasectomy and female sterilisation by fallopian tube occlusion or tubectomy.

It is performed on couples who have completed their family and are certain that they do not want another pregnancy.

Mechanism of action — Surgery to cause mechanical occlusion or resection of the fallopian tubes in females, or vas deferens in males, to prevent fertilisation.

Efficacy — Failure rate is 0.5% in female sterilisation and 0.1% in male sterilisation with perfect use.

Male sterilization

Vasectomy

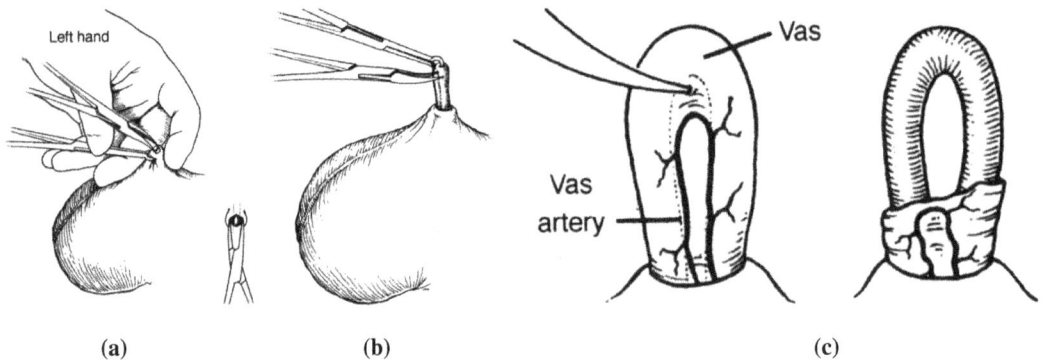

FIGURE 12.11 ■ (a) Holding the vas with ring locked forceps. (b) Loop for vas deferensee. (c) A segment of vas deferensee is resected and ligated on both sides.

The surgery can be performed under local anaesthesia and failure rate is very low 1/2,000. The operative technique is simple, with a short learning curve, and has a very low complication rate. However, it needs additional contraceptive protection for next three months and until azoospermia is evident on two samples in semen analysis. It may take 10–15 ejaculates to achieve this.

Advantages

- Simple and safe
- No effect on masculinity or virility
- No side effects of hormones
- Improves sexual life of couple, as no fear of unwanted pregnancy

Disadvantages

- Permanent method
- Regret

Female sterilisation

It can be performed 24–48 hours after normal delivery (puerperal), six weeks after delivery (interval) or concurrently with the termination of pregnancy.

It can be performed by various methods.

- Minilaparotomy
- Laparoscopy
- Vaginally
- Hysteroscopically (Essure)

Minilaparotomy — In this method a small incision is made and bilateral fallopian tubes are resected and ligated. The operation is technically easy and done during the same admission of delivery. Various methods have been described e.g. Pomeroy's technique, Uchida's method, Irving method, Madlener technique etc.

Modified Pomeroy's technique is popularly used. It involves resecting a segment of fallopian tube by making a loop and ligating the base with delayed absorbable suture. The cut ends eventually get sealed off and separated after few weeks.

Interval sterilisation is ideally performed during the proliferative phase of menstrual cycle, or anytime if sure that the woman is not pregnant. The commonest method is

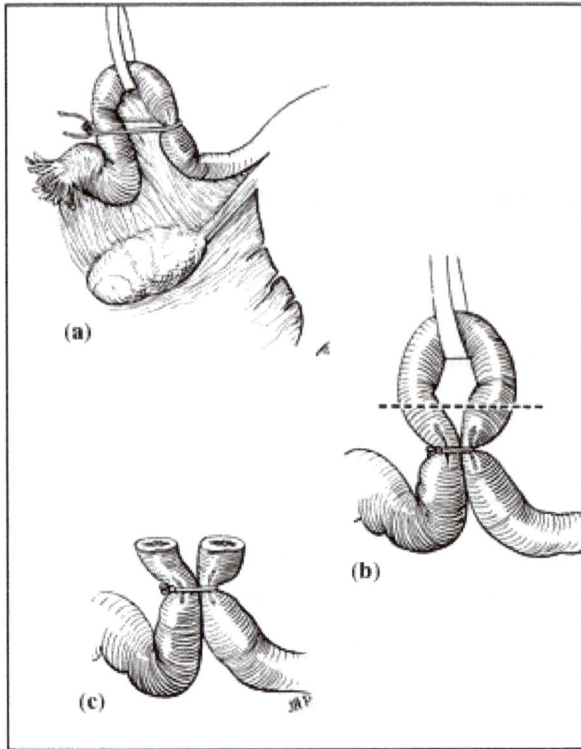

FIGURE 12.12 ■ Modified Pomeroy's technique.

Laparoscopic sterilisation. It is performed by application of silastic rings, Hulka or Filshie clip, or by the electrosurgical method of destroying the fallopian tubes.

During application of Filshie clips, a clip loaded applicator approaches the fallopian tube, grasps it in entire thickness about 2–3 cm from the cornual end and is clamped over the tube bilaterally.

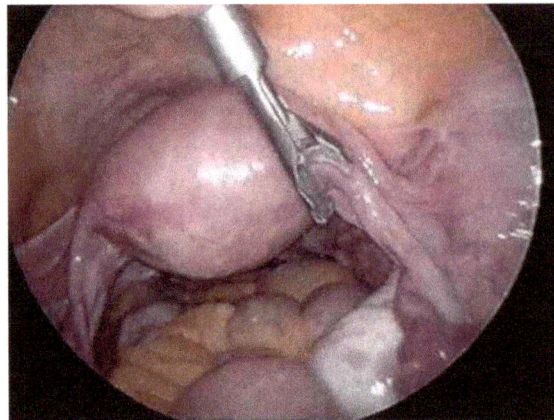

FIGURE 12.13 ■ Laparoscopic Filshie clip application.

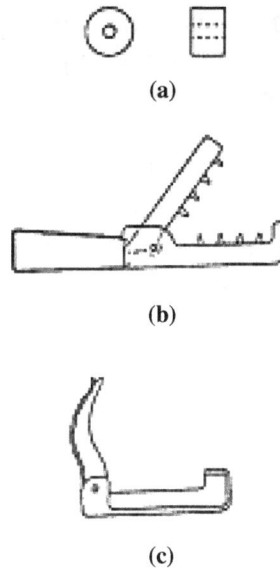

FIGURE 12.14 ■ (a) Fallope ring. (b) Hulka clip. (c) Filshie clip. Devices used for tubal occlusion.

Advantages

- Highly effective day surgery — Short operation, speedy recovery
- Immediate
- Permanent
- Does not affect breast feeding
- No long-term side effects

Disadvantages

- Permanent
- Irreversible
- Surgical procedure — Needs general anaesthesia, with very rare but serious risks. Small risk of vascular or viscous injury during laparoscopic entry.
- Needs trained doctor to perform
- Small risk of failure
- May regret later

Emergency Contraception

Methods used to prevent pregnancy following unprotected sexual intercourse are referred to as emergency contraception. Emergency contraceptive pills (ECPs) are sometimes called "morning after" pills or post-coital contraceptives.

Mechanism of action — is primarily by preventing or delaying ovulation or preventing implantation. Does not disrupt an existing pregnancy.

They are safe for all women — even women who cannot use ongoing hormonal contraceptive methods.

Although, in the past, combined oral contraceptive pills were used for EC, three methods are currently offered as standard ECs (Table 12.10).

They do not provide long-term contraception.

Return to fertility — no delay in return to fertility after ECs.

TABLE 12.10.   Summary of Key Points for Various EC Methods[15,16]

LNG (Levonelle One Step)	Progestin only — dedicated ECPs	1.5 mg LNG single dose	Within 72 hours of UPSI • 95% of expected when taken within 24 hours • 85% if taken within 25–48 hours • 58% if taken within 49–72 hours	Seek medical advice if they vomit within 3 hours of taking EC
Ella One Ulipristal acetate (UPA)	Progesterone receptor modulator	30 mg Ulipristal acetate single dose	Up to 120 hours of UPSI	Newer EC
IUCD	Cu-IUCD Or LNG containing IUCD	Any IUCD	Can be inserted up to 5 days after the first episode of UPSI or within 5 days of the earliest expected date of ovulation. (Most effective method — 99% effective)	— Not affected by liver enzyme inducing drugs. — Consider prophylactic antibiotics to cover for *Chlamydia trachomatis*

References

1. Guillebaud J. (2012) *Contraception Today*. Seventh Edition. Informa healthcare. 8–2.
2. Trussell J. (2011) Contraceptive Efficacy. In Hatcher RA, Trussell J, Nelson AL, *Contraceptive Technology: Twentieth Revised Edition*. New York, NY: Ardent Media.
3. Fritz MA, Speroff L (2010) *Clinical Gynaecologic Endocrinology and Infertility*, 8th edn. Lippincott Williams and Wilkins.
4. Johns Hopkins Bloomberg School of Public Health/Center for Communication Programs and World Health Organization (2011) *Family planning: a global handbook for providers*.
5. Baillargeon JP, McClish DK, Essah PA, *et al.* (2005) Association between the current use of low-dose oral contraceptives and cardiovascular arterial disease: a meta-analysis. *J Clin Endocrinol Metab* **90**(7):3863–3870.
6. FSRH Healthcare Statement (2014): Venous Thromboembolism (VTE) and Hormonal Contraception; Faculty of Sexual and Reproductive Healthcare.
7. Paseka J, Unzeitig V, Cibula D, *et al.* (2000) Liver function tests during administration of triphasic contraceptives containing Norgestimate. *Ceska Gynekol* **65**(6):420–424.
8. Hannaford PC, Selvaraj S, Elliott AM, *et al.* (2007) Cancer risk among users of oral contraceptives: cohort data from the Royal College of General Practitioner's oral contraception study. *BMJ* **335**(7621):651.
9. Hankinson SE, Colditz GA, Manson JE, *et al.* (1997) Prospective study of oral contraceptive use and risk of breast cancer (Nurses' Health Study, United States). *Cancer Causes Control*; **8**(1):65–72.
10. Vessey M, Yeates D. (2013) Oral contraceptive use and cancer: final report from the Oxford-Family Planning Association contraceptive study. *Contraception* **88**(6):678–683.
11. National Institute for Health and Care Excellence (2014). *CG30: Long-acting reversible contraception*. London, UK: NICE.
12. Buttini MJ, Jordan SJ, Webb PM. (2009) The effect of the levonorgestrel releasing intra-uterine system on endometrial hyperplasia: an Australian study and systematic review. *Aust NZ J Obstet Gynaecol* **49**(3):316–322.
13. Deans EI, Grimes DA. (2009) Intrauterine devices for adolescents: a systematic review. *Contraception* **79**(6):418–423.
14. Winner, B; Peipert, JF; Zhao Q *et al.* (2012) Effectiveness of Long-Acting Reversible Contraception. *N Eng J Med* **366**(21):1998–2007.
15. Li HW, Lo SS, Ho PC. (2014) Emergency contraception. *Best Pract Res Clin Obstet Gynaecol* **28**(6):835–844.
16. Faculty of Sexual and Reproductive Healthcare. CEU guidance, Emergency contraception, updated 2012.

Part III

CONCEPTION — WHERE LIFE BEGINS

Introduction

Life begins in the human with the fusion of two unique and complementary cells — the human oocyte, the largest cell in the human body measuring 1 mm across and barely visible to the naked eye; and the smallest cell in the human body, the human spermatozoon which is less than 60 microns. Fitness to survive and reproduce sexually in the human race has evolved in such a way that the spermatozoa are made in the testes carried by the human male and the oocytes are carried in the ovaries of the human female. Importantly, the journey of the spermatozoon and oocyte to develop into mature functional gametes before meeting to form a new life can be fraught with hurdles — from normal physiological insults (oxidative distress) and barriers (such as the cervical mucus) to diseased states in the male and/or female reproductive systems can lead to difficulties in conceiving. The following chapters will discuss the basic reproductive physiology of the gametes (spermatozoon and oocyte) and the problems associated with abnormal gametes production and development, including various pathophysiological processes afflicting the reproductive systems of the male and female which may lead to human infertility. Additionally, strategies to manage these problems will be presented.

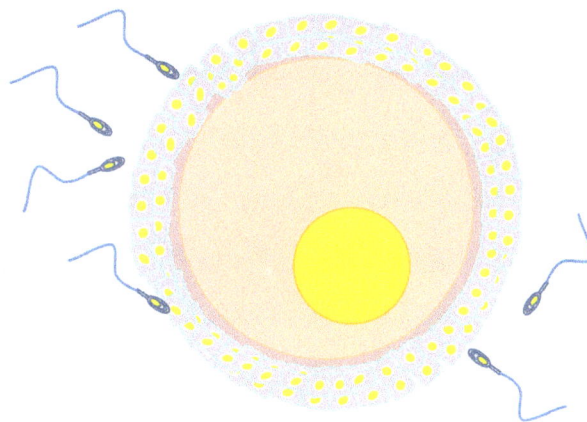

Meeting of the oocyte and spermatozoa.
Illustration by Z Huang, 2015

13

REPRODUCTIVE PHYSIOLOGY OF THE HUMAN SPERMATOZOON AND OOCYTE

Zhongwei Huang

Introduction

In sexual reproduction, the human male will produce the male gametes, spermatozoa, in the testes (extra-abdominal), and the human female will produce the female gametes, oocytes, in the ovaries (intra-abdominal). These gametes need to undergo a special cellular division known as meiosis, which will halve the number of chromosomes during their production and development in the gonads (testes or ovaries). During fertilisation, the spermatozoon will fuse with the oocyte and the two nuclei will form a diploid conceptus. This entire process happens differently in the human male and female, with the following sections highlighting the similarities in the process of gamete production and development in addition to discussing the differences between spermatogenesis, oogenesis and the maturation processes for spermatozoa and oocytes.

What is Common between Spermatogenesis and Folliculogenesis?

The gametes are formed from germline stem cells in the gonads. Upon formation of the gametes, the gametes need supporting cells to ensure its continued survival and these cells are known as the Sertoli cells in the testes and granulosa/thecal cells in the ovaries. The function of these cells is vital in sustaining, nurturing and ensuring proper development of the gametes to maturation. The development of the gametes involved the presence of steroid hormones (androgens and oestrogens) which will interact with gonadotrophins from the hypothalamus and anterior pituitary gland through positive and negative feedback pathways. Appropriate signals via the hypothalamic-pituitary — gonadal axis are necessary to ensure that normal spermatogenesis and ovarian folliculogenesis occur. This will be discussed in detail in the chapters on male and female infertility.

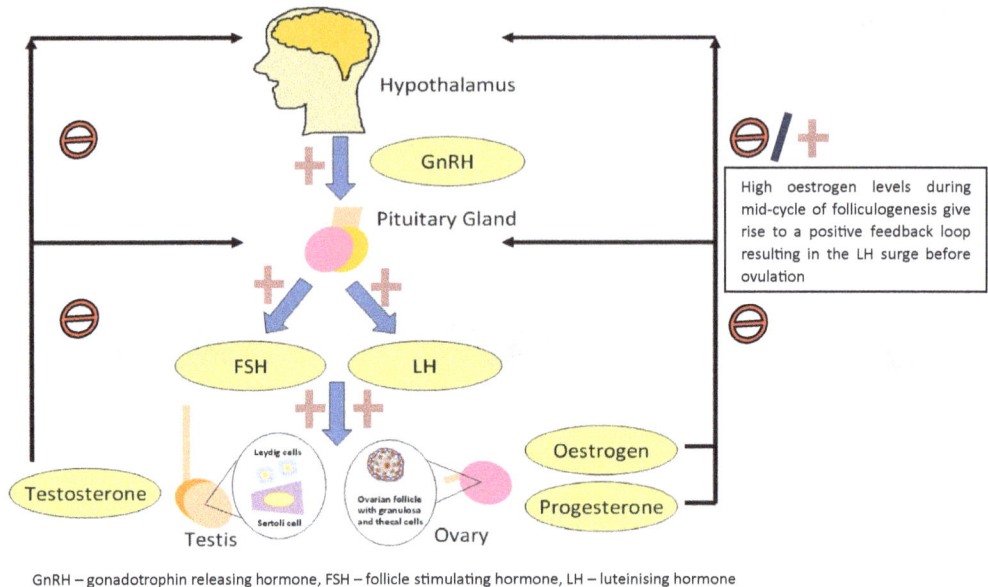

GnRH – gonadotrophin releasing hormone, FSH – follicle stimulating hormone, LH – luteinising hormone

FIGURE 13.1 ■ The hypothalamic-pituitary-gonadal axis. Illustration: Z Huang 2015.

Meiosis in the Spermatozoon and Oocyte

Meiosis is a special type of cell division in sexually reproducing organisms that results in four daughter cells each with half the number of chromosomes of the parent cell. In addition, it is also during meiosis that homologous paired chromosomes form crossover links where pieces of DNA are broken and recombined to produce new combinations of alleles. This is known as meiotic recombination, which is unique to sexual reproduction and allows the generation of genetic diversity.

Briefly, in spermatogenesis, spermatozoa are produced in the seminiferous tubules of the testes. The first stage of spermatogenesis involves the division of germline epithelium by mitosis. This results in the formation of spermatogonia, which then undergo mitosis before they undergo meiosis, a two-stage process that results in the formation of four haploid daughter cells. Follicle stimulation hormone (FSH) stimulates the first meiotic division of spermatogonia while luteinising hormone (LH) stimulates the Leydig cells to produce testosterone, which brings about the second meiotic division of spermatogonia. The maturation of spermatozoa requires them to undergo further differentiation and they are nourished by the Sertoli cells in the early stages of development.

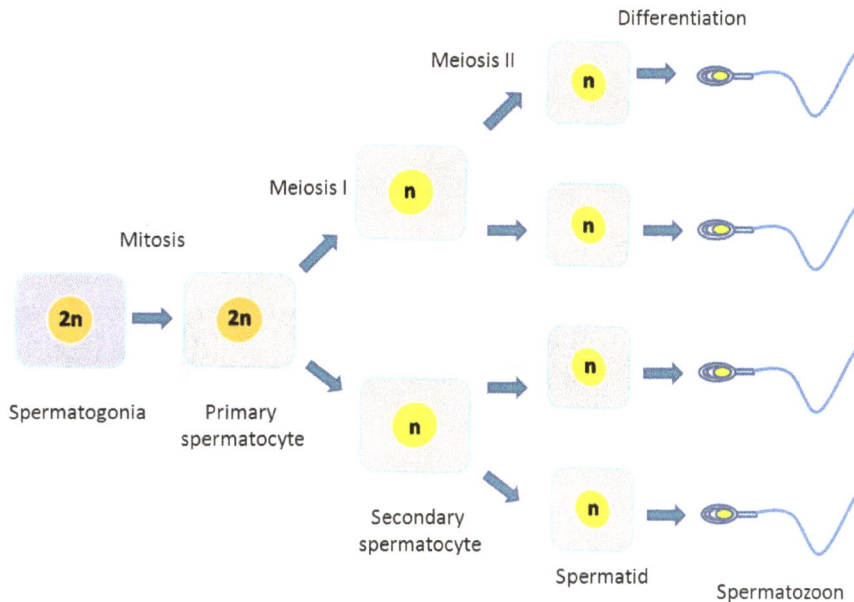

FIGURE 13.2 ■ Meiosis and spermatogenesis. Illustration: Z Huang 2015.

Oogenesis is the production of oocytes within the ovary and this commences during foetal development; a large number of oogonia are formed by mitosis which then undergo a period of growth. These oogonia begin the first stage of meiosis and become arrested in prophase I until puberty. At puberty, the oogonia are surrounded by supporting cells (granulosa cells) and are known as ovarian follicles. These ovarian follicles will develop each month in response to FSH stimulation, which will allow the completion of the first meiotic division to form two cells of unequal size — a small cellular structure with less cytoplasm known as a polar body (which degenerates subsequently), and a larger cell known as the secondary oocyte. The secondary oocyte begins the second meiotic division but is arrested in prophase II until it is ovulated under the influence of the LH surge. If fertilisation occurs after fusion with a spermatozoon, this will complete the second meiotic division with the release of the second polar body.

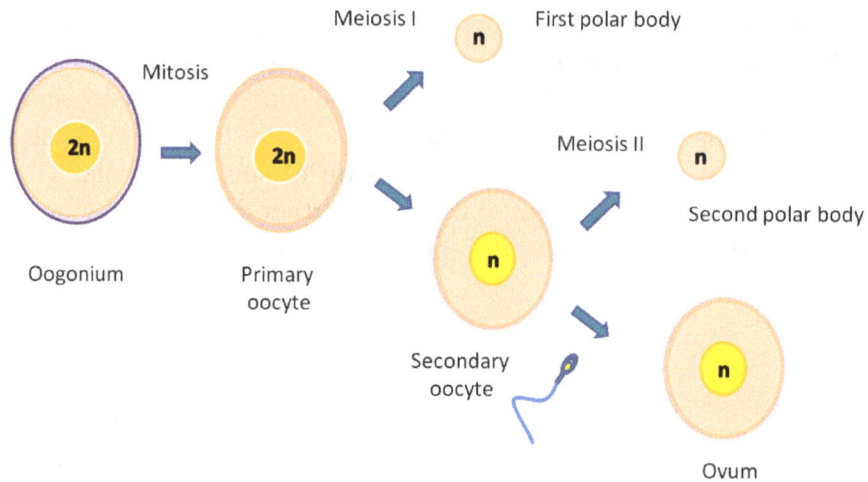

FIGURE 13.3 ■ Meiosis and oogenesis. Illustration: Z Huang 2015.

Differences Encountered between Spermatogenesis, Oogenesis and Folliculogenesis

The process of gametogenesis differs between the human male and female in many ways — in terms of site and duration of production, lifespan, number and when the gametes are released. The following table aims to highlight these pertinent differences in the human male and female.

	Human Male	**Human Female**
Process	Spermatogenesis	Oogenesis and Folliculogenesis
Site	Testis (extra-abdominal organ)	Ovaries (intra-abdominal organ)
Supporting cell(s)	Sertoli cells (maturation and nourishment of spermatogonia)	Granulosa cells (nutrition and endocrine function such as production of oestradiol)
	Leydig cells (production of testosterone)	Thecal cells (androgens production)
Time of initiation	At puberty	At foetal development in utero
Number of gametes produced	Throughout a man's lifespan (millions)	Fixed number of oocytes (about 400 oocytes) in a woman's lifetime

(Continued)

(Continued)

	Human Male	Human Female
Number of gametes formed per germ cell	4 spermatozoa	1 oocyte and 2 polar bodies
Process of meiosis	Uninterrupted	Arrested at prophase I and prophase II Needs initiating factor such as puberty and fertilisation to complete meiosis I and II, respectively
Duration of gametogenesis	Approximately 74 days	Oogenesis occurred since foetal development and then arrested in prophase I until puberty or when ovarian follicle recruited for ovulation (13 to 50 years)
Lifespan of gametes	Up to 80 hours in the fallopian tube	Up to 24 hours after ovulation
Duration of production	Life long	Ceased at menopause
Timing of release	On demand — usually millions	Once a month — one ovum is released (folliculogenesis occurred)

During coitus, the spermatozoa enter the female reproductive tract. Capacitation is an essential step in the spermatozoa to allow fertilisation to occur. The spermatozoon will swim towards the oocyte due to the release of chemical signals from the secondary oocyte via a process known as chemotaxis. To enter the oocyte membrane, the spermatozoa must penetrate the zona pellucida, and the acrosome vesicle in the spermatozoon fuses with the zona pellucida and releases digestive enzymes that soften the glycoprotein matrix.

The membrane of the oocyte and spermatozoon then fuse and the sperm nucleus (and centriole) enters the oocyte. To prevent polyspermy, the oocyte then undergoes biochemical changes via the cortical reaction. The cortical granules release enzymes that destroy the sperm-binding proteins on the zona pellucida. Now fertilised, the nucleus of the secondary oocyte completes meiosis II and the nuclei of both gametes fuse to form a diploid zygote.

References

1. Fritz MA, Speroff L. (2012) *Clinical Gynecologic Endocrinology and Infertility*, 8th edn, pp. 157–198, 243–268.
2. Johnson MH. (2013) *Essential Reproduction*, 7th edn, pp. 1–205.
3. Huang Z, Wells D. (2010) The human oocyte and cumulus cells relationship: new insights from the cumulus cell transcriptome *Mole Human Reprod*, **16**(10):715–725.
4. Huang Z, Wells D. (2011) *Molecular Aspects of Ovarian Follicular Development, Principles and Practice of Fertility Preservation*. Cambridge University Press, Editors J Donnez & S Kim, pp. 114–128.
5. Huang Z, Fragouli E, Wells D. (2012) Biomolecules of human female fertility — potential therapeutic targets for pharmaceutical design. *Curr Pharmaceut Design* **18**(3):310–324.

14

FEMALE INFERTILITY

Shakina Rauff, Lim Min Yu and Wong P. C.

Introduction

As public awareness of the burden of infertility heightens along with the advancement in assisted reproductive techniques available over the last three decades, more couples present with this problem seeking help. It is important to understand some of the definitions which will be used in this chapter. Infertility is generally defined as the inability to conceive despite regular unprotected sexual (vaginal) intercourse over a specific period of time, usually one year.

Primary infertility is the inability to conceive in a couple who have had no previous pregnancies.

Secondary infertility refers to the inability to conceive in a couple who have had at least one previous pregnancy, which may have ended up in a live birth, stillbirth, miscarriage, ectopic pregnancy or induced abortion.

Cycle fecundability is the probability that a cycle will result in a pregnancy, whereas fecundity means the probability that a cycle will result in a live birth.

Normal Conception

To understand the mechanisms and aetiologies underlying infertility, it is first necessary to comprehend the basic principles and processes involved in a normal conception. Disruption of this normal sequence can result in infertility.

In reproduction, the function of the ovary is to produce a cyclical release of an oocyte under the influence of pituitary hormones and steroids — a process known as ovulation. Ovulation is preceded by follicular development and maturation.

During follicular development, a cohort of dormant primordial follicles is mobilised to form a group of growing follicles. These follicles will progress through the pre-antral and antral stages, and usually only one dominant follicle among these will reach the pre-ovulatory stage, be fully mature and ovulate. This process takes place in response to rising FSH levels and the follicles developing FSH receptors. FSH initiates steroidogenesis and granulosa cell proliferation. The granulosa cells contain the enzyme aromatase, which converts androgens to oestrogen, and only the dominant follicle acquires sufficient aromatase to produce adequate quantities of oestradiol. This dominant follicle is destined to develop ahead of the others as it secretes an increasing amount of oestradiol (E2) while the rest undergo atresia. As the follicle develops, the theca cells develop LH receptors which stimulate androgen production which is, in turn, aromatised to more oestrogen. Oestradiol levels rise and reach a peak about 24–36 hours prior to ovulation.

The continuous production of E2 by the growing follicle leads to an LH surge by a positive feedback mechanism. The LH surge is necessary for oocyte maturation, resumption of the first meiotic division and preparation of the endometrium for implantation. The LH surge usually lasts about 48 hours from start to end and ovulation occurs ~24–36 hours after the LH surge. When ovulation occurs, the dominant follicle ruptures and the oocyte is released. The collapsed follicle forms a corpus luteum.

The next step in the course of conception involves the core event in reproduction — fertilisation or the fusion of the male and female gametes. Within 2–3 minutes of ovulation, the oocyte is within the fallopian tube (ampullary region) and has a fertilisable life span of ~24 hours. During intercourse, although millions of sperm are ejaculated into the vagina and near the cervix, only a few hundred will reach the fallopian tube. The sperm will undergo capacitation to bind with and penetrate the egg. Fusion of the male and female gametes produces a diploid zygote and the second meiotic division is complete. Further division of the zygote produces an embryo and forms a blastocyst by Day 5 post-fertilisation, which migrates from the fallopian tube to the uterine cavity.

The last step in achieving a pregnancy involves implantation, the process by which the embryo attaches itself to the endometrial side of the uterine wall and gradually penetrates the epithelium to reach the circulatory system of the mother. At this stage, the embryo is between Day 5–7 post-fertilisation and is a blastocyst. The hatched blastocyst produces human chorionic gonadotrophin (hCG) which maintains the corpus luteum and its production of progesterone and oestradiol. These hormones are required to support further growth of the pregnancy and prevent the onset of menstruation.[1]

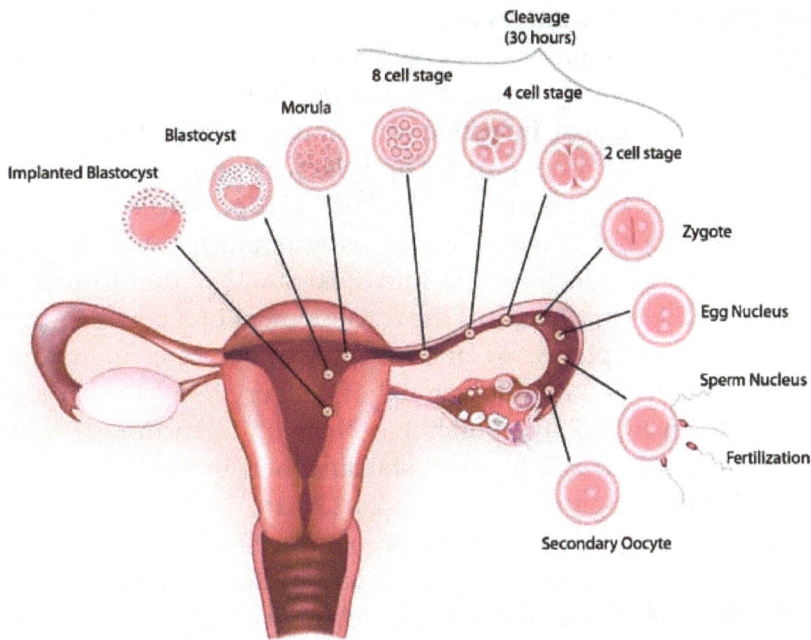

FIGURE 14.1 ■ Stages of oocyte development from fertilisation to implanted embryo.

Epidemiology of Infertility and How Fertile We Are

When compared to other mammals, for example the baboon, humans are not highly fertile. The cycle fecundity rate for normally fertile couples averages about 20% even when coitus is timed around the time of ovulation, the so-called "fertile period."

With the average cycle fecundity rate of 20%, the cumulative pregnancy rate for most healthy young couples will be 72% within six months i.e. 72% of couples will conceive within six months. The cumulative spontaneous pregnancy rate after one year is about 85% and after two years, the cumulative spontaneous pregnancy rate reaches 93%, after which there is very little increment.[2]

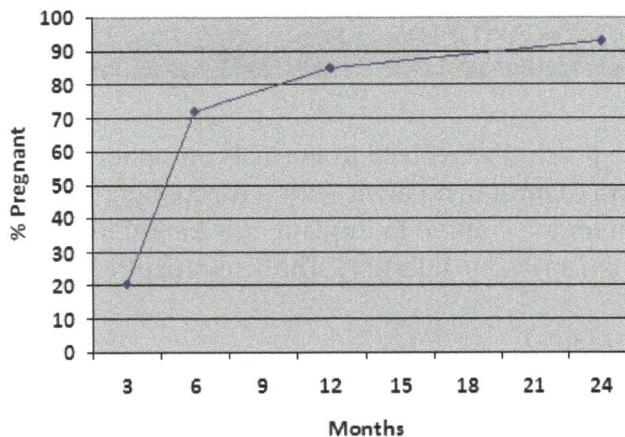

FIGURE 14.2 ■ Normal fecundity rate.

Therefore, infertility affects about 10–15% of couples and it is justified to start evaluating and investigating a couple after one year of unsuccessful attempting, as most (85%) of normally fertile couples would have conceived by then. An earlier referral for specialist investigation should be initiated if there are known causes of infertility in either partner or if the woman is more than 35 years old. In Singapore, infertility affects about 1 in 7 or ~15% of couples.

Singapore experienced a post-war baby boom between 1947 to 1964, after which the birth rate fell from the mid-1960s to 1987 due to fear that a rapidly growing population might retard the development of a newly independent country. Abortions were permitted and couples undergoing voluntary sterilisation were given benefits like reimbursement of delivery fees.[3] These measures were so effective that, since 1987, the policy has changed to encourage more babies. The impact of our falling fertility rate is startling, and in the last few years, the birth rate has fallen to a staggering low of 1.2 in 2011.[4]

The decline in fertility rate in Singapore can be attributed to several factors — couples are getting married later as many prefer to focus on their career and advancing their education first. Delayed childbearing can be the consequence of a later marriage, preference for a smaller family size and the widespread availability of contraception. As divorce rates are also on the rise, many may be reluctant to have children early or may not have more children due to marital problems.

The impact of female age on fertility cannot be underestimated and it is well known that female fertility declines with increasing age. This is mainly because women have a predetermined and fixed follicle number at birth and at puberty. The reproductive ability depends on the rate of depletion of this pool too. A woman's fertility potential peaks between 20–24 years, decreases little until the age of 30–32 years and thereafter regresses progressively and rapidly. Women between 35–39 years are 26–46% less fertile, and in those aged 40–45 years, fertility is up to 95% lower.[5] Age also affects the outcome of assisted reproductive techniques (ART) — success rates are lower as age rises.

Causes of Female Infertility

Following the processes involved in normal conception — which requires a mature egg and sperm to meet in a patent with a functioning fallopian tube and receptive endometrium for the embryo to implant, it is logical to conclude that any defect in one of the steps can lead to infertility. The causes of infertility in a couple are broadly:

- Male factor (35%)
- Tubal and pelvic pathology e.g. endometriosis (30–35%)

- Ovulatory dysfunction (20–40%)
- Unexplained (10–15%)
- Other uncommon problems like coital problems, sexual dysfunction and uterine factors (5%)

In the female, when male factors are excluded as a cause of infertility, the causes are in the following proportion: (Fig. 14.3).

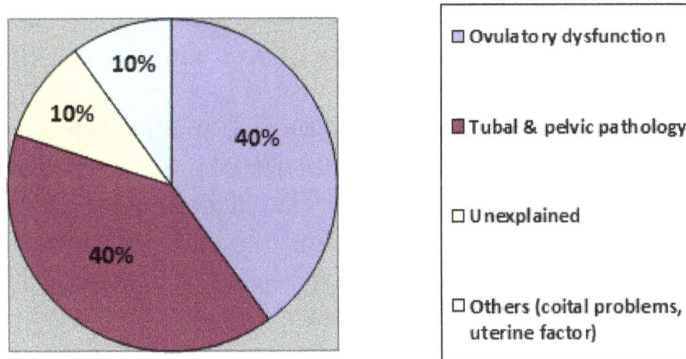

FIGURE 14.3 ■ Female cause of infertility.

Thus, the commonest causes of infertility in the female are tubal and pelvic pathology like endometriosis and anovulation. Of course, a patient may have a combination of factors or other contributing causes, too.[6]

Ovulation disorders can be classified into the WHO type I, II and III categories, with a separate group encompassing hyperprolactinaemia. Other endocrine disorders like hypothyroidism, Cushing's disease/syndrome or hyperandrogenism may also result in anovulation.[7]

WHO type I: hypothalamic pituitary failure or hypogonadotrophic hypogonadism e.g. anorexia nervosa, chronic illnesses, Kallman's syndrome, previous brain trauma or irradiation, excessive exercise and stress.

WHO type II: hypothalamic pituitary dysfunction or normo-gonadotrophic normo-gonadism. The cause of anovulation in this case is at the level of the gonads or the ovary and this is the commonest type of ovulatory disorder, with polycystic ovary syndrome as the most frequent reason.

WHO type III: ovarian failure or hypergondaotrophic hypogonadism e.g. Turner's syndrome, autoimmune premature ovarian failure, previous chemotherapy or radiotherapy.

Hyperprolactinaemia: raised prolactin levels can result in a hypo-oestrogenism and anovulation. This may be due to exogenous drugs, micro-/macro-prolactinoma etc.

Tubal and pelvic pathology comprises of tubal damage which may be anatomical or functional and pelvic pathology, the commonest reason being endometriosis.

Many events occur in the fallopian tubes — sperm transport and egg pick-up, sperm capacitation, fertilisation, zygote division and early embryo growth and transport of the embryo to the uterine cavity. Thus, tubal damage may result in occluded tubes or even if patency is maintained, the functional ability to permit these roles may be lost. The leading cause of tubal damage is pelvic inflammatory disease (PID) and this is strongly associated with *Chlamydia* infection. Hydrosalpinges can result from PID and these are not only a cause of tubal occlusion, but can also decrease the chances of successful ART treatment should the patient require it. Tubal injury can also result from other pelvic infections, especially if there is extensive contamination involved, like in a ruptured appendix or diverticulitis. Septic abortions can also be very destructive to tubal integrity.

Endometriosis can cause infertility by two main mechanisms: Firstly, pelvic endometriosis can cause significant distortion of the normal adnexal anatomy and this anatomical distortion can result in tubal damage via adhesions or impair ovum capture (post-ovulation) by the fimbrial end. Secondly, the disease process of endometriosis is linked with excessive release of prostaglandins, cytokines and chemokines. A chronic inflammatory state ensues that is detrimental to folliculogenesis, oocyte quality, fertilisation and implantation as ovarian function and endometrial receptivity are affected negatively. The more severe the stage of endometriosis, the greater the impact on fertility, difficulty in conceiving and the lower the success rate of ART treatment cycles.

Uncommon causes of female infertility include coital problems like female sexual dysfunction and vaginismus, as well as uterine abnormalities like submucous myomas, endometrial polyps or congenital malformations.

When routine investigations fail to identify a cause of infertility, the diagnosis of unexplained infertility is made which is a diagnosis of exclusion. In a woman, there must the minimal criteria that she is ovulating regulating, the tubes are patent and the uterine cavity is normal. This affects about 10–15% of women and couples, and management will be outlined further on in this chapter.

Clinical Evaluation of Female Infertility

When evaluating female infertility, the basic components of the reproductive journey must be remembered. Basically, around the time of ovulation, sperm should be deposited at or near the cervix and the sperm must be able to move up through the cervix, into the uterine cavity and through the fallopian tubes. Regular ovulation of a mature oocyte must occur and the fallopian tubes must be able to capture the ovulated egg. Capacitation of the sperm and fertilisation with the oocyte must follow and the tube must transport the resulting embryo to the uterine cavity where the endometrium has to be receptive for implantation to be successful. Thus, in the evaluation of female infertility, we attempt to test the integrity of each step and hopefully detect the underlying cause. Unfortunately, although investigations have improved greatly in the last 2–3 decades, there are still components of the cycle that are unable to be tested routinely, but that only a procedure like *in-vitro* fertilisation (IVF) may reveal.

The likelihood of achieving a pregnancy and live birth decreases with increasing maternal age and length of infertility and is higher if the couple has conceived before. Some causes of infertility have a better prognosis than others in terms of treatment success but this will only be known after an evaluation. Since the majority of couples will conceive within 1–2 years of trying to, evaluation and work-up should be offered to all couples who have failed to conceive after a year or more of regular (2–3×/week) unprotected intercourse.[8]

Earlier evaluation is justified in couples who have a known cause of infertility or risk factors. For example, an earlier referral for specialist investigation should be made within six months in women who have irregular or infrequent menstrual cycles, a history of pelvic infection or endometriosis, a history of procedures that might result in a reduction in ovarian reserve or if the woman's age is above 35 years old.

Ideally the couple should be seen together both at the initial consultation and subsequent visits because both partners should understand the reproductive norms and conception process. Furthermore, both partners will be affected by decisions about which investigations are to be performed and what treatment is to be planned.

History-Taking of the Female Patient

The aim of history-taking is to identify any symptoms that may suggest a specific cause of infertility and to detect any risk factors that may reduce fertility potential. This will help direct the evaluation of the factor(s) that are more likely to be responsible.

TABLE 14.1   History-Taking in Cases of Infertility

Features in History-Taking Required	Reason and Rationale
Age, number of years married, previous marriages and length of time actively trying to conceive	Gives an idea of the duration of infertility and the age of the woman is an important prognosticator of fertility potential
Previous obstetric history, gravidity, parity, pregnancy outcomes and associated complications, breastfeeding	To define if this is primary or secondary infertility problem and how a previous pregnancy may have affected the current situation. Include that with a previous partner if relevant

(Continued)

TABLE 14.1 (*Continued*)

Features in History-Taking Required	Reason and Rationale
Contraception history	Some forms of contraception e.g. Depo Provera are associated with a delay in return of fertility
Menstrual history including cycle length, menstrual flow pattern and associated dysmenorrhoea and its severity	Oligo-/amenorrhoea is indicative of anovulation; severe dysmenorrhoea may be a symptom of endometriosis; severe menorrhagia may be associated with uterine pathology like submucous fibroids
Coital frequency and any sexual dysfunction issues and dyspareunia	Low coital frequency and difficulty in intercourse minimises the chance of pregnancy and may be one of the main reasons why conception has not occurred
Past surgery, especially pelvic and hysteroscopic surgery, and its indication and outcome	Surgery for endometriosis or ectopic pregnancy or ovarian cystectomy may have an impact on tubal function or ovarian reserve. Ruptured appendicitis or bowel surgery may also affect tubal integrity. Hysteroscopic surgery suggests an abnormality of the uterine cavity
Past medical or chronic illnesses and gynaecological infections	PID or STDs may affect tubal status; uncontrolled thyroid disease can affect ovulation and fertility; history of malignancy and its subsequent treatment (chemotherapy or radiotherapy) may affect ovarian reserve
Current medications and drug allergies	Check compliance to medications for chronic diseases if relevant to ensure disease control optimal; some medications may have an impact on ovulation e.g. some anti-psychotics may cause hyperprolactinaemia
Previous abnormal Pap smears and treatment	Previous cervical surgery may have an impact on insemination techniques
Previous infertility investigation results, procedures and treatment done	Gives an idea of the extent of treatment that has been attempted and why the couple required it; the number of and details of previous ovulation induction or ART attempts should be well documented and an effort should be made to attain a medical report if the fertility treatment has been done elsewhere
Occupation and use of recreational drugs/tobacco smoking/alcohol etc.	These may reduce a woman's fertility

(*Continued*)

TABLE 14.1   (*Continued*)

Features in History-Taking Required	Reason and Rationale
Family history of birth defects, genetic disorders, early menopause	A history of inherited diseases should trigger a work-up for the couple before proceeding to fertility treatment. Genetic or chromosomal disorders may impact the type of treatment proposed as well.
Symptoms of galactorrhoea/ visual disturbances/ hirsutism/weight loss or gain (thyroid symptoms)/ menopausal symptoms/ pelvic pain	Endocrine disorders like hyperprolactinaemia, PCOS and hyperandrogenism and hypothyroidism affect fertility
Use of folic acid, previous vaccinations, previous chicken pox infection	Prior to pregnancy, it would be ideal if vaccinations are up to date

Physical Examination of the Female Patient

The aim of a thorough physical examination is to detect any signs that may suggest an abnormality which is a cause of infertility.

TABLE 14.2   Physical Examination

Features in Physical Examination to Note	Reason and Rationale
Weight/height and body mass index	Extremes of weight can affect ovulation and fertility
Blood pressure and pulse rate	Risk of hypertension higher in older women and this should be treated before embarking on fertility treatment
Thyroid enlargement	Functioning goitre may cause infertility if thyroid levels are not well-controlled
Breast examination: lumps and secretions	Galactorrhoea is a feature of hyperprolactinaemia
Acne, hirsutism, voice changes and acanthosis nigricans	These are features of androgen excess and insulin resistance which can result in anovulation
Abdominal-pelvic tenderness and masses and scars	To detect any pelvic pathology e.g. ovarian cysts or uterine fibroids and previous surgery
Vulvo-vaginal and cervical abnormalities	Check the hymenal status; any abnormal discharge, cervical polyps or cervicitis
Bimanual examination	Ensure uterine size is normal and mobile and to detect any adnexal masses; Pouch of Douglas tenderness or uterosacral ligament thickening/ nodularity may indicate endometriosis

Investigations of Female Infertility

General Screening Tests

Besides the tests targeted towards specific causes of infertility, there are some general screening tests that are recommended for all women concerned about their fertility. This is to ensure the woman has no problems that need to be addressed first, before embarking on any treatment.

A Pap smear should be done if it has not been performed within the recommended national screening time frame or if a previous Pap smear showed an abnormality. The date and result of the most recent Pap smear should also be documented.

Although most women in Singapore would have been immunised against Rubella in their childhood, a documented test of immunity (Rubella IgG) would be good to have. If the patient has never been vaccinated before or is found to be sero-negative, vaccination is highly recommended and pregnancy should be avoided for one month after vaccination. Likewise, if there is no history of chickenpox, a Varicella IgG should be done and vaccination offered if not immune. Similarly, avoid pregnancy for one month after each dose of vaccination.

If the blood group and Rhesus factor are not known, this should be done and women who are Rhesus negative should have an antibody screening as well. Thalassaemia is more prevalent in Southeast Asia and a thalassaemia screen should be offered — if the patient is found to be a thalassaemia carrier, her husband should then be screened too.

Women 40 years of age and older will require a mammogram if not done in the last year in line with the national screening guidelines, as well as an electro-cardiogram (ECG) as they are at higher risk of new onset cardiac disease than younger patients.

Specific Tests for Female Infertility[9,10]

The aim of the remaining investigations is to assess ovulation, ovarian reserve, tubal patency and uterine factors. The evaluation and investigations of the male will be covered in the chapter on "Male Infertility." Not all the tests are done at the initial visit — some will be performed after the initial investigations reveal an abnormality. In general, at the initial consultation, these tests will be ordered:

- Amenorrhoea panel (done on Day 2–3 menses): FSH, LH, E2, testosterone and prolactin
- Anti-müllerian hormone (AMH) level

- Serum progesterone level (done in the mid-luteal phase)
- Serum thyroid stimulating hormone (TSH) level
- Transvaginal ultrasonography of pelvis or TVUS (done on Day 2–3 menses)
- *Chlamydia* endocervical swab
- Semen analysis for the male partner (covered in Male Infertility section)

Some of these tests are specific for one problem, whereas others are useful in detecting various problems and as a screening tool. For example, serum progesterone is done as a test of ovulation but a TVUS can detect ovarian pathology like cysts or polycystic ovaries, uterine abnormalities like fibroids and also serve as a test of ovarian reserve by measuring the antral follicle count. The timing of some of the tests is crucial for interpretation and this will be explained in greater detail.

Tests of ovarian reserve

The peak number of oocytes is achieved *in utero* when the fetus is about 16–20 weeks and this maximum number is 6–7 million. At birth, this number falls to about 1–2 million and thereafter an irreversible decline in the number of oocytes begins such that by the onset of puberty, there are only 300,000 oocytes. Over the reproductive lifespan of a woman, which is about 35–40 years, about 400 oocytes will ovulate, although many more are recruited and undergo atresia during each menstrual cycle. By menopause, fewer than 1,000 follicles remain. As the follicular pool shrinks, the rate of atresia increases and the proportion of abnormal oocytes (the "quality" of the oocyte) increases as well, which explains why older women have a higher rate of miscarriage than younger women.

The ovarian reserve generally refers to the size and quality of the remaining ovarian follicular pool that has the potential to develop into antral follicles and a mature follicle. Although there is no screening test that can determine the quality of the oocyte or the exact number of eggs a woman has, an ovarian reserve test can aid in providing an estimate of the size of the follicular pool and to help prognosticate the response to fertility treatment.

Another aim of ovarian reserve testing would be to identify the individuals who have a diminished ovarian reserve, who may not respond as well to infertility treatment. Reduced ovarian reserve may be the result of previous ovarian cystectomy, oophorectomy or may be seen in patients with severe endometriosis. Sometimes there may not be a precipitating cause found. Ovarian reserve tests include both biochemical and ultrasonographic measurements. Biochemical tests include serum FSH, E2 and AMH, and ultrasonography measures the antral follicle count. Bear in mind that fertility varies greatly among individuals of similar age and that these tests only help to predict the response to ovarian stimulation and fertility treatment but do not predict the chances of a successful pregnancy.

Basal FSH and E2 concentrations (done on Day 2–3 menses): This is done early in the cycle as FSH levels can vary significantly across the menstrual cycle. A high baseline FSH level (>10 IU/L) is an early indication of reproductive aging, reduced ovarian reserve and reproductive potential. A single high basal FSH level should be repeated, as FSH levels can show marked inter-cycle and intra-cycle variation. Oestradiol value should be interpreted in conjunction with the basal FSH value — an early elevation of oestradiol (>220 pmol/L) level reflects advanced follicular development more characteristic of older women.

AMH levels: AMH is produced by the granulosa cells of pre-antral and small antral follicles, which correlates with the size of the residual follicular pool. AMH levels decline with age and are near undetectable approaching the menopause. Unlike FSH and E2, there is little inter- and intra-cycle variation in AMH levels. Women with lower AMH levels have poorer response in IVF stimulation cycles and egg yield is lower compared to those with normal AMH values. It has a higher sensitivity than FSH. AMH levels are categorised into good, average, poor or very poor.

Antral follicle count (AFC): Ultrasonography of the pelvis is done as a screening tool to ensure there are no occult uterine abnormalities e.g. fibroids/polyps, hydrosalpinges or ovarian pathology e.g. ovarian endometriomas or other cysts. It is performed in the early follicular phase as the likelihood of physiological ovarian cysts is lower, and to measure the antral follicle count before a dominant follicle develops. The number of antral follicles is proportional to the number of primordial follicles remaining and a low AFC is specific to predict low response to IVF ovarian stimulation and greater chances of having a lower oocyte yield.

Out of all the ovarian reserve tests available, AMH and AFC predict response to ovarian stimulation the best.

TABLE 14.3   Methods for Testing Ovarian Reserve

Test	Range of Normal Values	Remarks
FSH (Day 2–3)	3.5–12.5 IU/L	Values <1.5 with low E2 levels indicate hypogonadotrophic hypogonadism. Values >10 indicate reduced ovarian reserve.
E2 (Day 2–3)	90–716 pmol/L	Baseline E2 levels >220 with normal or raised FSH reflect advanced follicular development seen in older women
AMH	6.5–<19.8 pmol/L	AMH <1.5 indicates very low ovarian reserve; AMH 1.5–<6.5 indicates low ovarian reserve; AMH ≥19.8 reflects good ovarian reserve

Assessment of ovulation and regularity of the menstrual cycle

While a history of regular periods usually indicates that ovulation is taking place, a reliable marker to prove that ovulation has occurred is useful as well. Women with irregular periods may ovulate occasionally but this is unpredictable and not consistent.

Serum progesterone level. This test has to be appropriately timed. It should be performed in the mid-luteal phase when progesterone levels peak — which is ~7–8 days after ovulation and the resulting formation of a corpus luteum, which secretes this hormone. In a 28-day cycle, this test would be done on Day 21 i.e. seven days before the onset of the next menses. A level of >31.5 nmol/L is indicative that ovulation has occurred. In women with prolonged irregular menstrual cycles, a serum progesterone level is hard to time and is often not performed unless one is willing to repeat the level weekly until the onset of the next menses. This is often unnecessary and the general assumption would be that the patient is not ovulating regularly.

Urinary LH or ovulation predictor kits. These kits can be bought over the counter and are designed to detect the mid-cycle LH surge which occurs before ovulation. The LH surge starts and ends within a time frame of 48–50 hours and LH is rapidly excreted in the urine, which is tested by the woman in a method similar to a urine pregnancy test. Testing should be done daily, beginning 2–3 days before the surge is expected and when the test is positive, coitus can be timed accordingly. Ovulation predictor kits are non-invasive, widely available and can predict when ovulation will occur rather than retrospectively determine if ovulation has already occurred, which is the basis of the serum progesterone level test. The accuracy of ovulation predictor kits varies and some may be better than others.

Serial transvaginal ultrasonography (TVUS). Serial TVUS allows the process of ovarian follicle development to the pre-ovulatory phase to be visualised, as well as demonstrating evidence of post-ovulatory follicle rupture. This is known as monitoring of ovulation. The TVUS is performed every 2–3 days from the mid-follicular phase (about Day 12) until the immediate pre-ovulatory phase when the follicle reaches 18–20 mm and coitus timed accordingly. This test is more invasive and time-consuming than the above and is particularly useful when monitoring ovulation induction cycles.

Serum prolactin level. Women who have irregular or infrequent menses should have a serum prolactin measurement as hyperprolactinaemia is a fairly common cause of anovulation.

Serum TSH level. Menstrual irregularities are commoner in hypothyroid women and the risk of pregnancy loss is increased in women with overt or subclinical hypothyroidism.

Serum testosterone level. This may be slightly elevated in patients with PCOS or hirsutism and much higher values should provoke further investigations to look for other causes of androgen excess which can cause anovulation.

TABLE 14.4   Tests for Assessing Ovulation

Test	Range of Normal Values	Remarks
Progesterone	>31.5 nmol/L	This indicates ovulation.
Prolactin	70–510 mIU/L	Levels >1,000 should prompt further investigation for a prolactinoma. Levels <1,000 should be repeated.
TSH	0.45–4.5 mIU/L	Levels >4.5 should be investigated further for hypothyroidism and free T4 measured too.
Testosterone	0.22–2.90 nmol/L	Levels >5 warrant investigation into causes of androgen excess

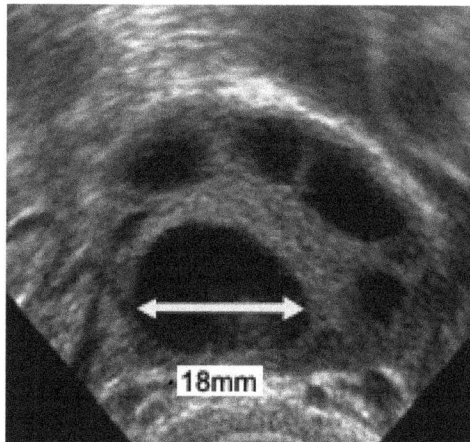

FIGURE 14.4 ■ TVUS showing ultrasound monitoring of an ovulation. The dominant follicle has reached 18 mm in size and is pre-ovulatory.

Tubal patency tests

The fallopian tubes allow the sperm and oocyte to meet and fertilise and the ciliary action in the mucosal portion enables embryo transport into the uterus — thus the tubes should be patent and function properly. Although there are no tests to prove effective tubal function, anatomical abnormalities that cause tubal occlusion can be established and sometimes treated.

At the initial consultation, not all women will be sent directly for a tubal patency test — low risk women need not. However, if there are risk factors gleaned from the history which suggest a possibility of tubal damage, then a tubal patency should be offered at the initial visit. Some of these risk factors include:

- History of pelvic inflammatory disease (PID)
- *Chlamydia* infection (past or current)
- History of septic miscarriage/abortion
- Ruptured appendix or other pelvic surgery with pelvic contamination
- History of tubal surgery
- History of ectopic pregnancy
- History of, or physical findings/investigations suggestive of, endometriosis

Of these, PID is the leading cause of tubal factor infertility and ectopic pregnancies. The risk of tubal infertility increases with number and severity of PID attacks as does the risk of ectopic pregnancy. The impact of PID on the fallopian tubes include anatomical distortion of the fallopian tube due to peri-tubal adhesions, fimbrial agglutination preventing ovum capture or hydrosalpinges causing tubal occlusion. It is possible that tubal function and the internal mucosa of the fallopian tube are affected by the infection and inflammatory changes although there is no test to prove this.

Although a basic ultrasonography of the pelvis is not a test of tubal patency, it is worthwhile to mention that moderate to large hydrosalpinges can sometimes be detected by ultrasound and further investigations should then be ordered to evaluate this further as outlined below. An ultrasound may also pick up other pelvic and adnexal pathology, like endometriomas or large lateral fibroids, which may affect tubal integrity and should thus be ordered before other radiological investigation for tubal patency.

Chlamydia swab test (endocervical swab). This is a useful screening tool as majority of patients with *Chlamydia* infection are asymptomatic and *Chlamydia* infection is associated with "silent PID" and tubal disease. It should be done for all women at the initial setting and is useful to help in deciding which women will require further evaluation of their tubal status. Furthermore, before undergoing any uterine instrumentation, women should be screened for *Chlamydia* infection, as instrumenting the uterus in untreated patients can precipitate an acute PID. If tested positive, both the woman and her partner should be treated.

Hysterosalpingography (HSG). This test is done during Day 7–10 of the menstrual cycle in the Radiology Department and involves injecting a radio-opaque contrast medium through the cervix into the uterus, while pelvic X-rays are taken at intervals during and after the injection. The main purpose of this test is to detect tubal patency, although the test will reveal the uterine outline and sometimes detect uterine anomalies e.g. bicornuate uterus. The passage of contrast into the tubes and spillage of contrast into the peritoneal cavity will be clearly demonstrable on the X-ray. Thus the HSG may demonstrate bilateral tubal patency, unilateral tubal patency or complete tubal occlusion. The site (proximal or distal tube) and sometimes the cause may be detected as well e.g. hydrosalpinges. An HSG is ordered at the initial consultation if the patient has the above risk factors or is keen to have intra-uterine insemination (IUI) treatment soon. A positive *Chlamydia* test done at the initial visit should prompt an HSG after treatment has been completed.

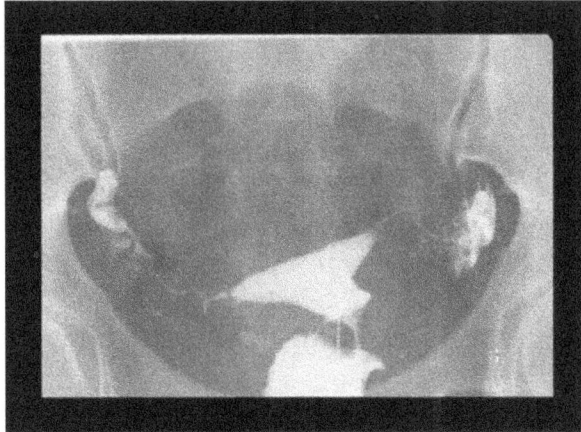

FIGURE 14.5 ■ Normal HSG showing the usual triangular configuration of the uterus and bilateral spillage of dye (blush) from patent fallopian tubes.

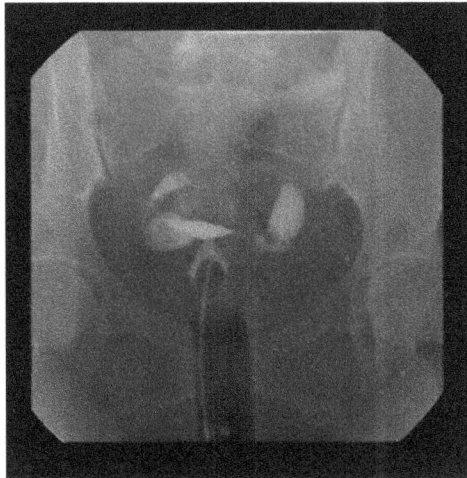

FIGURE 14.6 ■ HSG demonstrating bilateral hydrosalpinges with no spillage of contrast from either tube.

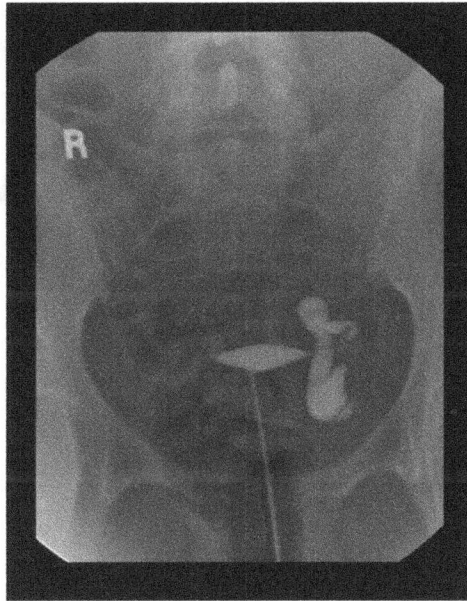

FIGURE 14.7 ■ Picture below and left: HSG demonstrating a left-sided hydrosalpinx and an absent right fallopian tube (a previous right salpingectomy had been done).

Sonohysterosalpingography or hysterosalpingo-contrast-ultra-sonography (HyCoSy). This test is also done during the first half of the menstrual cycle and is an effective alternative to HSG. The test utilises ultrasonography to assess tubal patency. A contrast solution is injected through the cervix and the ultrasound detection of the fluid accumulating in the Pouch of Douglas indicates the patency of at least one tube. Although HyCoSy is superior to HSG in picking up intra-uterine abnormalities e.g. submucous myomas or polyps, it does not give as much anatomical information about the tubes as HSG does.

Laparoscopy and dye hydrotubation. This is generally regarded as the "gold standard" for assessing the pelvis. The principle of this is to visualise the flow of methylene blue dye through the fallopian tubes during laparoscopy. Women who have other pelvic pathology detected at initial screening e.g. ovarian cyst, or who require a pelvic assessment e.g. if pelvic endometriosis is suspected, or who have an HSG which shows blocked tubes can be offered this procedure. Importantly, a laparoscopy also allows the chance to treat any pathology that may be present e.g. adhesiolysis, cystectomy, endometriotic ablation etc. Of course, laparoscopy is a surgical procedure with the attendant risks associated with surgery and general anaesthesia, so is not a first-line screening test or investigation. Laparoscopy does not assess the uterine cavity nor the internal luminal structure of the tube.

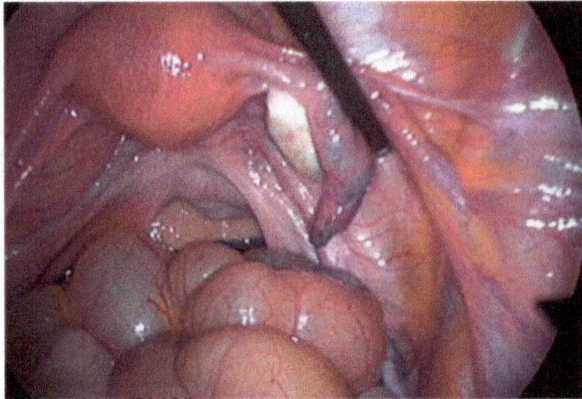

FIGURE 14.8 ■ Laparoscopy: normal uterus, tubes and right ovary (left ovary not seen). Hydrotubation has demonstrated good efflux of methylene blue dye through the fallopian tube, indicating a patent tube.

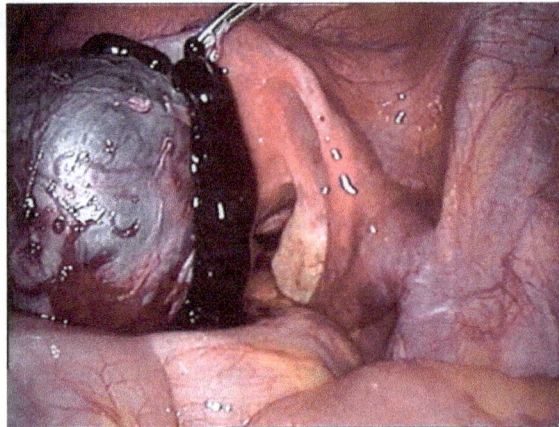

FIGURE 14.9 ■ Laparoscopy — Left ovarian endometrioma and normal right ovary.

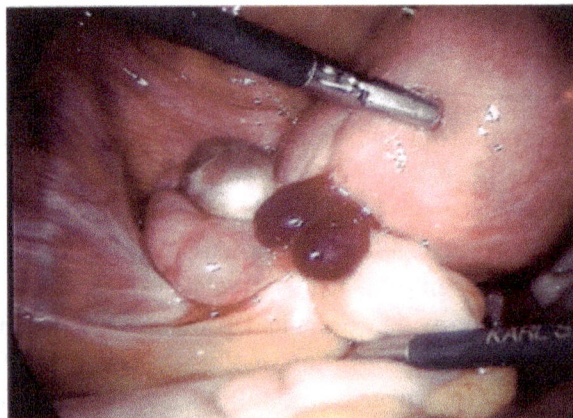

FIGURE 14.10 ■ Laparoscopy — Severe endometriosis with adhesions of the sigmoid colon to the uterus and left fallopian tube resulting in distorted tubal anatomy.

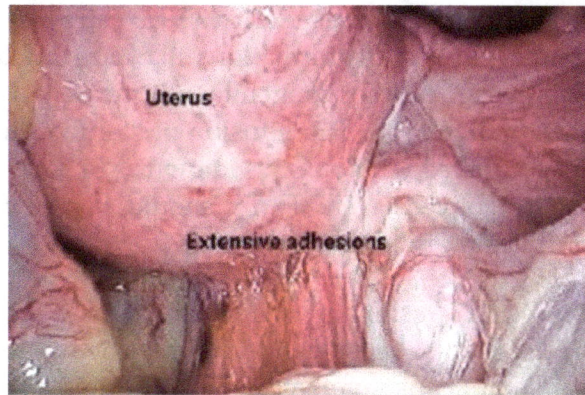

FIGURE 14.11 ■ Laparoscopy — Dense adhesions from endometriosis resulting in distorted tubal and uterine anatomy. Right ovarian endometrioma also present.

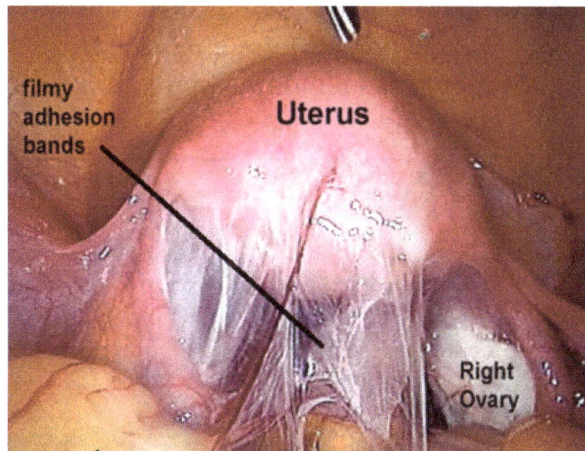

FIGURE 14.12 ■ Laparoscopy — Filmy adhesions from previous PID can also cause tubal distortion and result in tubal occlusion.

Assessment of uterine abnormalities

Uterine factors are a far less common cause of infertility. The anatomic abnormalities that can affect fertility and the success of fertility treatment are uterine polyps, submucous myomas, intrauterine adhesions/synechiae (Asherman's syndrome) and congenital anomalies like septated uterus. Some of these factors can cause recurrent pregnancy loss as well. The main methods of evaluating the uterine cavity are transvaginal ultrasonography (TVUS) with or without saline infusion sonography (SIS), HSG and hysteroscopy.

TVUS +/− SIS In experienced hands, TVUS is a reliable and easily available basic investigation tool to detect submucous myomas, endometrial polyps and to assess the endometrial thickness and regularity. TVUS can also complement HSG in diagnosing congenital uterine malformations like bicornuate uterus. The diagnostic accuracy of standard TVUS for congenital uterine malformations is increased with the availability of 3D TVUS. The infusion of sterile saline via a catheter into the uterine cavity combined with TVUS is known as SIS and is sensitive in picking up intrauterine pathology as well. TVUS should be the first-line investigation to screen for uterine abnormalities.

HSG. Besides being a test mainly for tubal patency, HSG can also define the size and shape of the uterus, detect congenital uterine malformations and sometimes pick up larger submucous myomas and intrauterine adhesions.

Hysteroscopy. This is not recommended as a routine test for all women but for further evaluation of endometrial abnormalities detected on initial screening e.g. an endometrial polyp detected on standard TVUS. It is the gold standard for both diagnosis and treatment of intrauterine pathology and can be done in an outpatient setting or in the operating theatre if more extensive treatment is required e.g. hysteroscopic resection of a submucous fibroid or lysis of intrauterine adhesions.

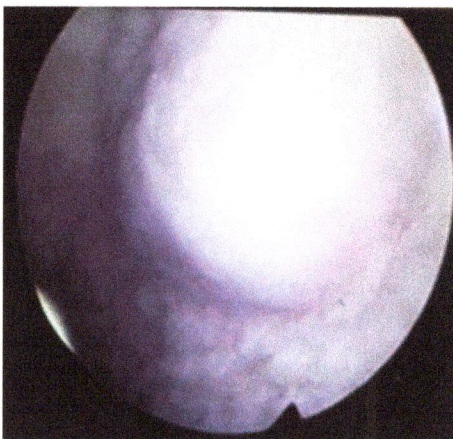

FIGURE 14.13 ■ Outpatient hysteroscopy picture of a submucous fibroid causing significant endometrial cavity distortion.

What if all the investigations return as normal?

When the routine tests of ovulation, tubal patency, assessment of the uterine cavity and semen results all return as normal and a cause of infertility cannot be identified, the couple has unexplained infertility — this is a diagnosis of exclusion and affects about 15% of couples. The management strategies for unexplained infertility will be discussed further on in the chapter. It is important to realise that there are limitations to the tests currently available and not every detail or step in the conception process has an investigation labelled to it.

Treatment Options

General Advice

The couple should be given advice on maintaining a healthy lifestyle. In particular, they should be given advice on weight management, smoking, alcohol and drug intake. If the woman has not had a recent (<3 years) cervical smear, one should be performed. Women should take folic acid periconceptually. The recommended dose is 0.4 mg daily, unless there is a specific risk factor, such as a previous child affected with neural tube defect, mother on anticonvulsants etc., when the dose should be 5 mg/day.

Weight management: The ideal BMI range in the Asian population is 18–23. Couples should be advised that underweight women are at risk of hypothalamic anovulation, and at the other end of the spectrum, overweight women may also suffer from ovulatory dysfunction. Steps should therefore be taken to either gain or lose weight as appropriate. Referral to a dietician for healthy eating advice should be considered. Regular exercise should be encouraged, although those who are underweight and exercise excessively increase the risk of amenorrhoea, and should be advised accordingly.

Smoking is known to be detrimental in both men and women who are trying to conceive, and there are the general health effects as well. Couples who smoke should also be given advice on the effects of second-hand smoke and how this can be harmful to a baby if they do succeed in falling pregnant, so they should make efforts to stop smoking.

Alcohol should be stopped or limited to seven units per week, and if they are using any illicit drugs, they should be advised to stop.

Anovulation

WHO group I

Women who have hypogonadotrophic hypogonadism will require exogenous gonadotrophins in order to ovulate. Follicle stimulating hormone (FSH) and Luteinising Hormone (LH) can be obtained from purified human menopausal urine (human menopausal gonadotrophin or HMG), or there are recombinant preparations also available. As these drugs are parenteral only, daily injections are self-administered, and the patient is monitored for ovarian response by ultrasound scan and serum oestradiol levels. The aim of treatment is to have one dominant follicle recruited, and when the follicle is deemed to be mature, ovulation is triggered by means of an injection of human chorionic gonadotrophin (hCG), which mimics the LH surge. An alternative for patients with hypogonadotrophic hypogonadism where pituitary function is normal is to use gonadotrophin releasing hormone (GnRH) in a pulsatile fashion. This needs to be delivered via syringe pump, but this is cumbersome and therefore not widely offered or accepted.

WHO group II

In overweight and obese women who are anovulatory, weight loss has been shown to increase the chances of return to spontaneous ovulation. Some women may resume ovulation even before they reach their ideal BMI, especially if they previously had regular cycles when their BMI was in the healthy range. There is evidence that losing 5% of body weight can result in the return of spontaneous ovulation. Even if ovulation does not occur, weight loss will make her more likely to respond to drug treatment. Morbidly obese women may require referral for bariatric surgery. The patient must be counselled that becoming pregnant while obese increases the risk of pre-eclampsia and gestational diabetes, with consequent increased maternal and neonatal morbidity.

Clomiphene is the first-line drug for ovulation induction. It is low cost, easy to use and has few side effects. It is an anti-oestrogen and works at the level of the pituitary. It enhances gonadotrophin production, leading to follicular development. It is given as a five day course, starting on Day 2 or 3 of the menstrual cycle. The initial starting dose is 50 mg, with cycle monitoring by ultrasound recommended to confirm follicular development and to exclude multifollicular development. The dose may be increased in 50 mg steps to 150 mg. The product license in the UK is for six months, arising from data that suggests an increased risk of ovarian cancer. Although the original data has not been confirmed, the license limit stands. Many patients will take more than six cycles of treatment, and they should be informed of the concerns about adverse effects. Many of them would consider that the benefits of taking more than six cycles of clomiphene outweigh the risks.

Tamoxifen has a similar mechanism of action but tends to be used less often. It may be considered if women experience side effects on clomiphene, particularly if their endometrium appears to be thin while taking clomiphene.

Gonadotrophins may also be used to induce ovulation. They are administered parenterally, and cost substantially more than clomiphene. Therefore, they are usually second-line treatments, where ovulation induction has been unsuccessful with the maximum dose of clomiphene. As with oral agents, the aim of treatment is unifollicular development with the lowest possible dose.

Ovarian drilling is an alternative treatment to gonadotrophins in clomiphene-resistant women. This is performed laparoscopically, and in some women this will help the resumption of spontaneous ovulation. The presumed mechanism of action is that the intra-ovarian androgen balance is altered, so that inhibition of antral follicles is released. The risks are that of laparoscopic surgery, of post-operative adhesion formation and of ovarian failure secondary to excessive electrosurgery.

WHO group III

Women with primary ovarian failure will require oocyte donation in order to conceive. This may prove challenging, as most units do not have a ready bank of oocyte donors. Women who are willing to be oocyte donors would need to undergo controlled ovarian hyperstimulation followed by oocyte retrieval (see section below on IVF for further details), and these processes have side effects and risks. After oocyte retrieval, the donated eggs would be fertilised with the sperm of the partner of the egg recipient. The recipient would need to have hormonal treatment to prepare her endometrium for embryo transfer. Alternatively, adoption should be discussed with women who have ovarian failure.

Hyperprolactinaemic anovulation

If serum prolactin is extremely elevated (>1,000 mU/L), imaging by CT or MRI should be organised to exclude a macroprolactinoma (>10 mm). If there is a macroprolactinoma with symptoms such as visual disturbance, surgical treatment may be necessary. This may be due to a prolactin secreting adenoma, or drug induced e.g. phenothiazines. Women with a microprolactinoma can be treated with a dopamine agonist, such as bromocriptine or cabergoline. This is usually sufficient to allow the menstrual cycle to resume. Both drugs are safe to continue during pregnancy should the woman conceive. For cases of drug-induced hyperprolactinaemia (e.g. antipsychotics such as haloperidol and risperidone), alternative medicines that do not cause this side effect should be explored.

Tubal Factor

Women with tubal factor infertility have the option of tubal surgery or IVF. The surgical options for tubal factor infertility include adhesiolysis, tubo-tubal anastomosis, salpingostomy, fimbrioplasty and salpingectomy. Peritubal adhesions are often the result of inflammation, which may arise after infection, following previous surgery, or as a consequence of endometriosis. Adhesions may either block the fimbrial ends, or they may distort the normal tubo-ovarian anatomy. External adhesions may be lysed surgically, but intratubal adhesions are not easily corrected with surgery.

The test of tubal patency should localise the site of tubal blockage. A proximal obstruction may be more difficult to correct surgically than a more distal obstruction. A proximal obstruction may need to be excised, with reanastomosis of healthy tubal tissue. If the fimbrial end is obstructed by adhesions, division of these adhesions may restore tubal patency. However, if there is an extensive obstruction, then sometimes a new opening has to be created. This is known as neosalpingostomy. Tubal surgery may be performed by laparotomy, laparoscopy or, if the local expertise allows, robotically. The chance of successful pregnancy after tubal surgery is about 25% per year. While this may be lower than the success rate of one cycle of IVF, tubal surgery would allow the possibility of conceiving more than once without further treatment. There is an increased risk of ectopic pregnancy and women undergoing tubal surgery should be advised to seek medical advice early should they conceive, in order to locate the pregnancy.

The availability and cost of IVF have to be taken into consideration when counselling women with tubal disease about their treatment options.

Hydrosalpinges

Studies show that IVF success rates are up to 50% lower in women with hydrosalpinges. Women with known hydrosalpinges should be counselled that these should be removed or occluded prior to IVF treatment, as this has been associated with an improved pregnancy rate. Studies suggest that hydrosalpinx fluid has a deleterious effect on the embryo, the endometrium or both.

Endometriosis

Treatment of endometriosis can be considered under two categories: for endometriosis-associated pain, and for endometriosis-associated infertility. In this section, treatments for fertility will be discussed, as treatment for pain will be discussed in the chapter on endometriosis.

Treatment of endometriosis to improve spontaneous pregnancy rate

A Cochrane review of drugs to suppress ovarian function (oral contraceptive pill (OCP), GnRH analogues, danazol) to improve fertility in minimal to mild endometriosis found that they were not effective and should not be offered for this indication alone.

In minimal to mild endometriosis, a Cochrane review showed that surgical treatment with division of adhesions and excision or ablation of endometriotic lesions increases spontaneous pregnancy rates. There are no controlled studies comparing reproductive outcomes after surgery versus expectant management in moderate to severe endometriosis. If there is an endometrioma requiring surgical treatment, the endometrioma capsule should be excised rather than drained and electrocoagulated, because this increases spontaneous pregnancy rates.

With regard to post-operative medical therapy after surgery for endometriosis, this has not been shown to improve spontaneous pregnancy rate and therefore should not be prescribed for this purpose.

Medically assisted reproduction and adjunctive treatments in endometriosis-related infertility

Controlled ovarian stimulation followed by intrauterine insemination (IUI) increases pregnancy rates in women with minimal to mild endometriosis, compared to IUI alone, as well as compared to expectant management.

If there is concomitant male factor or tubal factor infertility, or other treatments have failed, then assisted reproductive technologies such as IVF are recommended. There does not seem to be a difference in the success rates of IVF for endometriosis when compared with other indications, e.g. tubal factor.

A Cochrane review concluded that in women with endometriosis, medical treatment with GnRH analogue for 3–6 months before starting IVF can improve pregnancy rates.

In women undergoing surgery before IVF, complete removal of visible endometriotic lesions in women with mild to moderate endometriosis prior to IVF may increase pregnancy rates.

With regard to endometriotic ovarian cysts, there is no evidence that surgery before IVF improves pregnancy rates, even with cysts more than 3 cm diameter. Cystectomy may be considered to improve access to follicles for oocyte retrieval, or to reduce endometriosis related pain. Women should be warned about the risk of reduced ovarian function after surgery and the potential need for oophorectomy during surgery.

Uterine Factor

If a uterine septum has been diagnosed, hysteroscopic resection is associated with an improvement in pregnancy outcomes. If the woman has intrauterine polyps, or a submucous leiomyoma that interferes with the endometrial cavity, hysteroscopic resection may be considered.

Unexplained Infertility

Expectant management

As spontaneous pregnancy is still possible in unexplained infertility, advising couples to continue having regular unprotected intercourse without any active medical treatment is one treatment option. A study in Holland showed that more than 80% of couples with unexplained infertility became pregnant within five years of trying. 74% of pregnancies were conceived spontaneously. Factors to consider would include the woman's age, the duration of infertility and the occurrence of a previous pregnancy.

Assisted reproduction

After an unsuccessful trial of expectant management, assisted reproduction such as intra-uterine insemination (IUI) or *in vitro* fertilisation (IVF) may be considered.

IUI

Intrauterine insemination is thought to increase the chance of pregnancy by transferring the most motile sperm into the uterus, to bring them closer to the oocyte. If the woman has ovulatory cycles, natural cycle monitoring may be performed by ultrasound scan, to track the growth of the dominant follicle. A follicle is considered mature if it is approximately 17 mm or larger diameter. If she is anovulatory, ovulation induction may be performed using Clomiphene or gonadotrophins as above. Ovulation may be triggered by the use of an injection of HCG when the follicle is mature. The male patient's semen is prepared by successive centrifugation and washing so as to have a concentrated pellet of motile spermatozoa for insemination. The semen is then drawn up into a specialised intrauterine catheter, the catheter is inserted transcervically and the insemination performed.

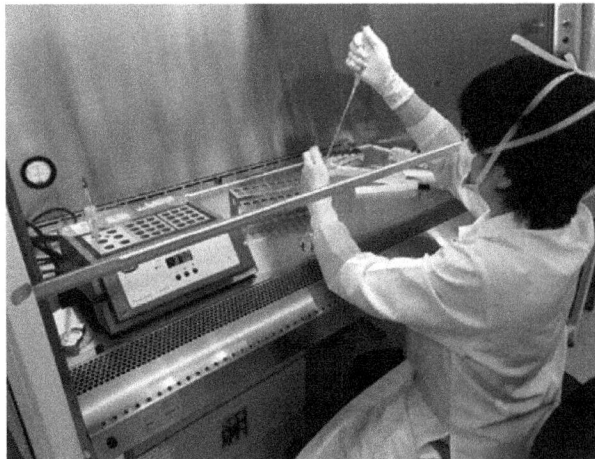

FIGURE 14.14 ■ Preparation of semen for IUI.

The success rate of IUI ranges from 8–10% per cycle in couples with unexplained infertility. A Cochrane review of patients with unexplained infertility treated with IUI showed a live birth rate of 23% versus 16% for expectant manage-ment over a six month period.

IVF

In vitro fertilisation was first described in the 1970s. Louise Brown was the world's first IVF baby, born in 1978, and the first IVF baby in Singapore was born in 1983. The team of doctors in Singapore was led by the late Prof SS Ratnam. Since then, there have been more than five million babies born worldwide as a result of IVF.

Stimulation

Women undergo controlled ovarian stimulation, using gonadotrophin injections. These may either be purified urinary gonadotrophins, or recombinant. In order to prevent a premature LH surge leading to premature ovulation, they also require other medications. There are two methods, firstly using a GnRH agonist before gonadotrophin stimulation, so as to cause downregulation of GnRH receptors in the pituitary gland. GnRH agonists would be continued alongside the gonadotro-phin. The alternative method is to introduce a GnRH antagonist during the stimu-lation cycle, which is a competitive inhibitor of the GnRH receptors. Women are closely monitored during their stimulation, with frequent ultrasound scans to measure the number and mean diameter of follicles. Some ART centres will also measure serum oestradiol levels as a measure of stimulation response. Ovulation is triggered when there are at least 3–4 follicles that are about 17–18 mm mean diameter. Final maturation and ovulation can be induced either by an injection of HCG, or if a GnRH antagonist was used to prevent premature ovulation, a dose of GnRH agonist can be given, leading to an increase in the endogenous levels of FSH and LH, thereby causing ovulation to be induced.

Oocyte retrieval

Oocyte retrieval is performed in the operating theatre, with the patient under seda-tion or a general anaesthetic. A needle guide is attached to the transvaginal ultra-sound probe, and the needle is passed into each follicle under ultrasound guidance. The needle is connected to a suction pump and the follicular fluid is aspirated from each follicle. Embryologists examine the follicular fluid to identify oocytes.

Mature oocytes are then prepared for fertilisation. IVF insemination involves adding spermatozoa to each oocyte, then examining under the microscope for fer-tilisation. If there is a male factor involved, for example severe oligospermia, embryologists may perform intracytoplasmic sperm injection (ICSI) instead. A sin-gle sperm is selected and injected into each oocyte.

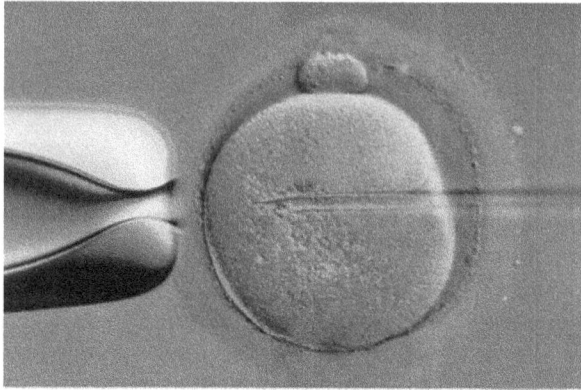

FIGURE 14.15 ■ ICSI.

The embryos are maintained in culture medium, and their development is monitored on a daily basis. Embryos are selected for transfer, and if there are excess embryos of sufficient quality, they may be frozen and stored, so that they can be subsequently thawed and transferred.

Embryo transfer

This is performed in the operating theatre. Many centres utilise ultrasound guidance to aid in embryo transfer. The embryo(s) are loaded in a soft tip catheter specially designed for the purpose. The catheter is inserted transcervically, and the embryos are released near the uterine fundus.

Success rates

The woman's age is probably the most significant predictor of successful outcome. Other factors include the general health of the patient, especially obesity and cigarette smoking, ovarian reserve and a concurrent male factor. The highest live birth rates are in women under the age of 35 years. There is some variation between different countries and regions (see Table 14.5). The chance of live birth is the highest during the first three cycles of IVF, but appears to decrease with subsequent cycles. In one study of cumulative live birth rates in the Netherlands, 90% of pregnancies were achieved within the first three treatment cycles.[11]

TABLE 14.5   Live Birth Rate Per IVF Cycle Started in Women Under 35

Country/Region (Source)	Live Birth Rate (%)
UK, 2012 (HFEA)	32.8
USA, 2012 (CDC)	40.5
Europe, 2010 (ESHRE)	26.1
Australia and New Zealand, 2012 (ANZARD)	24.8

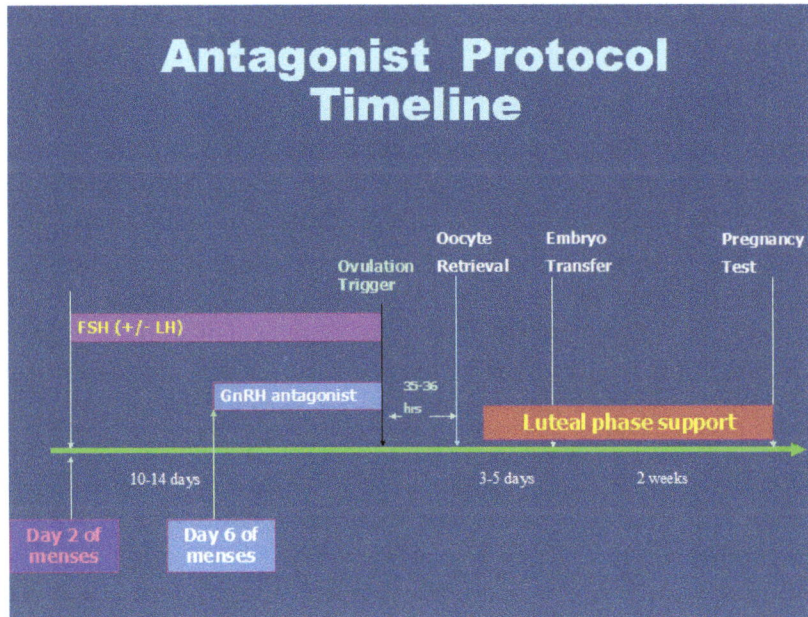

FIGURE 14.16 ■ Summary of IVF cycle (antagonist protocol).

Complications

Oocyte retrieval

At oocyte retrieval, the risks include bleeding, infection and visceral injury. Steps taken to reduce this include proper cleansing of the vagina pre-procedure and careful notation of the pelvic blood vessels e.g. internal iliac arteries and veins, the bladder and bowel during transvaginal ultrasound scan, taking care to avoid these structures during follicular aspiration.

Multiple pregnancy

The rate of multiple pregnancies is approximately 20–25% with assisted reproductive therapies, compared to a spontaneous incidence of about 1%. With IVF, this is a result of multiple embryos being transferred per cycle, in an attempt to increase the pregnancy rate. As there is a dramatic increase in perinatal morbidity and mortality, leading to increased healthcare costs such as neonatal intensive care because of premature birth, and the total lifetime costs of complications such as cerebral palsy, globally there has been a move toward elective single embryo transfer as this reduces the chance of multiple pregnancy. In Singapore, the maximum number of embryos that may be transferred at any one time is two, although it is the policy in our unit to offer elective single embryo transfer to women under the age of 35 undergoing their first IVF cycle.

OHSS

Ovarian hyperstimulation syndrome is an iatrogenic complication whereby there is a third space shift of fluid following ovarian stimulation. It occurs most commonly after gonadotrophin injections, but has also been described with oral agents such as clomiphene. HCG is the triggering factor for this syndrome. Women complain of bloatedness, abdominal pain and poor appetite. They may also complain of dyspnoea. They may have ascites and enlarged ovaries on ultrasound scan. More rarely, they may also develop a pleural effusion. Because of fluid shift, they may develop haemoconcentration and are at increased risk for venous thromboembolism. Mild OHSS may occur in up to 30% of patients undergoing IVF. Severe OHSS may be life threatening. Those at increased risk are women with PCOS, younger patients, those with a low BMI, and who have had many follicles during the stimulation cycle. OHSS is usually managed expectantly, with analgesia, fluid replacement and thromboprophylaxis. Some women require ascitic tapping if they are symptomatic.

Poor response

Older women and those with a reduced ovarian reserve (e.g. from previous ovarian surgery) may not respond adequately to gonadotrophin stimulation. They need to be counselled about abandoning the cycle of treatment, or if they wish to continue, that there is a chance that there will be no oocytes at retrieval and hence no embryos to transfer. Subsequently, the alternatives of oocyte donation or adoption should be discussed with patients with poor or no response.

References

1. Lashen H. (2004) Normal conception. In: Luesly DM, Baker PN (eds), *Obstetrics and Gynaecology: An Evidence-based Text for MRCOG*. Edward Arnold Ltd., London. Chapter 52.1; pp. 563–565.

2. Lashen H. (2004) Female infertility. In: Luesly DM, Baker PN (eds) *Obstetrics and Gynaecology: An Evidence-based Text for MRCOG.* Edward Arnold Ltd., London, Chapter 52.2, pp. 566–567.

3. Wong T, Yeoh BSA. Fertility and the family: an overview of pro-natalist population policies in Singapore. *Asia MetaCentre Research Paper Series No. 12.* Website: http://www.populationasia.org/Publications/RP/AMCRP12.pdf.

4. Singapore economic indicators. Singapore fertility rate, births per woman. Source: The World Bank. Website: http://www.theglobaleconomy.com/Singapore/Fertility_rate/.

5. Speroff L, Fritz MA. (2005) *Clinical Gynecologic Endocrinology and Infertility,* 8th edn. Lippincott Williams & Wilkins, Philadelphia. Chapter 27, Female infertility, p. 1140.

6. Speroff L, Fritz MA. (2005) *Clinical Gynecologic Endocrinology and Infertility,* 8th edn. Lippincott Williams & Wilkins, Philadelphia. Chapter 27, Female infertility, p. 1156.

7. Lashen H. (2004) Female infertility. In: Luesly DM, Baker PN (eds) *Obstetrics and Gynaecology: An Evidence-based Text for MRCOG.* Edward Arnold Ltd., London. Chapter 52.2, pp. 567–568.

8. Speroff L, Fritz MA. (2005) *Clinical Gynecologic Endocrinology and Infertility,* 8th edn. Lippincott Williams & Wilkins, Philadelphia. Chapter 27, Female infertility, pp. 1158–1160.

9. Speroff L, Fritz MA. (2005) *Clinical Gynecologic Endocrinology and Infertility,* 8th edn. Lippincott Williams & Wilkins, Philadelphia. Chapter 27, Female infertility, pp. 1147–1182.

10. Lashen H. (2004) Female infertility. In Luesly DM, Baker PN (eds) *Obstetrics and Gynaecology: An Evidence-based Text for MRCOG.* Edward Arnold Ltd., London. Chapter 52.2, pp. 569–570.

11. Witsenburg C, Diebeb S, Van der Westerlaken L, *et al.* (2005) Cumulative live birth rates in cohorts of patients treated with *in vitro* fertilization or intracytoplasmic sperm injection. *Fertil Steril* **84**: 99–107.

15

MALE INFERTILITY

Joe Lee and Wong P. C.

Introduction

Infertility is defined as the inability of a couple to achieve pregnancy after one year of frequent unprotected sexual intercourse. The prevalence of infertile couples is approximately 15%, out of which male factors alone account for 30% of cases, female factors alone 35%, combination of both male and female factors 20% and 15% cases are unexplained. In male factor infertility, the deficiency may be with sperm production or sperm transportation.

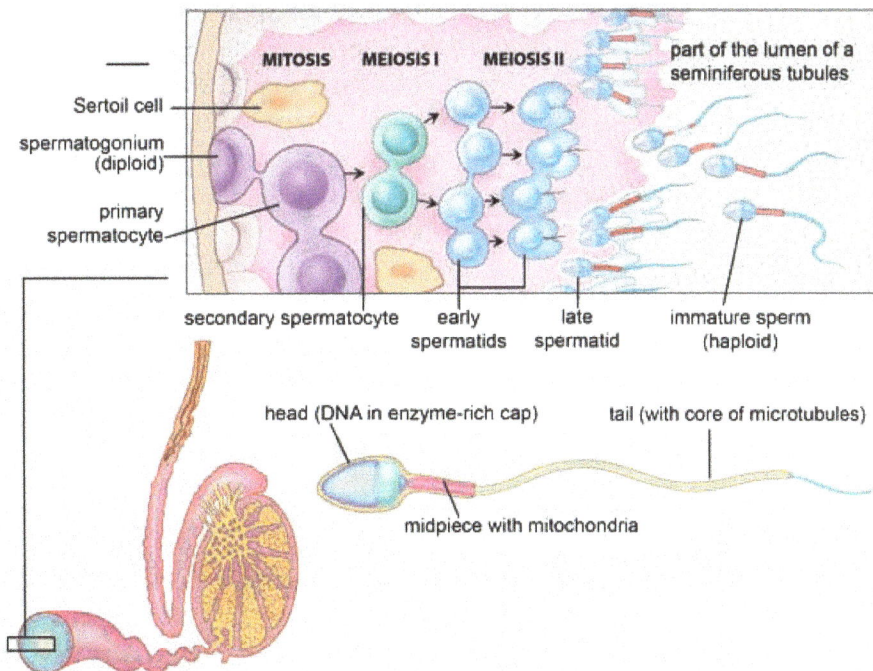

FIGURE 15.1 ■ Physiology of sperm production and transportation.

Sperm is produced in the testes and matures in the epididymis. Sperm production is regulated by the hypothalamic-pituitary-gonadal axis. The hypothalamus secretes gonadotropin releasing hormone (GnRH) in a pulsatile pattern which stimulates the release of follicle stimulating hormone (FSH) and luteinising hormone (LH) from the pituitary gland.

The testicle is made up of 200–350 pyramids filled with seminiferous tubules and covered by the tunica albuginea. The seminiferous tubules are composed of Sertoli cells and germ cells, with Leydig cells found in the interstitium between the seminiferous tubules. FSH stimulates Sertoli cells which facilitate germ cell differentiation, while LH stimulates the Leydig cells which produce testosterone. The Sertoli cell function is moderated by intra-testicular testosterone and the Sertoli cells also secrete inhibin which provides a negative feedback on the hypothalamus.

The precursors to spermatozoa are the germ cells, which first become spermatogonia under the stimulation of FSH. After mitotic divisions, the spermatogonia will become primary spermatocytes, which then undergoes meiosis to become secondary spermatocytes. After a second meiosis, the secondary spermatocytes will become spermatids, which now have a haploid chromosome number. The spermatids will next undergo the process of spermiogenesis to form the acrosome and flagella. The mature spermatid is then released from the Sertoli cells into the lumen of the seminiferous tubules as immature spermatozoa, where they will successively pass through the tubuli recti, rete testes, ductuli efferentes and into the epididymis. The entire developmental process from spermatogonia to spermatozoa takes approximately 74 days.

As the spermatozoa move from the head to tail of the epididymis, they mature and acquire their fertilisation capacity. From the epididymis, the mature spermatozoa enter the vas deferens, which joins the seminal vesicles distally at the ejaculatory duct. During ejaculation, the spermatozoa are mixed with fluids from the seminal vesicles, prostate and bulbourethral glands to form semen.

The main bulk of the semen is formed by secretions from the accessory ducts with the spermatozoa contributing only a negligible volume. The prostatic component of the semen contains liquefaction factors like prostate specific antigens (PSA), zinc, citric acid, phosphatase and spermine. Spermine is responsible for the characteristic odour of semen. PSA is a protease that helps to liquefy the coagulum of human semen about 10–20 min after ejaculation. The seminal vesicle fluid contains specific substances such as fructose and prostaglandins.[1]

Semen Analysis

The most important test used to determine male fertility is semen analysis. The semen is usually collected into a clean glass container by masturbation after 2–3 days of abstinence and examined within two hours. Care should be taken to deliver the specimen at close to body temperature if the specimen is collected at the patient's home. The normal pH of semen is between 7.2–8.0. Absence of fructose produced by the seminal vesicles should lead one to consider ejaculatory duct obstruction, seminal vesicle dysfunction or absence of the vas deferentia and seminal vesicles.

The normal parameters for semen analysis have been standardised by the World Health Organization[2] (see Table 15.1).

TABLE 15.1   WHO* 5th Semen Reference Value

Measurement	Lower Limit Normal	95% Confidence
Volume	1.5 ml	1.4–1.7 ml
Total sperm number	39 million	33–46 million
Concentration	15 million/ml	12–16 million/ml
Vitality	58%	55–63%
Progressive motility	32%	31–34%
Total motility	40%	38–42%
Normal morphology	4%	3–4%

Data from >4,500 healthy fertile men who created pregnancy with their partner in ≤12 months.

According to WHO criteria, one test is sufficient if the semen analysis results are normal. If the first test shows abnormal results, a repeat test should be done.

Oligospermia or low sperm count is defined as spermatozoa <15 million/mL. Asthenospermia or low sperm motility is defined as <32% motile spermatozoa. Teratozoospermia or low normal morphology is defined as <4% normal forms. Azoospermia is an extreme form of oligospermia where no spermatozoa are seen.

OATS (oligoasthenoteratozoospermia syndrome) is a term used to describe a situation when all three abnormalities occur simultaneously.

Causes of Male Factor Infertility

The causes of male factor infertility can be divided into pre-testicular, testicular and post-testicular. Men with azoospermia can be further classified into those with obstructive azoospermia (OA) and non-obstructive azoospermia (NOA).

Pre-Testicular Causes

In pre-testicular causes of male infertility, there is failure to stimulate appropriate spermatogenesis in the testes. This can be related to congenital or acquired conditions that disrupt the hypothalamic-pituitary axis.

The three main categories of hypogonadism include:

(a) Primary (hypergonadotrophic) hypogonadism due to testicular failure
(b) Secondary (hypogonadotrophic) hypogonadism due to insufficient gonadotropin-releasing hormone (GnRH) and/or gonadotropins (FSH and LH)
(c) Androgen insensitivity (end-organ resistance)

Primary (hypergonadotrophic) hypogonadism is considered under testicular causes.

In secondary (hypogonadotropic) hypogonadism, there is a failure of GnRH secretion which leads to decreased release of FSH and LH. This condition can be linked to **Kallmann syndrome** (associated with anosmia, cleft palate, deafness, cryptorchidism and colour-blindness), or may be idiopathic. Pulsatile GnRH and HCG in combination with FSH can be used to stimulate spermatogenesis in this group of patients.

Pituitary insufficiency can lead to infertility due to low FSH and LH. Acquired causes include intra-cranial tumours, infarction, previous radiation and infection.

Prolactin stimulates breast development and suppresses FSH and LH production. Patients with hyperprolactinaemia may have gynaecomastia and should be further investigated with an MRI of the brain to identify any functional prolactinoma. Dopamine agonists like bromocriptine and cabergoline are used to suppress prolactin levels in patients with microprolactinomas. This helps to increase testosterone and improve spermatogenesis.

Testicular Causes

In testicular causes, there is failure of spermatogenesis which can be caused by chromosomal, autosomal disorders or acquired conditions[3] (Table 15.2).

TABLE 15.2   Causes of Testicular Deficiency (from EAU)

Factors	Causes
Congenital	Anorchia
	Testicular dysgenesis/cryptorchidism
	Genetic abnormalities (karyotype, Y chromosome deletions)
Acquired	Trauma
	Testicular torsion
	Post-inflammatory forms, particularly mumps orchitis
	Exogenous factors (medications, cytotoxic or anabolic drugs, irradiation, heat)

(Continued)

TABLE 15.2 (*Continued*)

Factors	Causes
	Systemic diseases (liver cirrhosis, renal failure)
	Testicular tumour
	Varicocele
	Surgery that may compromise vascularisation of the testes and lead to testicular atrophy
Idiopathic	
Unknown aetiology	Unknown pathogenesis

Klinefelter's syndrome is the commonest sex chromosome abnormality encountered in male factor infertility. The affected male has a 47, XXY karyotype. The testes of an adult with Klinefelter's syndrome are usually small, firm and devoid of germ cells. They are usually azoospermic, with primary testicular failure and raised gonadotropins. Testicular biopsies often show hyalinisation of the seminiferous tubules, although close to 20% of men with mosaic Klinefelter's syndrome may have isolated foci of spermatogenesis amenable to sperm retrieval and assisted reproductive techniques (ART).

Y chromosome microdeletion The long arm of the Y chromosome is important in male fertility. Azoospermic factors a, b and c (AZFa, AZFb and AZFc) are regions on the Y chromosome whereby deletion is associated with poorer prognosis, as there are several spermatogenesis candidate genes in these regions. Before sperm retrieval, a male who is found to have AZFa and AZFb microdeletions will be counselled not to proceed with surgery as the likelihood of finding sperm in such cases is close to 0%.

Non-chromosomal disorders resulting in testicular causes of male infertility include previous radiation and torsion. These conditions cause irreversible damage to the germ cells in the seminiferous tubules which can render the male infertile.

Intra-testicular obstruction can occur in 15% of men with obstructive azoospermia, usually after inflammatory or traumatic episodes. Orchitis and trauma can result in intra-testicular obstruction by means of intra-tubular fibrosis.

Varicocele refers to abnormal dilatation of veins forming the pampiniform plexus of the scrotum, which drains blood from the testes. They are believed to form due to incompetent valves of the internal spermatic veins. The clinically detectable varicoceles can be graded from I–III (refer to Clinical Varicocele Classification[4] Table 15.3).

TABLE 15.3   Clinical Varicocele Classification

Classification	Definition
Clinical (Palpable):	
Grade III (Large)	Easily visible
Grade II (Medium)	Palpable at rest (without Valsalva manoeuvre), invisible.
Grade I (Small)	Palpable with Valsalva manoeuvre only
Subclinical (not palpable):	
Grade 0	Vein larger than 3 mm on ultrasound; Doppler reflux on Valsalva manoeuvre

15% of men in the general population have varicoceles. The proportion is higher at 35% for men with primary infertility and 75% for men with secondary infertility. It is more common on the left side and occasionally bilateral. Isolated right varicocele is fairly rare although most men with varicoceles are still able to father children.

The exact mechanism whereby varicoceles impair testicular function is not fully understood. Theories include raised scrotal temperature, hypoxia from venous stasis, dilution of intra-testicular substrates such as testosterone, disruption of the hypothalamic-pituitary-gonadal axis, and reflux of renal and adrenal metabolites down the spermatic vein. Higher testicular temperatures have been observed to affect spermatogenesis and sperm function but the pathophysiology of varicocele on male fertility is most likely multi-factorial.

Men with clinical varicoceles (Grade I–III) should consider varicocelectomy, but men with subclinical varicoceles (Grade 0) are unlikely to benefit. After surgery, 40–70% of patients show improved semen parameters, with up to 40% achieving pregnancy.

Cryptorchidism is a common congenital abnormality found in 5% of newborn boys. At three months of age, spontaneous testicular descent can occur, and the number can drop to 1%. The cause of undescended testes is multifactorial, with possible contributions from disrupted endocrine regulation during early pregnancy and genetic defects. Germ cells tend to degenerate in the undescended testis after the first year of life and 40% of men with bilateral cryptorchidism are eventually azoospermic.

Nonetheless, there is no age limit for bilateral orchidopexy. Correction, even in adult life, can lead to appearance of spermatozoa in the ejaculate. In general, men with undescended testes are at increased risk of developing germ cell tumours in the affected testes and should always be evaluated with a scrotal ultrasound to exclude testicular masses and microcalcifications. While fertility is usually unaffected in men with unilateral cryptorchidism, the fertility of men with bilateral undescended testes are often affected by testicular dysgenesis.

Post-testicular Causes

In post-testicular causes, the problem lies in sperm delivery through the ductal system. Genital duct obstruction can occur at the testis, epididymis, vas deferens or ejaculatory ducts.

Congenital bilateral absence of vas deferens (CBAVD) often manifests as epididymal obstruction, where the distal aspect of the epididymis is absent. This condition is often associated with cystic fibrosis. Patients with bilaterally deficient vas need to be screened for cystic fibrosis genes and genetic counselling should be rendered when necessary.

Acquired epididymal and ductal obstruction can result from insults arising from infections (*Chlamydia*, gonorrhoea, tuberculosis), previous procedures such as vasectomy, hernia repair and sperm retrieval, extrinsic compression from prostatic cysts and luminal obstruction by ductal calculi.

Vas deferens obstruction is most commonly seen in patients who have undergone vasectomy. 2–6% of these men may request vasectomy reversal later in life. Vasal obstruction can also occur after a herniorrhaphy with mesh repair, where the vas is entrapped by a fibroblastic response.

Ejaculatory duct obstruction (EDO) accounts for 1% of obstructive azoospermia. Patients may notice a decreasing ejaculate volume or total absence of ejaculate. Pain is sometimes present during ejaculation. In complete obstruction, semen volume is usually <1.5 ml, seminal fructose is usually absent and the semen has an acidic pH. This can be caused by infection, ductal calcification or congenital cysts. The seminal vesicles are usually dilated with an anterior–posterior diameter >15 mm on transrectal ultrasonography.

Retrograde ejaculation occurs when semen that is usually directed down the urethra refluxes backwards towards the bladder. Aetiologies include diabetic neuropathy, previous bladder neck surgery or transurethral resection of prostate, multiple sclerosis, spinal cord injury and use of medications such as alpha-agonists. These patients are usually able to experience an orgasmic sensation without seminal emission. The confirmatory test for this condition is a post-ejaculatory urine analysis looking for spermatozoa. Retrograde ejaculation can be managed with drug therapy, using alpha agonists such as ephedrine sulphate or tricyclic antidepressants such as imipramine.

History

In clinical evaluation of the infertile male, a detailed fertility history is required. It is important to ascertain how long the duration of infertility has been. If the currently infertile male has successfully impregnated a female partner before, the underlying aetiology of infertility is most likely acquired. Delayed puberty, previous cancers requiring chemotherapy or radiation and childhood surgeries to treat conditions such as undescended testes are significant as these are known to impact fertility. A history of smoking, alcohol abuse, and occupational exposures to toxic substances may suggest environmental causes. Family history of subfertility or cystic fibrosis leads one to suspect genetic causes. Spinal cord injury or use of certain medications may affect ejaculation.

The sexual history should include frequency of sexual intercourse and masturbation. Overly frequent or infrequent intercourse can affect the couple's fertility outcome adversely. Patient's libido, erectile function and ability to have normal vaginal intercourse must not be overlooked. Ensure that ejaculation occurs deep within the vagina and not outside as seen in cases of severe premature ejaculation or hypospadias. Lubricants are usually spermicidal and vegetable oil based substances can sometimes be used in place of them.

Physical Examination

During inspection, one should identify the presence of secondary male sexual characteristics such as facial, body and pubic hair, laryngeal enlargement, deepening of voice, body habitus and genital development. Presence of gynaecomastia may imply underlying endocrine disorders.

The penis should be stretched during palpation to detect abnormalities such as plaques and severe phimosis. The location of the urethral meatus should be normal. In severe hypospadias, ejaculate delivery may occur outside the vaginal canal.

Both testes should be examined for location, size, consistency and symmetry. A normal testicle is approximately 2.5 × 4 cm and 15–20 ml in volume. Atrophic testes may be seen in previous maldescent or endocrinopathies. Since infertile males are at higher risk of developing testicular cancers, they need to be examined for testicular masses. With the testes steadily held with one hand, the other examining hand should palpate the epididymis lying posteriorly to detect any fullness, induration or tenderness. An obstructed epididymis will feel enlarged while a chronically infected and scarred epididymis will feel hard and irregular.

Both vas deferentia need to be palpated to ensure they are not absent. The inguinal region is examined to identify any hernias or scars suggestive of past inguinal surgery. At this point, patient should be asked to stand up, to allow palpation for varicoceles near the spermatic cords. Patient can be asked to perform a Valsalva manoeuvre while standing to facilitate detection of a Grade I varicocele.

A digital rectal examination is recommended to evaluate the prostate. While the seminal vesicles are normally not palpable, they may be felt in ejaculatory duct obstruction.

Other Investigations

Besides semen analysis, other laboratory tests are used to investigate the infertile male whenever appropriate.

Urinalysis and Urine Cultures

These tests are used to evaluate for lower genitourinary tract infections, which can present with pyuria or a positive urinary culture.

Endocrine Evaluation

A complete hormonal evaluation of male infertility should include serum FSH, LH, testosterone and prolactin. Raised FSH and/or LH with low testosterone is usually seen in primary testicular failure, while low LH with low testosterone is seen in hypogonadotrophic hypogonadism. Prolactin is important in the presence of hypogonadism to exclude hyperprolactinaemia.

Genetic Testing

Karyotype analysis is useful in evaluating men for underlying chromosomal disorders such as Klinefelter's syndrome. Specific microdeletions of AZF regions on the Y chromosome can be done as a prognostic test before patient undergoes surgical sperm retrieval. Patients with complete deletion of AZFa and AZFb will have a very low chance of success.

Scrotal Ultrasound

A scrotal ultrasound is recommended in infertile males. Besides confirming the presence of varicoceles, scrotal ultrasound can ascertain the presence of intra-testicular masses or testicular microcalcifications which may affect the decision for sperm retrieval and other reproductive treatments.

Transrectal Ultrasound

Infertile men with low ejaculate volumes <1.5 ml should be further evaluated with a transrectal ultrasound for ejaculatory duct obstruction. These patients can be identified by a dilated seminal vesicle (>15 mm anterior–posterior distance). Stones, midline prostatic cysts and persistent utricle can be visualised on ultrasound.

Vasography

This is an intraoperative investigation which is done by injecting contrast into the lumen of the vas under an image intensifier. The purpose is to identify discrete sites of obstruction where vaso-vasostomy may be beneficial.

Diagnostic Testicular Biopsy

In azoospermic males with normal hormonal parameters and fructose, testicular biopsy can be done to identify the state of spermatogenesis. This can also be done as part of a sperm retrieval procedure. Histology showing maturation arrest or Sertoli cell only syndrome helps to prognosticate treatment outcomes.

Treatment

Surgical

Varicocelectomy

Varicocelectomy is recommended in cases of clinical varicocele where there is oligospermia and infertility duration of two years or more. There are various approaches to performing varicocelectomy. The subinguinal approach is the commonest, where the spermatic cord is isolated after it has left the superficial inguinal ring. This is done through a small groin incision. Individual veins are ligated between sutures and cut. Care is taken to avoid injury to the testicular artery which may lead to testicular atrophy. The Doppler ultrasound can be used intra-operatively to identify the testicular artery whenever there is doubt. Magnification to improve visualisation of the veins can be achieved by using surgical loupes or an operating microscope. In the inguinal approach, the spermatic cord is isolated further upstream at the level of the inguinal canal, where there are usually less veins. Some muscle-splitting is required in this approach. Varicocelectomy can also be performed laparoscopically when the cost-effectiveness is justifiable.

After a successful varicocelectomy, 60–70% of men who had clinically palpable varicoceles will see an improvement in semen parameters after at least three months. Follow-up studies have shown a higher rate of spontaneous pregnancy in this group compared to the group with untreated varicoceles.

After varicocelectomy, it is not uncommon to observe persistently dilated and palpable veins distal to the level of ligation, even when there is no longer venous reflux. This may be due to venous thrombosis or loss of elasticity of the veins from chronic stretching and does not necessarily imply recurrence.

Complications of varicocelectomy include testicular arterial injury leading to testicular atrophy, scrotal haematoma and post-operative hydrocele.

Vaso-vasostomy or vaso-epididymostomy

Also known as vasectomy reversal surgery, since this is most commonly per-formed for men who are seeking fertility again after previous vasectomies. In vaso-vasostomy, the two ends of the cut vas are dissected and reanastomosed using 9/O or 10/O nylon sutures. If the distal vas is too short, a direct anastomosis to the epididymis or vaso-epididymostomy will be performed. All these specialised microsurgical procedures have to be done with the aid of an operating microscope. Intra-operatively, fluid expressed from the distal vas are examined for sperm. A thin watery fluid usually implies patency as compared to a white toothpaste-like fluid which usually contains debris and non-viable sperm fragments. The success rate of vasectomy reversal is close to 90% in the three years after vasectomy. This figure drops to 80% at 10 years after vasectomy and 70% after 15 years or more. This is due to the secondary epididymal obstruction that can develop over time.

Transurethral resection of ejaculatory ducts (TURED)

For men diagnosed with ejaculatory duct obstruction, TURED is indicated. The obstruction is usually caused by a midline prostatic cyst which can be visualised on transrectal ultrasonography along with dilated seminal vesicles. The TURED procedure is similar to how transurethral resection of the prostate (TURP) is per-formed for benign prostatic hyperplasia (BPH). Using a resectoscope with a cut-ting loop, deep resections are made to the verumontanum to expose the ducts and release the trapped ejaculate. The complications associated with TURED include bladder neck injury causing retrograde ejaculation, or urinary reflux into the ejaculatory ducts, seminal vesicles and vas causing epididymitis.

Sperm retrieval

In azoospermic males, sperm can be retrieved either by aspiration or extraction from surgically removed testicular tissue. Both aspirations and extractions can be done conventionally without magnification or microsurgically with the aid of an operating microscope.

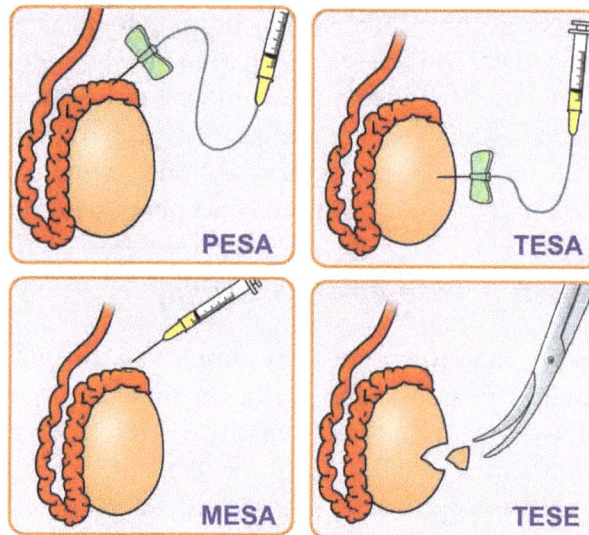

FIGURE 15.2 ■ Methods of sperm retrieval.

Percutaneous epididymal sperm aspiration (PESA) can be done under local anaesthesia in the office setting. The epididymis is palpated and a butterfly needle is inserted blind into the body of the epididymis. Negative suction is created using a syringe and aspirate collected. The limitation of this procedure is that it does not allow multiple site samplings and there is risk of secondary epididymal obstruction post-procedure.

Microsurgical epididymal sperm aspiration (MESA) requires general anaesthesia and an operating microscope. The epididymis is exposed to reveal the underlying tubules. After the epididymal tubule is incised, a small needle is used to aspirate the epididymal fluid. This approach is more targeted and less likely to cause collateral injuries to the testis.

Testicular sperm aspiration (TESA) can also be done under local anaesthesia in the office setting. This approach to sperm retrieval can be attempted after a negative PESA or when there is a known obstruction between the testis and epididymis.

Testicular sperm extraction (TESE) are conventionally performed under local anaesthesia with sedation or under general anaesthesia. During this procedure, a median raphe scrotal incision is usually made, through which the underlying testis is exposed. The tunica albuginea is incised to reveal the underlying seminiferous tubules which are excised with dissecting scissors. If necessary, multiple quadrants of the testis can be sampled using multiple stab incisions.

Microdissection testicular sperm extraction (Micro-TESE) is the preferred method of sperm extraction, as magnification allows the testis to be examined more closely. In this procedure, the testes are usually delivered through a median raphe incision. A transverse incision is made over the avascular plane of the tunica albuginea to reveal the seminiferous tubules. The surgeon will examine the seminiferous tubules under the microscope, targeting the biopsies at tubules that are visibly more dilated and likely to contain sperm. The target tubules are teased free with micro-forceps and micro-scissors. To facilitate sperm search, the tubules can be further minced using mechanical or enzymatic digestion. This approach minimises the amount of testicular tissue lost and is especially beneficial in men with small testicular volume and borderline testosterone levels, where further loss of testicular tissue may lead to testosterone deficiency syndrome requiring long-term testosterone replacement therapy.[5]

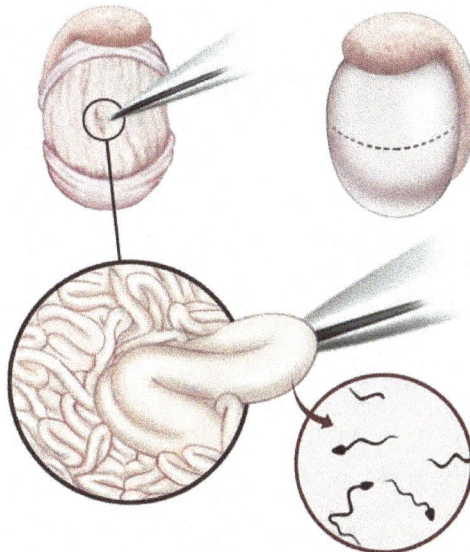

FIGURE 15.3 ■ Microdissection testicular sperm extraction (Micro-TESE).

Electroejaculation

This less common form of sperm retrieval is usually used in men with ejaculatory dysfunction due to spinal cord or neurological disorders. Under general anaesthesia, an electrode is inserted per rectally and placed at the posterior seminal vesicles. Repeated delivery of direct electrical stimulation will allow the seminal vesicles to contract and empty their contents. The semen ejaculated is collected per urethrally.

Sperm retrieval in retrograde ejaculation

When sperm aspiration or extraction is not amenable for a patient with retrograde ejaculation, sperm retrieval can be done by first alkalinising the urine with either oral agents or direct instillation of an alkaline medium into the bladder using a urethral catheter. After the patient has ejaculated, a second catheterisation is immediately done to drain out the spermatozoa.

Medical

Medical treatment of male factor infertility has not been a major success, although dietary supplements consisting of anti-oxidants such as Vitamin C and E have been shown to improve sperm quality to a certain extent, presumably by decreasing the number of free radicals. Some studies have shown zinc, selenium and fish oil to be useful. Supplements can be used in idiopathic situations where there are no definitive interventions that can be applied.

References

1. Griswold MD. (1995) Interactions between germ cells and Sertoli cells in the testis. *Biol Reprod* **52**(2):211–216.
2. World Health Organization, Department of Reproductive Health and Research. WHO Laboratory Manual for the Examination and Processing of Human Semen, 5th edn, pp. 223–226.
3. Jungwirth A, Giwercman A, Tournaye H, *et al.* (2012) European Association of Urology Working Group on male infertility. European Association of Urology guidelines on Male Infertility: the 2012 update. *Eur Urol* **62**(2):324–332.
4. Practice Committee of the American Society for Reproductive Medicine. (2014) Society for Male Reproduction and Urology. Report on varicocele and infertility: a committee opinion. *Fertil Steril* **102**(6):1556–1560.
5. Ishikawa T1, Nose R, Yamaguchi K, *et al.* (2010) Learning curves of microdissection testicular sperm extraction for nonobstructive azoospermia. *Fertil Steril* **94**(3):1008–1011.

16

RECURRENT PREGNANCY LOSS

Zhongwei Huang and Mahesh Choolani

Introduction

Recurrent pregnancy loss is a distressing condition to couples. However, this condition has several definitions which may impact the way clinicians initiate investigations and manage this problem appropriately.

The Royal College of Obstetricians and Gynaecologists (RCOG) defined recurrent pregnancy loss as the loss of three or more consecutive pregnancies before viability and include three or more first-trimester pregnancy losses.[1] The RCOG also includes one or more second-trimester pregnancy losses until 24 weeks of gestation in its definition. The American Society of Reproductive Medicine (ASRM) defines two or more failed clinical pregnancies as recurrent pregnancy loss and a clinical pregnancy is defined as a pregnancy documented by ultrasonography or histopathological examination.[2]

Epidemiology

Epidemiological studies have shown that 15% of pregnancies identified on ultrasonography usually end in pregnancy loss. Two thirds of these pregnancies are lost in the first and early second trimesters and one third is lost later in gestation. Amongst all conceptions, 40% result in occult losses at less than six weeks' gestation, 13% at less than 12 weeks' gestation and 1% of these conceptions are lost at 12 weeks and above in gestation, thereby resulting in 30% of all conceptions progressing to successful live births.

Three or more pregnancy losses affect 1–2% of women in the reproductive age group, with two or more losses affecting around 5% of these women.[3] The spontaneous pregnancy loss rate rises to about 25% and 35% after two and three consecutive pregnancy losses respectively.

Maternal age has been associated with pregnancy loss. With advancing maternal age, the number and quality of oocytes decrease, resulting in rising age-related pregnancy loss as detailed: 12–19 years, 13%; 20–24 years, 11%; 25–29 years, 12%; 30–34 years, 15%; 35–39 years, 25%; 40–44 years, 51%; and ≥45 years, 93%. Advancing paternal age is also associated with miscarriage and risk is highest in couples in which the woman is ≥ 35 years and man ≥ 40 years.

Unfortunately, a history of live birth followed by consecutive pregnancy losses does not reduce the risk of further losses subsequently. In addition, retrospective studies on being underweight or obese has been associated with recurrent pregnancy loss. Current evidence is insufficient to associate maternal cigarette smoking and caffeine consumption to sporadic pregnancy loss. Heavy alcohol consumption is known to be toxic to the embryo and fetus, hence moderate consumption of five or more units of alcohol have been associated with sporadic pregnancy loss.

Causes

The plausible causes of recurrent pregnancy loss are weakly associated — only approximately 50% of early recurrent pregnancy losses have a putative cause due to karyotype/genetic abnormalities, structural uterine abnormalities, anti-phospholipid syndrome, some thrombophilias, immunological factors, endocrinological disorders and infective agents.

Parental Genetic Factors/Chromosomal Abnormalities

Approximately 2% to 5% of couples with recurrent pregnancy loss have one of the partners who carry balanced structural chromosomal anomalies i.e. Robertsonian translocation. Couples with chromosomal anomalies are at increased risk of pregnancy loss which is influenced by the size and the genetic content of the rearranged chromosomal segments. However, in these couples, there is still a possibility of a 70% live birth rate in a subsequent pregnancy. Notably, 1% of offspring from couples with balanced translocations have unbalanced translocations. Therefore, in consideration of the above, where the 1% pregnancy loss rate is close to the loss rate in normal pregnancies after invasive prenatal diagnosis, parental karyotyping is no longer thought to be cost-effective. Although in women with a history of subfertility, recurrent pregnancy loss and a balanced translocation, observational studies have demonstrated that preimplantation diagnosis combined with assisted reproductive techniques has better pregnancy outcomes, despite lower rates of embryo transfer and shorter time to a successful pregnancy.[4]

Embryonic/Foetal Chromosomal Abnormalities

Chromosomal abnormalities of the embryo account for 30–57% of pregnancy loss, and this risk increases with advancing maternal age, accounting for 70% of early pregnancy loss while only 20% of pregnancy loss between 13 to 20 weeks' gestation is due to chromosomal abnormalities.[5] However, it is important to note that, as the number of miscarriages increases, the risk of euploid pregnancy loss increases.

Structural uterine abnormalities

Congenital uterine anomalies such as unicornuate, didelphys, bicornuate, septate or arcuate uterus are noted to be in 4.3% (2.7–16.7%) of the general population of fertile women versus 12.6% (1.8–37.6%) of women with two or more pregnancy losses.[6] A high incidence of pregnancy loss occurred in patient with septate (44.3% loss), bicornuate (36% loss) or arcuate (25.7% loss) uteri, therefore correction (especially of septate uteri) in women with recurrent pregnancy loss is likely to be beneficial, leading to live birth rates of 83.2% (77.4–90.9%).[2] However, no randomised controlled trials have proven hysteroscopic surgery to be effective for the above indications.[7]

Cervical Weakness

This condition is a recognised factor of second trimester losses, but exact incidence remains unknown and diagnosis is based on a history of second trimester pregnancy loss with spontaneous rupture of membranes or painless cervical dilatation. Cervical cerclage has potential risks related to surgery and should only be considered in women who are likely to benefit, such as women with a singleton pregnancy and a history of one second-trimester miscarriage attributable to cervical factors. In such instances, an ultrasound-indicated cerclage should be offered if a cervical length of 25 mm or less is detected by trans-vaginal scan before 24 weeks of gestation.

Acquired Uterine Anomaly

Fibroids, intrauterine adhesions (Asherman's syndrome) and uterine polyps are also associated with recurrent pregnancy loss. However, no conclusive evidence or data from randomised controlled trials are available to suggest that surgical treatment will reduce the risks of pregnancy loss. The general consensus is that surgical correction of significant uterine cavity defects can still be considered in women with recurrent pregnancy loss.[2]

Anti-Phospholipid Syndrome (APS)

All women with recurrent first-trimester pregnancy losses and all women with one or more second-trimester pregnancy losses should be screened before the next pregnancy for anti-phospholipid antibodies. The prevalence of APS is noted to be 15% in women with recurrent first-trimester pregnancy losses. A single unexplained loss of a morphologically normal fetus after 10 weeks' gestation, or preterm delivery of a normal fetus before 34 weeks because of severe pre-eclampsia or placental insufficiency, also warrant screening for APS. To diagnose APS, it is mandatory that the woman has two positive tests at least 12 weeks apart for either lupus anticoagulant or anti-cardiolipin antibodies, of immunoglobulin G and/or immunoglobulin M class, present in a medium or high titre over 40 g/l or ml/l, or above the 99th percentile.[1]

Anti-phospholipid antibodies can cause pregnancy morbidity through the following mechanisms, which include inhibition of trophoblastic function, differentiation and the activation of complement pathways at the maternal-foetal interface resulting in a local inflammatory response. In later pregnancy, thrombosis of the utero-placental vasculature can occur, resulting in placental insufficiency. *In vitro* studies have demonstrated that the effect of anti-phospholipid antibodies on trophoblast function and complement activation is reversed by heparin {summarised in Ref. 1}.

Pregnant women with APS should therefore be considered for treatment with low-dose aspirin plus heparin to prevent pregnancy loss. Corticosteroids and intravenous immunoglobulin therapy have not been shown to improve the live birth rate of women with recurrent pregnancy loss associated with anti-phospholipid antibodies when compared with other treatment modalities. Their use may provoke significant maternal and foetal morbidity, such as increased risk of gestational hypertension, diabetes and premature birth.[1,2]

Inherited Thrombophilias

Factor V Leiden mutations, activated protein C resistance, prothrombin gene G20210A mutation and protein S deficiency are significantly associated with recurrent pregnancy loss, be it first or second trimester foetal loss. Methylenetetrahydrofolate mutation, protein C and anti-thrombin deficiencies were not associated with foetal loss. A plausible mechanism in women who have recurrent pregnancy loss and late pregnancy complications is likely due to the increased risks of thrombosis of the utero-placental circulation.

In the absence of APS, however, neither aspirin nor heparin demonstrated any substantial benefits in improving the live birth rates of women with either idiopathic or thrombophilia-associated recurrent pregnancy loss, in high quality large randomised controlled trials.[8–11]

Endocrinological Factors

Polycystic ovarian syndrome (PCOS) is associated with insulin resistance, hyperinsulinaemia and hyperandrogenaemia. The prevalence of insulin resistance is increased in women with recurrent pregnancy loss when compared with matched fertile controls,[12] and an elevated free androgen index appears to be a prognostic factor for subsequent foetal loss in women with recurrent pregnancy loss.[13] Hence, PCOS is linked with recurrent pregnancy loss especially in women with demonstrable hyperinsulinaemia and high androgen free index. Weight loss and prescription of metformin in women with abnormal glucose tolerance tests have been suggested to have a role in reducing pregnancy loss.[14–16]

Higher pregnancy loss rates have been associated with the presence of antithyroid antibodies which are due to either autoimmune causes or mild thyroid insufficiency.[17,18] A small study suggested that women with anti-thyroid antibodies but normal thyroid function tests may benefit from levothyroxine treatment.[19] However, well controlled thyroid disorders and diabetes are not risk factors for recurrent pregnancy losses, hence are not recommended for routine screening in the absence of symptoms.[1,2]

Hyperprolactinemia is linked to recurrent pregnancy loss due to alterations in the hypothalamic-pituitary-ovarian axis resulting in impaired folliculogenesis, oocyte maturation and a short luteal phase. Women with more than two pregnancy losses and noted to have high prolactin levels demonstrate higher live birth rates when compared to placebo when treated with bromocriptine.[20]

Immunological Factors

Cytokines are immune molecules that control both immune and other cells with responses generally divided into either T-helper-1 (Th-1) type, with production of the pro-inflammatory cytokines interleukin 2, interferon and tumour necrosis factor alpha (TNFα); or as T-helper-2 (Th-2) type, with production of the anti-inflammatory cytokines interleukins 4, 6 and 10. Normal pregnancy is associated with primarily a Th-2 cytokine response, whereas women with recurrent pregnancy loss have a predominantly Th-1 cytokine response, as the maternal immune system interacts with an allogeneically dissimilar embryo.

Peripheral and uterine natural killer (NK) cells have been associated with recurrent pregnancy loss.[21,22] Interestingly, peripheral blood NK cells are demonstrated to be phenotypically and functionally different from uterine NK (uNK) cells.[23] It was observed that uNK cells may play a role in trophoblastic invasion and angiogenesis in addition to being an important component of the local maternal immune response to pathogens.[24] However, there was no clear evidence that altered peripheral blood NK cells are definitively related to recurrent miscarriage.[25,26] A large study[27] examining the relationship between uNK cell numbers and future pregnancy outcome reported that raised uNK cell numbers in women with recurrent miscarriage was not associated with an increased risk of pregnancy loss. These findings suggest that much remains to be studied in the immunology of reproduction, and these interesting biological factors may still remain relevant as we await new research data and breakthroughs.

Available studies and data on cytokine polymorphisms, human leucocyte antigen (HLA) typing, HLA-G polymorphisms, blocking or anti-paternal antibody levels and embryo-toxic or decidual cytokine profiles are still insufficient to draw definite links with recurrent pregnancy loss. Further research is required to affirm these findings.

Infections

There are no convincing data that infections can cause recurrent pregnancy loss. An infective agent must be capable of persisting in the genital tract and avoiding detection, or must cause sufficient symptoms to disturb the woman before it can be implicated in the aetiology of recurrent pregnancy loss. *Ureaplasma urealyticum*, *Mycoplasma hominus*, toxoplasmosis, rubella, cytomegalovirus, herpes and listeria infections do not fulfil these criteria, but can result in pregnancy loss. Although RCOG does not recommend routine TORCH screening[1] and ASRM does not recommend the routine use of antibiotics due to the lack of any prospective studies linking any infectious agent to recurrent early pregnancy loss,[2] every woman with recurrent pregnancy loss should be assessed individually and investigations can be considered.

Investigations

Investigations for couples with two or more clinical pregnancy losses can be initiated, although the RCOG recommends that investigations be offered to couples with three or more recurrent pregnancy losses. These criteria do not include ectopic or molar pregnancies. Women with recurrent first-trimester and second-trimester pregnancy losses should be looked after by a health professional with the necessary skills and expertise, ideally within a recurrent pregnancy loss clinic.

Karyotyping

Cytogenetic analysis should be performed on products of conception of the third and subsequent pregnancy losses.[1] Parental peripheral blood karyotyping of both partners, given the low yield of abnormality, cost, and limited prognostic value, should be performed in couples with recurrent pregnancy losses, when testing of products of conception reports an unbalanced structural chromosomal abnormality.

Knowledge of the karyotype of the products of conception allows an informed prognosis for a future pregnancy outcome to be given.[1] The risk of miscarriage as a result of foetal aneuploidy decreases with an increasing number of pregnancy losses.[28] If the karyotype of the miscarried pregnancy is abnormal, there is a better prognosis for the next pregnancy.[29]

Anatomical Assessment

All women with recurrent first-trimester pregnancy loss and all women with one or more second-trimester pregnancy losses should have a pelvic ultrasound to assess uterine anatomy.[1] Suspected uterine anomalies may require further investigations to confirm the diagnosis, using sonohysterography, hysterosalpingogram, magnetic resonance imaging, three-dimensional pelvic ultrasound, hysteroscopy or laparoscopy. The latter two surgical modalities may fulfil dual roles of diagnosis and treatment of any uterine anomalies.

Anti-Phospholipid Antibodies and Thrombophilia Assessment

All women with recurrent first-trimester and all women with one or more second-trimester pregnancy losses should be screened before pregnancy for anti-phospholipid antibodies. This test should be positive twice or more at least 12 weeks apart for lupus anticoagulant, anti-cardiolipin or anti-β2 glycoprotein-1 antibodies, of immunoglobulin G and/or immunoglobulin M class, in titres >99th centile.[1,2]

Women with second-trimester pregnancy losses should be screened for inherited thrombophilias including factor V Leiden, factor II (prothrombin) gene mutation and protein S, due to the strong association between second trimester pregnancy loss and the mentioned inherited thrombophilias.[1,30]

Thyroid Assessment

Thyroid function tests for TSH and thyroid peroxidase (TPO) antibodies may be assessed in women with clinical manifestations or a personal history of thyroid disease, as there is evidence of an increased risk of pregnancy loss in women with subclinical hypothyroidism[31] and in euthyroid women with TPO antibodies.[32,33] Screening of asymptomatic women for subclinical thyroid conditions remains controversial.

Evaluation for ovarian reserve, diabetes screening, progesterone levels and microbiological cultures/infectious diseases screen are not routinely offered, but can be considered on a case by case basis based on the clinician's individual assessment and patient's profile.

HLA genotyping, cytokine profiling and NK cell measurement are under active research, and further studies are required to push the frontiers of reproductive immunology to understand how immunological mechanisms act in pregnancy loss, such that novel therapies can be proffered to women with this distressing condition.

Management

The primary objective in managing recurrent pregnancy loss is dependent on the most likely aetiology.

In couples diagnosed with abnormal parental karyotypes, a referral to a clinical geneticist should be made. Genetic counselling on the prognosis of future pregnancies and the need for familial chromosome studies can be discussed, with subsequent reproductive options such as prenatal diagnosis test, gamete donation or adoption.[1]

Women with recurrent pregnancy losses who are diagnosed with APS are offered aspirin and heparin in the next pregnancy to improve pregnancy outcomes. Women with inherited thrombophilia (as ascribed before) are prescribed anticoagulants to improve maternal outcomes (for example, prevention of venous thromboembolic events). There is insufficient evidence to evaluate the benefit of heparin in women with recurrent first-trimester pregnancy loss and inherited thrombophilia. However, heparin therapy can improve the live birth rate of women with inherited thrombophilia who have suffered from second-trimester pregnancy loss.

Hyperprolactinemia in women with recurrent pregnancy loss should be treated with bromocriptine prior to getting pregnant, as it is associated with a higher pregnancy success.[20]

Women with PCOS and recurrent pregnancy loss — Weight loss and addition of metformin can be beneficial to improve the success of subsequent pregnancies.[14-16]

Women with recurrent pregnancy loss and identified with thyroid problems are advised to be treated. Even euthyroid women with high serum thyroid peroxidase antibody concentrations may benefit from treatment with thyroid hormone during pregnancy, as administration of levothyroxine (median dose 50 mcg daily) to early pregnant euthyroid women with positive thyroid peroxidase antibodies decreased the miscarriage rate from 13.8% to 3.5% (RR 1.72, 95% CI 1.13–2.25) in a randomised control trial.[31]

Observational studies suggest that hysteroscopic surgery for uterine anomalies such as septate uteri can be effective in reducing pregnancy loss.[2] Cervical cerclage for cervical weakness can be considered.

No definitive causative factors can be found in 50–60% of couples with recurrent pregnancy loss — these couples are identified to have idiopathic recurrent pregnancy loss. Three quarters of these women will achieve a live birth in subsequent pregnancies, given tender loving care which involves regular reassurance, scans and psychological support in a dedicated early pregnancy assessment unit.[34,35] Aspirin, progestogens and human chorionic gonadotropin supplementation in this group of women have not been demonstrated to reduce the risk of pregnancy loss.[35–37]

Novel therapies, such as immunotherapies,[38,39] are not routinely offered to women with recurrent pregnancy loss — such treatment may be used in the setting of a clinical trial regulated by an Institutional Review Board. In addition, oral glucocorticoids are not usually administered because of uncertain efficacy and concerns on possible complications, such as preterm premature rupture of membranes, gestational diabetes, and maternal hypertension,[40,41] although intrauterine glucocorticoid treatment (which is under investigation) may be safer.[42]

Prognosis of Future Pregnancies

Detection of foetal cardiac activity in early pregnancy is reassuring of subsequent viable delivery, but the greatest risk of recurrent loss occurs during the period up to the time of the previous pregnancy loss. The pregnancy loss rate in those women with a history of recurrent pregnancy loss still remains above that of the general population. When these women conceive again, they may be at higher risk for developing foetal growth restriction and premature delivery.

Increasing maternal age and a higher number of miscarriages at the initial visit are associated with a significant decrease in the likelihood of having a live birth. Overall, more than two-thirds of women with recurrent pregnancy loss can still have a live birth subsequently.

Conclusion

The management of recurrent pregnancy loss remains a challenge to clinicians. Couples who suffer from recurrent pregnancy loss are distressed by this complex condition, as more than 50% of recurrent pregnancy loss has no apparent causative factor. A systematic approach to the management of such couples, in addition to continuous supportive and tender loving care in a dedicated recurrent pregnancy loss clinic, is pertinent. There is a dire need to conduct high quality and methodologically rigorous trials within possible means, to enhance the evidence base that is much required for this upsetting condition which is lacking in efficacious therapies.

TABLE 16.1 Summary Table on Recurrent Pregnancy Loss

Cause	Contribution to Recurrent Pregnancy Loss	Recommended Investigation	Recommended Management	Probably Effective/ Unknown	Under Evaluation
Parental genetic factors/ chromosomal anomalies	2–5%	Parental karyotype	Referral to geneticist, preimplantation diagnosis	—	—
Embryo genetic factors/ chromosomal anomalies	30–57%	Karyotype of products of conception	As above	—	—
Structural uterine defects	12.6%	Ultrasound/MRI	—	Surgical correction of defects (e.g. hysteroscopically)	—
Acquired uterine anomalies	—	Ultrasound	—	Hysteroscopic correction of significant uterine cavity defects	—
Cervical weakness	—	Ultrasound indicated based on history	—	Cervical cerclage	—
Anti-phospholipid syndrome	15%	Positive (twice or more at least 12 weeks apart) for lupus anticoagulant, anti-cardiolipin or anti-β2 glycoprotein-1 antibodies, of immunoglobulin G and/or immunoglobulin M class, in titres >99th centile	Aspirin and heparin once pregnant	—	—

(*Continued*)

TABLE 16.1 (*Continued*)

Cause	Contribution to Recurrent Pregnancy Loss	Recommended Investigation	Recommended Management	Probably Effective/ Unknown	Under Evaluation
Inherited thrombophilias	—	Factor V Leiden mutations, activated protein C resistance, prothrombin gene G20210A mutation and protein S	—	Heparin for maternal reasons	—
Endocrinological factors	—	(1) Hyperinsulinaemia and glucose intolerance in PCOS (2) TSH and thyroid peroxidase antibodies (3) Prolactin	—	(1) Weight loss/ Metformin (2) Levothyroxine (3) Bromocriptine	—
Infections	—	TORCH screening (case by case basis)	—	Antibiotics	—
Immunological factors	—	—	—	—	(1) Corticosteroids — intra-uterine (2) Immunoglobulin Test for peripheral/ uterine natural killer cells, cytokines profile, HLA typing under evaluation/ further research

References

1. Royal College of Obstetricians and Gynaecologists, United Kingdom. (2011) The Investigation and Treatment of Couples with Recurrent First-trimester and Second-trimester Miscarriage. Green-top Guideline No. 17.

2. The Practice Committee of The American Association of Reproductive Medicine. (2012) Evaluation and treatment of recurrent pregnancy loss: a committee opinion. *Fertil Steril* **98**(5): 1103–1111.

3. Stirrat GM. (1990) Recurrent Miscarriage. *Lancet* **336**: 673–675.

4. Fisher J, Colls P, Escudero T, Munne S. (2010) Preimplantation genetic diagnosis (PGD) improves pregnancy outcome for translocation carriers with a history of recurrent losses. *Fertil Steril* **94**: 283–289.

5. Hogge WA, Byrnes AL, Lanasa MC, Surti U. (2003) The clinical use of karyotyping spontaneous abortions. *Am J of Obstet Gynecol* **189**: 397–400.

6. Grimbizis GF, Camus M, Tarlatzis BC, (2001) Clinical implications of uterine malformations and hysteroscopic treatment results. *Human Reprod Update* **7**: 161–174.

7. Kowalik CR, Mol BW, Veersama S, Goddijn M. (2011) Critical appraisal regarding the effect on reproductive outcome of hysteroscopic metroplasty in patients with recurrent miscarriage. *Arch Gynaecol Obstet* **282**: 465.

8. Laski CA, Spitzer KA, Clark CA, *et al.* (2009) Low molecular weight heparin and aspirin for recurrent pregnancy loss: results from the randomized, controlled Heaps Trial. *J Rheumatol* **36**: 279–287.

9. Kaandorp SP, Goddijn M, van der Post JA, *et al.* (2010) Aspirin plus heparin or aspirin alone in women with recurrent miscarriage. *NEJM* **362**: 1586–1596.

10. Clark P, Walker ID, Langhorne P, *et al.* (2010) SPIN: The Scottish Pregnancy Intervention Study: a multicenter randomized controlled trial of low molecular weight heparin and low dose aspirin in women with recurrent miscarriage. *Blood* **115**: 4162–4167.

11. Visser J, Ulander VM, Helmerhorst FM, *et al.* (2011) Thromboprophylaxis for recurrent miscarriage in women with or without thrombophilia. HARBENOX: a randomized multicenter trial. *Thrombosis and Haemostasis* **105**: 295–301.

12. Craig LB, Ke RW, Kutteh WH. (2002) Increased prevalence of insulin resistance in women with a history of recurrent pregnancy loss. *Fertility Sterility* **78**: 487–490.

13. Cocksedge KA, Saravelos SH, Wang Q, *et al.* (2008) Does free androgen index predict subsequent pregnancy outcome in women with recurrent miscarriage? *Human Reprod* **23**: 797–802.

14. Cocksedge KA, Li TC, Saravelos SH, Metwally M. (2008) A reappraisal of the role of polycystic ovary syndrome in recurrent miscarriage. *Reproduct Biomedi Online* **17**: 151–160.

15. Clark AM, Ledger W, Galletly C, *et al.* (1995) Weight loss results in significant improvement in pregnancy and ovulation rates in anovulatory obese women. *Human Reprod* **10**: 2705–2712.

16. Zolghadri J, Tavana Z, Kazerooni T, *et al.* (2008) Relationship between abnormal glucose tolerance test and history of previous recurrent miscarriages, and beneficial effect of metformin in these patients: a prospective clinical study. *Fertil Steril* **90**: 727–730.

17. Arredondo F, Noble LS. (2006) Endocrinology of recurrent pregnancy loss. *Seminars in Reprod Medi* **24**: 33–39.

18. Stagnaro-Green A, Glinoer D. (2004) Thyroid autoimmunity and the risk of miscarriage. *Best Pract Res Clin Endocrinol Metab* **18**: 167–181.

19. Vaquero E, Lazzarin N, De Carolis C, *et al.* (2000) Mild thyroid abnormalities and recurrent spontaneous abortion: diagnostic and therapeutic approach. *Am J Reprod Immunol* **43**: 204–208.

20. Hirahara F, Andoh N, Sawai K, *et al.* (1998) Hyperprolactinemic recurrent miscarriage and results of randomized bromocriptine treatment trials. *Fertil Steril* **70**(2): 246–252.

21. Dosiou C, Giudice LC. (2005) Natural killer cells in pregnancy and recurrent pregnancy loss: endocrine and immunologic perspectives. *Endocr Rev* **26**: 44–62.

22. Quenby S, Nik H, Innes B, *et al.* (2009) Uterine natural killer cells and angiogenesis in recurrent reproductive failure. *Human Reproduction* **24**: 45–54.

23. Moffett A, Regan L, Braude P. (2004). Natural killer cells, miscarriage, and infertility. *Br Medi J* **329**: 1283–1285.

24. Le Bouteiller P, Piccinni MP. (2008) Human NK cells in pregnant uterus: why there? *Am J Reprod Immunol* **59**: 401–406.

25. Wold AS, Arici A. (2005) Natural killer cells and reproductive failure. *Curr Opin Obstet Gynecol* **17**: 237–241.

26. Rai R, Sacks G, Trew G. (2005) Natural killer cells and reproductive failure – theory, practice and prejudice. *Human Reprod* **20**: 1123–1126.

27. Tuckerman E, Laird SM, Prakash A, Li TC. (2007) Prognostic value of the measurement of uterine natural killer cells in the endometrium of women with recurrent miscarriage. *Human Reprod* **22**: 2208–2213.

28. Ogasawara M, Aoki K, Okada S, Suzumori K. (2000) Embryonic karyotype of abortuses in relation to the number of previous miscarriages. *Fertil Steril* **73**: 300–304.

29. Carp H, Toder V, Aviram A, *et al.* (2001) Karyotype of the abortus in recurrent miscarriage. *Fertil Steril* **75**: 678–682.

30. Rey E, Kahn SR, David M, Shrier I. (2003). Thrombophilic disorders and foetal loss: a meta-analysis. *Lancet* **361**: 901–908.

31. Negro R, Schwartz A, Gismondi R, *et al.* (2010) Increased pregnancy loss rate in thyroid antibody negative women with TSH levels between 2.5 and 5.0 in the first trimester of pregnancy. *J Clin Endocrinol Meta* **95**: E44–E48.

32. Chen L, Hu R. (2011) Thyroid autoimmunity and miscarriage: a meta-analysis. *Clin Endocrinol (Oxf)* **74**: 513–519.

33. Thangaratinam S, Tan A, Knox E, *et al.* (2011) Association between thyroid autoantibodies and miscarriage and preterm birth: meta-analysis of evidence. *Br Med J* **342**: d2616.

34. Quenby SM, Farquharson RG. (1993) Predicting recurring miscarriage: what is important? *Obstet Gynecol* **82**(1): 132–138.

35. Kaandorp S, Di Nisio M, Goddijn M, Middeldorp S. (2009) Aspirin or anticoagulants for treating recurrent miscarriage in women without antiphospholipid syndrome. *Cochrane Database Syst Rev* **21**(1): CD004734.

36. Haas DM, Ramsey PS. (2013) Progestogen for preventing miscarriage. *Cochrane Database Syst Rev* **10**: CD003511.
37. Quenby S, Farquharson RG. (1994) Human chorionic gonadotropin supplementation in recurring pregnancy loss: a controlled trial. *Fertil Steril* **62**: 708–710.
38. Clark DA, Coulam CB, Stricker RB. (2006) Are intravenous immunoglobulins (IVIG) efficacious in early pregnancy failure? A critical review and meta-analysis for patients who fail *in vitro* fertilization and embryo transfer (IVF). *J of Assis Reprod Gen* **23**(1): 1–13.
39. Wong LF, Porter TF, Scott JR. (2014) Immunotherapy for recurrent miscarriage. *Cochrane Database Syst Rev* **10**: CD000112.
40. Larkin CA, Bombardier C, Hannah ME, *et al.* (1997) Prednisone and aspirin in women with autoantibodies and unexplained recurrent foetal loss. *NEJM* **337**: 148–153.
41. Regan L, Rai R. (2000) Epidemiology and the medical causes of miscarriage. *Baillieres Best Pract Res Clin Obstet Gynaecol* **14**: 839–854.
42. Ogasawara M, Aoki K. (2000) Successful uterine steroid therapy in a case with a history of ten miscarriages. *Am J Reprod Immunol* **44**: 253–255.

Part IV

EARLY PREGNANCY

Introduction

The early pregnancy period is often a time of anxiety and nervous anticipation for the expectant mother. Some women may worry about the effect their lifestyles may have on the recently diagnosed pregnancy, and to what extent alcohol, smoking or medicine consumption may influence embryo and foetal development. Others may not be aware of their pregnancy until a complication arises that prompts investigation and the diagnosis. Common early pregnancy symptoms such as musculoskeletal pain, gastrointestinal symptoms and emesis may cause varying degrees of distress. A percentage of women may encounter vaginal bleeding and pelvic pain in the early stages of pregnancy, important presentations that prompt further evaluation of the pregnancy. Occasionally pregnancy failures, extra-uterine pregnancies and molar pregnancies (part of the spectrum of gestational trophoblast disease) may be diagnosed and require specific management. Once a pregnancy is confirmed to be correctly located and viable though, there are several ways in which prenatal caregivers can help the expectant mother to prepare for a healthy pregnancy and delivery. Prenatal care consists of ensuring the mother provides the foetus with the optimal environment for normal development and growth, early detection of medical or obstetric complications, and surveillance for foetal genetic and structural anomalies, much of which is achieved in the early stages of prenatal care. This series of topics cover the pertinent issues highlighted here.

17

BLEEDING IN EARLY PREGNANCY

Mary Rauff

Introduction

The teaching for a long time has been that any woman in the reproductive age group is deemed pregnant until proven otherwise. The diagnosis is made if she presents to the doctor having missed her period. By inference, this means that bleeding is a phenomenon that is not expected in pregnancy.

It is quite surprising, but as many as 20% to 30% of pregnancies are associated with bleeding, mostly occurring in the first trimester.

In this chapter, the term "early pregnancy" is used synonymously with "first trimester", and "miscarriage" with "abortion." Abortion is medically defined as the spontaneous or induced loss of a pregnancy before viability. Owing to the connotation that abortion is a deliberate termination of a pregnancy, the use of the term "miscarriage" is sometimes preferable when the loss is spontaneous.

Causes of Bleeding in the First Trimester

(1) Intrauterine pregnancies — Blighted ovum
Threatened miscarriage
Inevitable miscarriage
Incomplete miscarriage
Complete miscarriage
Missed miscarriage
Trophoblastic disease — molar pregnancy, partial mole and choriocarcinoma

(2) Ectopic pregnancies — usually tubal in origin but may occur in the uterine cornu, LSCS scar, cervix and intra-abdominal.

(3) Non-pregnancy causes coexisting with a pregnancy — cervical lesions e.g. polyps, cancer, erosion; vaginal varices or infections, haematuria.

Diagnosis of Pregnancy

Traditionally, pregnancy has been confirmed using the qualitative measurement of the beta Human Chorionic Gonadotropin (hCG) levels. Prior to the use of monoclonal antibodies to beta hCG, a pregnancy could only be detected when the urine levels of hCG were more than 625 IU/L. However, with the advent of very sensitive monoclonal antibodies, it is possible to detect hCG levels as low as 25 IU/L.

The assay of serum progesterone levels has been found to be useful in having some predictive value as to the likely outcome of the pregnancy which presents with bleeding. A level of 35 and above is associated with a more hopeful outcome than a lower level.

Ultrasound detection of a pregnancy using the transvaginal probe has eased the confirmation of pregnancy. An intra-uterine gestational sac may been seen when the hCG levels are >1,500 IU/L — this would correspond to about 4 to 5 weeks of amenorrhea. Between 5 to 6 weeks, a yolk sac is seen and a foetal pole thereafter. If foetal heart activity is seen, the foetus is at least six weeks and, of course, alive.

These two developments have led to increased sensitivity in the diagnosis of pregnancy — a pregnancy can now be diagnosed much earlier and more accurately than what was possible only 15 years ago. It has also increased the number of patients with apparent pregnancy losses as they may have positive hCG "biochemical pregnancies" followed by a bleeding episode, withnothing seen on ultrasound.

Aetiology of Miscarriages

Foetal Causes

More than 80% of spontaneous miscarriages occur in the first trimester, and at least half of these abortuses have a chromosomal anomaly. There is usually bleeding into the utero-placental junction, detaching the placental attachment to the decidua basalis. This is followed by uterine contractions and expulsion of the gestational sac and the placenta. If one were to open up the intact gestational sac, there would be no foetus inside **(blighted ovum)**, or a small macerated foetus.

95% of chromosomal abnormalities are a result of aberrations in maternal gametogenesis, while the rest are paternal in origin. Autosomal trisomies are the most commonly identified abnormalities. Others are the presence of a single X chromosome (as in Turner's syndrome), triploidies (usually manifesting as a partial mole) or tetraploidies.

Severe structural abnormalities of the foetus can theoretically cause miscarriages but these are very unlikely to occur in the first trimester.

Maternal Causes

Insulin dependent Diabetes Mellitus,[1,2] presence of thyroid antibodies in the absence of hypothyroidism,[3] Inherited Thrombophilias and Immune mediated disorders have all be proven to be associated with increased spontaneous miscarriage rates.

Frequent and increased doses of alcohol intake and excessive caffeine intake (more than 500 mg or 5 cups of coffee a day) in the first trimester have been associated with significantly increased miscarriage rate.[4,5]

Infections are an uncommon cause of first trimester miscarriages.[6]

Nutrition, as evidenced by severe weight loss following hyperemesis gravidarum in early pregnancy, is rarely associated with miscarriage.

Management of Bleeding in Early Pregnancy

If a woman presents with bleeding in early pregnancy either at the A&E or the clinic, the doctor should go through the following steps:

(1) Check her LMP and perform a speculum examination to ascertain whether the cervical os is open or closed.
(2) Perform a transvaginal ultrasound to confirm that the pregnancy is intrauterine, date the pregnancy and check for foetal viability.

Patient Pregnancy Test Positive with Bleeding and No Pain

The diagnosis will be as follows:

(a) If the cervical os is closed, the foetus is intrauterine with a crown-rump length (CRL) which corresponds to dates, with a foetal heart, she has a **threatened miscarriage**.

(b) If the cervical os is closed, the foetus is intra-uterine with a CRL which is more than 7 mm and no foetal heart, she is most likely to be having a **missed miscarriage.**

(c) If the cervical os is closed and there is an intrauterine gestational sac with no foetal pole, her dates could be wrong or she could have **blighted ovum.**

(d) If the cervical os is opened, regardless of the state and viability of the foetus, she is having an **inevitable miscarriage.**

(e) If there is no intrauterine pregnancy seen, check for the presence of a **molar pregnancy** in the uterus or an **ectopic pregnancy.**

Patient Pregnancy Test Positive with Bleeding and Cramping Pain Similar to Dysmenorrhoea

The diagnosis will be as in the section "Patient Pregnancy Test Positive with Bleeding and No Pain" but the prognosis for the pregnancy continuing is generally poor even if a foetal heart is present. The separation of the placenta (bleeding) will trigger abdominal cramps and cervical dilation followed by expulsion of the products of conception.

Patient Pregnancy Test Positive with Bleeding, Cramps, Passage of Blood and Possibility Some Tissue

The diagnosis will be as follows:

(a) The cervical os is opened and there may be tissue in the uterus or at the os, she is having an **incomplete miscarriage.**

(b) The cervical os is opened and the uterine cavity is empty, the adnexa should be checked for any **ectopic pregnancy**.

(c) The cervical os is closed and the bleeding and cramps have decreased. Transvaginal ultrasound scan shows an empty uterine cavity with a thin endometrium and no adnexal masses are seen, this would mean a **complete miscarriage.**

Management

Threatened Miscarriage. The treatment is conservative as vaginal spotting or bleeding may occur in 20% to 25% of women in the first trimester. Miscarriage may occur in 50% of patients but it is considerably less if foetal heart is seen.[7]

There is really no effective treatment for threatened abortion. Bed rest and the use of progestogens — parenteral and/or oral — have been the mainstay of management.

A repeat ultrasound evaluation of the pregnancy in one or two weeks is the only sure way of determining if the foetus is alive. If the bleeding progresses to become heavier, or there is development of abdominal cramps, there may be a necessity for the woman to come back earlier.

One should always be wary about the diagnosis of a threatened miscarriage as an ectopic pregnancy is also a possibility.

Inevitable Miscarriage. The treatment may be expectant or it may be aided with the use of prostaglandins.

If there is watery discharge and the scan reveals no liquor in the gestational sac, one may want to hasten miscarriage with prostaglandins rather than wait for the onset of pains and risk the onset of infection.

If uterine contractions follow soon after the rupture of membranes, there may not be a need for active management.

It would be useful to obtain the products of conception (POC), passed for histology in case the woman may have had a partial mole. The management of the latter will be dealt with in the chapter on Gestational Trophoblastic Disease.

Complete Miscarriage. When the foetus and the placenta are delivered together, the miscarriage is usually complete. A complete abortion is usually possible when the pregnancy is less than 10 weeks.

The diagnosis is made when the bleeding and the pain subside quite dramatically after the passage of the POC, and the cervix is found to be closed on vaginal examination. A confirmatory transvaginal scan will reveal very little or no POC in the endometrial cavity.

No treatment is required. The woman should be seen in one to two weeks to ensure that the bleeding has stopped. This would provide confirmation of the diagnosis.

Incomplete Miscarriage. As opposed to complete abortion, either the whole or part of the placenta and gestational sac is undelivered. Speculum or digital examination will reveal bleeding from the opened cervical os and sometimes tissue in the genital tract.

The placenta may be at the cervical os causing severe pain and even syncope from a vasovagal attack. The placental tissue will be seen on speculum examination and removal of the placental tissue with a polyp or sponge forceps will bring instant relief to the patient.

If the woman is stable, expectant therapy is a possible option.[8] Medical management with Misoprostol or surgical evacuation of the uterus are other options. Evacuation of the uterus is recommended if the bleeding is heavy or if there is infected POC. In the latter, evacuation should be carried out after at least one dose of antibiotics, followed by antibiotic cover.

Missed Miscarriage. This occurs when the foetus fails to develop and dies in utero. No miscarriage occurs and POC is retained for many days or weeks until the woman has her next ultrasound scan. Some women present with bleeding per vaginam, with or without pain, and the foetal demise is found on ultrasound. The woman may or may not find a decrease in her symptoms of pregnancy when she presents to the doctor.

Many will spontaneously miscarry, although some women prefer a termination. Termination may be done medically with the use of prostaglandins such as Misoprostol or Cervagerm pessaries administered vaginally. Surgical termination is the other option. This is done electively with preoperative cervical dilation with prostaglandins followed by vacuum aspiration under General Anaesthesia (GA).

Surgical treatment has the disadvantage of being an operation — an invasive treatment with its attendant risks of anaesthesia and uterine perforation. However, it is predictable and finished quickly.

Medical treatment with Misoprostol (vaginal or oral) or Cervagerm pessaries may obviate the need for a surgical procedure, but if there is heavy or continued bleeding, evacuation of the uterus will be necessary.

Ectopic Pregnancy, Gestational Trophoblastic Disease and non-Pregnancy causes of bleeding will be dealt with in other chapters of this book.

References

1. Greene MF. (1999) Spontaneous abortions and major malformations in women with Diabetes mellitus. *Semin Reprod Endocrinol* **17**:127.
2. Craig TB, Ke RW, Kutteh WH. (2002) Increase prevalence of insulin resistance in women with a history of recurrent pregnancy loss. *Fertil Steril* **78**:487.
3. Lakasing L, Williamson C. (2005) Obstetric complications due to autoantibodies. *Best Prac Res Clin Endocrinol Metab* **19**:149.
4. Armstrong BG, McDonald AD, Sloan M. (1992) Cigarette, coffee and alcohol consumption and spontaneous abortion. *Am J Public Health* **82**:85.
5. Cnattingius S, Signorello LB, Anneren G, *et al.* (2000) Caffeine intake and the risk of first-trimester spontaneous abortion. *N Engl J Med* **343**:1839.
6. American College of Obstetricians and Gynecologists. (2001) Management of recurrent early pregnancy loss. Practice Bulletin No. 24.
7. Tongsong T, Srisomboon J, Wanapirak C, *et al.* (1995) Pregnancy outcome of threatened abortion with demonstrable foetal heart activity: a cohort study. *J. Obstet Gynaecol* **21**:331.
8. Blohm F, Friden BE, Milsom I, *et al.* (2005) A randomized double blind trial comparing misoprostol or placebo in the management of early miscarriages. *BJOG* **112**:1090.

18

ACUTE ABDOMEN IN GYNAECOLOGY

Fong Yoke Fai

Acute abdominal pain is a common presenting complaint in women. Differential diagnoses can be grouped into broad systems including gynaecologic, urologic, gastrointestinal, vascular and musculoskeletal (Table 18.1). Gynaecologists are frequently called to assess if the abdominal pain is gynaecological or non-gynaecological in origin.

While many investigations may be available to the physician, it is important to start with a thorough history and physical examination. These are essential in narrowing possible diagnoses and focus the work-up.

When assessing the patient with abdominal pain, it is critical to identify life-threatening conditions that require immediate surgical intervention, such as severe haemorrhage from a ruptured ectopic pregnancy.

This chapter will discuss gynaecologic causes of acute abdomen.

Visceral and Somatic Pain

Acute abdominal pain may be of somatic or visceral origin, or both.[1]

Visceral pain originates from receptors located on serosal surfaces: in the mesentery, and within the walls of hollow viscera (e.g. vagina or ureters). Examples of visceral sources of pain include distention of an organ capsule, inflammation, infection, ischaemia, haemorrhage or neoplasm. Visceral pain is characterised by

TABLE 18.1 Differential Diagnosis of Acute Abdominal Pain in a Female Patient

Gastrointestinal	Gynaecology	Urologic
Appendicitis	Ectopic Pregnancy	Cystitis
Bowel obstruction	Pregnancy complications	Neoplasm
Constipation	Ovary cyst	Urethritis
Diverticulitis	Salpingitis	Pyelonephritis
Faecal impaction	Torsion of adnexa	Calculi
Gastroenteritis	Rupture of ovarian cyst	
Hirschsprung's disease	Endometriosis	**Vascular**
Incarcerated hernia	Abortion	Ischaemic bowel
Intussusception	Pelvic inflammatory disease	Neoplasm
Incarcerated hernia	Endometritis	
Intussusception	Dysmenorrhoea	**Musculoskeletal**
Irritable bowel syndrome	Neoplasm	Abdominal wall haematoma or infection
Meckel's diverticulitis		Trauma
Neoplasm		Herniated disc
Perforated viscous		Arthritis
Regional ileitis (Crohn's disease)		Strain or sprain
Ulcerative colitis		Hernia
Volvulus		Neoplasm

a deep, dull, vague sensation. It is accompanied by malaise and autonomic signs such as pallor, sweating, nausea/vomiting.

The localisation of visceral pain can be difficult because significant overlap of pathways within spinal segments, as well as within visceral and somatic structures, can result in referred pain.[2]

Somatic pain can originate from the abdominal and pelvic muscles, fascia, parietal peritoneum, subcutaneous tissue and the skeletal system.

Somatic mechanisms causing acute abdominal pain are often related to inflammation of the parietal peritoneum. The pain is steady and aching in character, and actions that place tension on the peritoneum, such as palpation or movement, consistently increase it. Hence the patient with peritonitis lies quietly in bed, avoiding any movement.

In addition to being constant with sharp exacerbations, somatic pain is well-localised with involuntary guarding and rebound tenderness. Diseases that lead to chemical stimulation of pain receptors in the peritoneum include: leakage of purulent matter into the peritoneal cavity, intraperitoneal bleeding, necrosis of an intra-abdominal structure or inflammation due to infection.

Differential Diagnoses

It is important to consider differential diagnoses of various aetiologies in any female patient with acute abdominal pain (Table 18.2).

TABLE 18.2   Gynaecological Differentials of an Acute Abdomen

Gynaecological	Obstetric: For Antenatal or Labouring Patients
Ectopic pregnancy	Uterine rupture
Ovarian cyst rupture/Torsion of adnexa	Uterine scar dehiscence/rupture (for women with previous Caesarean section)
Acute pelvic inflammatory disease/Tubo-ovarian abscess	Placental abruption

History

A thorough pain history should address:

- **Location**: Site of pain? Where does it radiate? Any change of location over time?
- **Onset** and **duration**: How long has the pain been? How did the pain originate? Was its onset sudden or gradual?
- **Character**: Description of pain (e.g. dull, sharp, colicky, waxing and waning)? Is the pain cyclic? What seems to make the pain better or worse?
- Any **prior history** of pain
- **Systems review**
  Identify associated symptoms that can help narrow the differential diagnosis. The presence of vaginal discharge, vaginal bleeding, a recent history of dyspareunia, or dysmenorrhoea is suggestive of pelvic pathology. For example, a purulent vaginal discharge suggests the presence of a sexually transmitted infection; cramping and vaginal bleeding are commonly seen with ectopic pregnancy or threatened miscarriage; and dyspareunia and dysmenorrhoea are features of endometriosis. Anorexia, nausea, and vomiting are often seen in appendicitis, but can be seen with any inflammatory pelvic process.

- **Gynaecologic/obstetrical history**
  Last menstrual period: a missed period suggests that the patient may be pregnant.
  Menstrual history
  Sexual history, contraception, history of sexually transmitted diseases
  Results of cervical cancer screening
  Obstetric history: outcomes of previous pregnancies.
- **Past medical and surgical histories**
  A history of pelvic organ surgery, pelvic inflammatory disease, or prior ectopic pregnancy are risk factors for ectopic pregnancy.[3]
  Any history of abdominal surgery increases the risk of bowel obstruction.
  Adnexal pathology is a risk factor for adnexal torsion.
- **Family history**: Family history may be relevant (e.g. a history of coagulation disorders or malignancies).
- **Social history**: Any substance abuse, history of domestic violence, or high-risk behaviour.

Physical Examination

General. Does the patient appear comfortable, or is she doubled up in pain?

Vital Signs. Any marked hypotension, tachycardia, a focused history and a directed physical examination are performed concurrently to facilitate emergency treatment. Fever suggests an infectious aetiology, but low grade fever may be observed with necrosis associated with adnexal torsion.

Abdominal Examination

Inspection for distention, masses, erythema, ecchymosis, scars and hernias.

Palpate the abdomen to assess for peritoneal signs: areas of tenderness, masses and organomegaly. The flank, inguinal area, and lower back should be examined for ecchymosis, tenderness, and lymphadenopathy. Palpation with sudden release of pressure will demonstrate rebound tenderness.

Auscultation is performed to evaluate the presence and character of bowel sounds. Absent or decreased bowel sounds suggest an ileus due to peritonitis. Increased bowel sounds suggest gastroenteritis or early intestinal obstruction. In the anxious patient, the stethoscope can be used for gentle palpation for more reproducible findings.

Percussion can be useful to identify distention versus ascites, and to detect organomegaly or masses.

Pelvic Examination

A speculum is inserted to evaluate the vagina for any abnormal discharge and to evaluate the cervix for abnormal bleeding, polyps, masses, or evidence of infection. Cervical specimens are obtained for testing for *Chlamydia* and gonorrhoea, and a sample of the vaginal discharge is obtained for microscopic examination.

After the speculum is removed, a bimanual examination is performed.

The introital and pelvic floor muscles are palpated for abnormal tenderness or trigger points.

The size and symmetry of the uterus are determined; symmetrical enlargement suggests intra-uterine pregnancy (or adenomyosis), while irregular enlargement is more indicative of leiomyomas, although asymmetric enlargement can also be caused by bowel or adnexal masses adherent to the uterus.

The cervix and uterus should be assessed for tenderness to palpation and movement. Significant cervical or uterine motion tenderness usually implies there is pelvic inflammation present. Cervical motion tenderness is a sensitive sign of pelvic inflammatory disease, but not as specific. Cervical motion tenderness also occurs in about half of women with ectopic pregnancy and about a quarter of those with acute appendicitis.[4]

The adnexae are evaluated for tenderness or masses. Ovarian neoplasms and ectopic pregnancies are generally not painful unless bleeding, ruptured, or torted. A fixed, painful adnexal mass is suggestive of an endometrioma or tubo-ovarian abscess. A rectovaginal examination is performed to assess the pouch of Douglas for masses or tenderness.

Investigations

All women of reproductive age, regardless of reported sexual history or contraception, should undergo a **pregnancy test** during evaluation of abdominal or pelvic pain.

If the patient is pregnant, quantitative beta hCG testing and Rh(D) typing may be indicated and the status of the pregnancy should be determined (i.e. ectopic, intra-uterine, threatened miscarriage etc.). A positive pregnancy test does not exclude a non-gynaecologic cause of abdominal pain.

Tests that may be useful when evaluating for gynaecologic pathologies include:

Full blood count with differential: An elevated white blood cell count may be due to infection, inflammation or necrosis related to adnexal torsion.

Urinalysis, with culture if urinalysis shows haematuria or pyuria.

Nucleic acid amplification tests for *Chlamydia* and gonococcus.

Imaging

Ultrasound examination has been the initial imaging modality in the evaluation of pelvic pain in women.

Gynaecologic pathologies identifiable with the aid of ultrasound include: ovarian neoplasms and torsion, uterine leiomyomas, pelvic abscess, intra-uterine and ectopic pregnancy.

Abdominal/pelvic *computed tomography* (*CT*) and/or *magnetic resonance imaging* (*MRI*) can be used for further evaluation in cases of diagnostic uncertainty.

X-rays of the abdomen or pelvis are rarely useful in the diagnosis of gynaecologic pathology.

When indicated, imaging modalities that do not use ionising radiation, such as ultrasound and MRI, are preferred in pregnant women.

Laparoscopy. Laparoscopy is sometimes indicated in the evaluation of acute pelvic pain, especially when the diagnosis is not clear after less invasive evaluations and the differential diagnoses include potentially life-threatening or organ-threatening disorders. Examples are appendicitis and ovarian torsion.

Ectopic Pregnancy

Ectopic pregnancy is the presence of a pregnancy outside the uterus. It is the leading cause of pregnancy-related death in the 1st trimester.

Ectopic pregnancies can occur in multiple sites. The distribution is as follows:[5]

Sites of Ectopic Gestation	Incidence
Fallopian tube (Tubal)	
Ampullary segment	70.0%
Isthmic segment	12.0%
Fimbrial end	11.1%
Interstitial and cornual	2.4%
Abdominal	1.3%
Ovarian	3.2%
Other uncommon sites including: Cervical Ectopic, Scar ectopic (over previous hysterotomy, CS scars)	

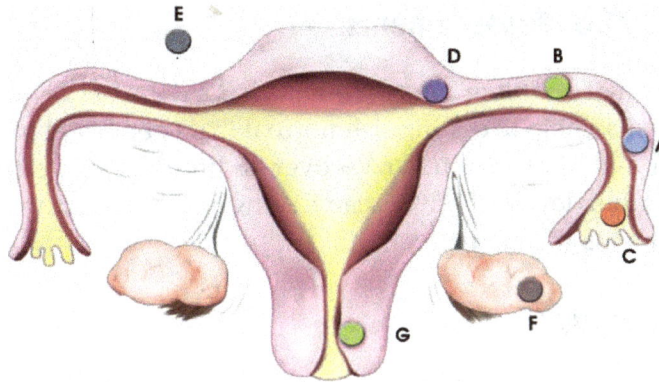

FIGURE 18.1 ■ Sites of ectopic pregnancy. (A) Ampullary, (B) Isthmic, (C) Fimbrial, (D) Interstitial, (E) Abdominal, (F) Ovarian, (G) Cervical.

Risk factors for ectopic pregnancy include previous pelvic inflammation (PID, endometriosis, previous surgery), IUCD use, assisted reproduction, smoking, previous ectopic pregnancy.

The presentation of symptomatic patients with a tubal ectopic pregnancy may be acute or subacute. In acute presentations, patients typically present with acute abdomen with intraperitoneal haemorrhage and haemodynamic shock. The initial assessment is as described in the earlier part of this chapter. The following will go on to elaborate on investigations and management specific to ectopic pregnancies.

Serum hCG

hCG is a glycoprotein secreted by syncytiotrophoblasts and consists of two non-covalently linked α and β subunits. The α subunit is identical to follicle stimulating hormone and luteinising hormone, while the β subunit is specific to hCG. Most commercially available monoclonal antibody based urine pregnancy tests can detect β-hCG concentrations above 25 IU/L, with a sensitivity of 99–100%.

Single β-hCG Measurement

A single serum β-hCG concentration has been used as a discriminatory level to detect an ectopic pregnancy. With a transvaginal ultrasound scan, failure to visualise an intra-uterine gestational sac if β-hCG concentrations are 1,500 IU/L or more may indicate an abnormal intrauterine pregnancy, a recent miscarriage or an ectopic pregnancy.

Serial β-hCG Measurements

As the normal doubling time for β-hCG is 2.2 days, serial quantitative assessments of β-hCG may help to distinguish normal from abnormal pregnancies. An increase in serum β-hCG of less than 66% over 48 hours is suggestive of an ectopic pregnancy.[6] Falling levels of β-hCG can distinguish between an ectopic pregnancy and a spontaneous miscarriage.

Ultrasonography

In the presence of an intrauterine pregnancy, a concomitant ectopic pregnancy is very rare (1:30,000). The earliest a normal intrauterine gestational sac (approximately 2 mm) can be seen is four weeks on a transvaginal scan and five weeks with a transabdominal scan.

The various ultrasound features of ectopic pregnancies are as follows:

Empty uterus and an adnexal mass
Varying amount of fluid in the pouch of Douglas
Presence of an ectopic gestational sac (with either yolk sac or foetal pole)
A pseudo-gestational sac in the uterus

Management of Ectopic Pregnancies

Surgical treatment

All of the surgical procedures for the treatment of ectopic pregnancy can be accomplished via laparoscopy or laparotomy. The main factors determining the approach are:

(1) Haemodynamic condition of the patient.
(2) Size and location of the ectopic gestation. Laparotomy should be considered where the patient is haemodynamically unstable, there is suspicion of extensive

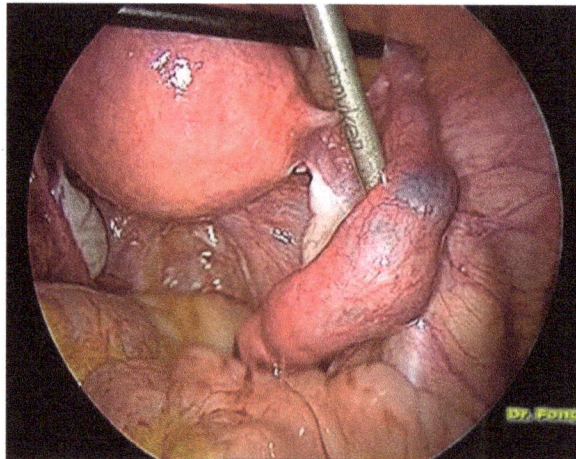

FIGURE 18.2 ■ Ampullary ectopic pregnancy visualised during laparoscopy.

abdominal and pelvic adhesions making laparoscopy difficult, or the ectopic is cornual.

Surgical procedures that can be performed for a tubal ectopic pregnancy include salpingectomy and salpingostomy.
In the presence of a healthy contralateral tube there is no clear evidence that salpingostomy should be used in preference to salpingectomy.[7]
Salpingectomy is still the most common method for treatment of ectopic pregnancy. It can be performed via laparotomy or laparoscopy.
Salpingectomy is indicated for women with:
> Ruptured tubal pregnancy
> Recurrent ectopic pregnancy in a tube already treated conservatively
> Previous sterilisation and reversal of sterilisation on the same tube
> Previous tubal surgery for infertility

Salpingostomy is the primary treatment of choice for tubal ectopic pregnancy in the presence of contralateral tubal disease and where the patient wishes to retain her potential for future fertility.

Medical treatment of ectopic pregnancy with methotrexate

Medical treatment has a role in ectopic gestations detected early, with the desire to retain fertility and minimising surgical morbidity. The most frequently used drug is methotrexate, a potent folic acid antagonist. Methotrexate is administered intramuscularly, and up to 90% of the drug is secreted unchanged into the urine within 48 hours, hence impaired renal function can result in prolonged exposure to high levels of methotrexate and its metabolic products.

The key for successful and safe medical treatment of ectopic pregnancy is proper selection of patients.

Indications

Initial pre-treatment plasma β-hCG not exceeding 5,000 IU/L
> Ultrasound findings of:
> — Absence of yolk sac/foetal heart
> — Adnexal mass < 3.5 cm
> — No free fluid in Pouch of Douglas

Good understanding and compliance for subsequent follow up visits for symptom and serum β-hCG monitoring
> Hemodynamic stability

No contraindications to MTX such as:

Breastfeeding
Immunodeficiency
Peptic ulcer disease
Active pulmonary disease
Renal/hepatic insufficiency
Coexisting viable intrauterine pregnancy
Hypersensitivity/drug allergy

 Serum β-hCG levels should be checked four and seven days after the first dose of methotrexate, and a further dose given if β-hCG levels have failed to drop by more than 15% between Day 4 and 7. The level of serum β-hCG is likely to increase between Day 1 and Day 4 after treatment.

Reproductive outcomes

In patients who underwent radical surgery treatment, recurrent ectopic pregnancy rate is 10–15%.

Adnexal Pathologies Resulting in Acute Abdomen

Adnexal masses (ovarian cysts/tubal cysts) may also cause acute onset of pain in the presence of a cyst accident such as torsion, rupture, or haemorrhage. Torsion usually gives rise to acute onset sharp constant pain caused by ischaemia of the cyst. Tissue may subsequently be infarcted if there is a delay in the treatment. Bleeding may also occur into the cyst and cause pain as the capsule becomes distended. Intraperitoneal bleeding may result from rupture of the cyst, most commonly from a ruptured, bleeding corpus luteum.

 The classic presentation of ovarian torsion is the acute onset of moderate to severe pelvic pain, often with nausea and possibly vomiting, in a woman with an adnexal mass. Fever may be a marker of adnexal necrosis, particularly in the setting of leukocytosis.

 In a patient who presents with an acute abdomen with a working diagnosis of an acute cyst accident, as a minimum, urine should be tested for infections and pregnancy. Blood should be obtained for a full blood count, blood grouping and cross match if patient is haemodynamically unstable.

Imaging

Ultrasound reporting of an adnexal mass — pay attention to location, dimensions, nature of contents (low echo, clear fluid), vascularity of the mass. Features suggestive of malignancy on ultrasound include: (1) Multilocular, (2) Evidence of solid areas, (3) Evidence of metastasis, (4) Presence of ascites, (5) Bilateral lesions.

CT has no significant advantage over ultrasound in cyst assessment, but can be useful in the presence of obvious extrapelvic disease to assess tumour bulk prior to treatment. MRI has a marginal advantage over CT in assessing the character of the cyst, but both have no benefit over good transvaginal ultrasound and should not be used routinely.

Surgical Management of Acute Cyst Accidents

Role of laparoscopy — Diagnostic and therapeutic

Indications for laparoscopy: (1) No evidence suggestive of malignancy, (2) favourable pelvis: no/minimal adhesions, no ascites/peritoneal nodules, (3) cosmesis.

Conservative intervention

For adnexal torsion: untwisting the adnexa, followed by a procedure with no adverse effect on fertility (e.g. cystectomy).

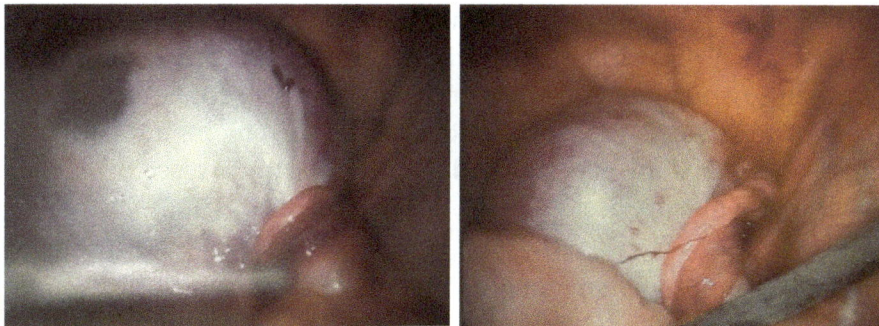

FIGURE 18.3 ■ Intensity of ovarian torsion.

For symptomatic/bleeding/ruptured adnexal (Ovarian/Tubal) cysts: Adnexal Cystectomy, haemostasis (bleeding corpus luteum). Ovariopexy can be considered, especially in young females who have ovarian torsion with normal ovaries (to prevent future recurrence).

In the reproductive age groups, surgeons should aim to remove the cyst intact with limited trauma to the residual ovarian tissue. Complete excision is preferred over aspiration and "ablation", while thermal ablation results in incomplete destruction of cyst wall, which increases recurrence risk. Underlying ovarian cortex may be also be damaged by heat with use of electrocautery on ovarian tissue.

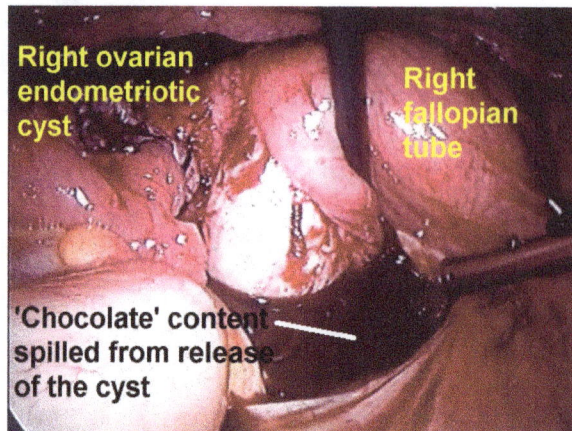

FIGURE 18.4 ■ Laparoscopic view of a ruptured ovarian endometriotic cyst with spillage of cyst contents.

Radical intervention

During adnexal torsion, necrotic/non-viable appearance after untwisting ischae-mic adnexa may require adnexectomy (oophorectomy/Salpingo-oophorectomy). However, caution is needed as the surgeon's intra-operative assessment can be poor. Simple untwisting of adnexa that initially appeared to be necrotic may allow ovarian function to return. When surgery is indicated for benign ovarian disease, preservation of ovarian tissue via cystectomy or enucleation of a solid tumour from the ovary is generally preferable to complete oophorectomy. When the ovary cannot be salvaged or insufficient viable tissue remains after attempts at conserva-tion, oophorectomy is performed. Oophorectomy is also considered if a patient is near to the menopause.

Indications for oophorectomy in benign conditions include:

Benign ovarian neoplasms that are not amenable to treatment by a lesser proce-dure (e.g. cystectomy, enucleation, partial oophorectomy)
Risk-reducing salpingo-oophorectomy
Tubo-ovarian abscess unresponsive to antibiotics
Definitive surgery for endometriosis

Conclusion

- The history and physical examination should be thorough, but tailored to the patient's clinical presentation

- Women presenting in shock or with peritoneal signs may require immediate surgical intervention
- A pregnancy test should be obtained in all women of reproductive age presenting with acute abdominal pain. Other laboratory testing and imaging studies should be based upon history and clinical examination findings

References

1. Lamvu G, Steege JF. (2006) The anatomy and neurophysiology of pelvic pain. *J Minim Invasive Gynecol* **13**:516.
2. Cervero F, Laird JM. (1999) Visceral pain. *Lancet* **353**:2145.
3. Barnhart KT, Sammel MD, Gracia CR, *et al*. (2006) Risk factors for ectopic pregnancy in women with symptomatic first trimester pregnancies. *Fert Sertil* **86**:36.
4. Quan M. (1992) Diagnosis of acute pelvic pain. *J Fam Pract* **35**:422.
5. Bouyer J, Coste J, Fernandez H, *et al*. (2002) Sites of ectopic pregnancy: a 10 year population-based study of 1800 cases. *Human Reprod* **17**:3224–3230.
6. Kadar N, Caldwell BV, Romero R. (1981) A method of screening for ectopic pregnancy and its indications. *Obstet Gynecol* **58**:162–166.
7. Royal College of Obstetricians and Gynaecologists. (2004) *The Management of Tubal Pregnancy*. Guideline No. 21. RCOG, London.

19

GESTATIONAL TROPHOBLASTIC DISEASE

Pearl Tong and A. Ilancheran

Introduction

The incidence of gestational trophoblastic disease (GTD) varies according to geographical regions. The incidence is higher in some parts of Asia, the Middle East and Africa; for example it can be as high as 1,299 per 100,000 pregnancies in Indonesia, whilst the incidence is the lowest in Paraguay, at 23 per 100,000 pregnancies. There are two known risk factors for developing GTD — extremes of maternal age, and history of a previous GTD. The risk of recurrence for a patient who has had a previous molar pregnancy is 1%, whereas it rises to 25% if she has had two or more previous molar pregnancies. The term GTD encompasses all the tumours that arise from the products of conception. They range from hydatidiform moles (complete and partial), which are non-invasive, to invasive entities (which are collectively classed as gestational trophoblastic neoplasia (GTN), such as invasive mole, placental site trophoblastic tumour and choriocarcinoma. There are several features that are unique about GTD — diagnosis can be particularly challenging. Unless one bears this differential diagnosis in mind, it can be easily missed, but cure rates remain very high, over 90% even for stage IV disease. It is one condition which is exquisitely sensitive to chemotherapy, and the only cancer for which chemotherapy can be initiated without any histological evidence.[1,2]

Types of GTD

Hydatidiform Moles

There are two types in general, complete and partial moles. They arise from abnormal fertilisation processes between the ovum and sperm.

Clinical presentation

Usually, suspicion arises based on investigation of abnormal bleeding per vaginum and a positive pregnancy test. Classical features of a complete mole, as outlined above, are uncommonly seen in the local setting when early booking scans are usually done. However, in unbooked cases or low resource settings, these presentations are relatively common.

Due to the markedly elevated levels of HCG, patients with complete moles can have other symptoms, such as severe vomiting, hence presenting like a case of hyperemesis gravidarum. Early onset of high blood pressure and proteinuria (<20 weeks' gestation), suggestive of pre-eclampsia, must immediately bring to mind the possibility of a complete mole. They can also present with symptoms of thyrotoxicosis, such as tremors or palpitations. There may also be acute abdominal pain, arising from accidents pertaining to the enlarged ovaries, such as torsion or rupture of the theca lutein cysts.

Physical examination looking for signs of anaemia or thyrotoxicosis, such as tremors, tachycardia, warm peripheries, dehydration from vomiting, hyperreflexia from hypertension, or abdominal tenderness. A pelvic mass may be felt, typically from uterine enlargement greater than that expected for the calculated gestational age; and enlarged theca lutein cysts in the ovaries. A speculum examination to evaluate the amount and nature of blood loss per vaginum is usually performed.

Partial moles mainly present as an early pregnancy failure, as either incomplete miscarriage or missed abortion. There are no clear distinguishing ultrasound featurues and the HCG levels may not be high. The diagnosis is only made after the products of conception are sent for histological assessment. This underscores the fact that, to avoid missing any molar pregnancies, all tissues removed during dilatation and curettage for pregnancy related conditions should be submitted for pathological assessment.

Women who present with persistent abnormal vaginal bleeding after any pregnancy (molar or non-molar) should have a pregnancy test to exclude GTN. Similarly, a high index of suspicion is necessary in women of reproductive age who present with acute respiratory or neurological symptoms, as these may be

TABLE 19.1 Features of Complete and Partial Mole

	Complete Mole	Partial Mole
Aetiology	Mostly paternal origin, from duplication of 2 haploid sperm	Triploidy, with extra set of chromosomes derived paternally
Karyotype	46 XX (90%), 46 XY (10%)	69 XXY, XYY
Histology	DIFFUSE hydatidiform swelling of chorionic villi and trophoblastic hyperplasia ABSENT foetal or embryonic tissue	Scalloping of chorionic villi and trophoblastic stromal inclusions, only FOCAL areas of hydatidiform swelling of chorionic villi and trophoblastic hyperplasia Foetal or embryonic tissue PRESENT.
Classical clinical presentation	Generally due to very high levels of circulating Human Chorionic Gonadotropin (HCG) — Abnormal vaginal bleeding (typically described as "prune juice" appearance), can be prolonged and heavy, leading to anaemia — Pre-eclampsia — Hyperthyroidism — Hyperemesis gravidarum — Uterine size larger than dates — Theca lutein cysts — Phenomena of trophoblastic embolisation	Generally presents as a missed/incomplete miscarriage, either as abnormal vaginal bleeding or an ultrasonography finding — Not uncommonly a HISTOLOGICAL finding after evacuation of uterus done
Classical ultrasonography presentation	Snow storm appearance of endometrium — multiple vesicles seen distending the endometrial cavity. Enlarged ovarian cysts (theca lutein cysts) — bilateral, multilocular and often large (>6 cm)	Non-specific ultrasonography findings: — May mimic that of missed miscarriage (foetal pole without foetal heartbeat) — Focal cystic spaces in placenta tissue — Increase in transverse diameter of intra-uterine gestational sac
Risk of progression to invasive entities	15% risk of local uterine invasion (invasive mole) 4% risk of choriocarcinoma	2–4% risk of persistence

evidence of GTN in the lungs or brain. These events may occur remotely from the antecedent pregnancy. A simple pregnancy test may help clinch the diagnosis.

Investigations

Investigations should be tailored to the history and physical findings elicited. It must be borne in mind that most of these patients would be managed surgically. Measurement of serum levels of HCG has been the traditional method of diagnosing GTN. While very high levels are suspicious, there is no pathognomonic value of HCG to make the diagnosis. However, it is the tumour marker par excellence in the follow-up of patients with GTN, to assess response to treatment and diagnose recurrence. Other blood tests that should be done include a full blood count to look at the haemoglobin level, keeping in mind cross matching of blood to standby in case of heavy bleeding, and renal panel to look for any electrolyte abnormalities. The blood group rhesus status of the patient should be known, as anti-D prophylaxis may be required for cases of a partial mole (not necessary for complete mole as there is poor vascularisation of chorionic villi and absence of anti-D antigen in these cases). A thyroid function check is recommended, even if the patient is asymptomatic, due to the risk of thyroid storm occurring intra-operatively. This can be prevented by administering medications such as beta blocking agents prior to induction of anaesthesia.

Ultrasound remains the most important diagnostic modality in GTN. In complete moles, the uterus shows the absence of a gestational sac but the cavity is filled with cystic spaces — the typical "snowstorm" appearance. Its value is more limited in PHM with no definite diagnostic features. More recently, high resolution vaginal ultrasound, with colour Doppler, has been used to diagnose GTN involving the uterine myometrium (invasive mole and choriocarcinoma).

Chest X-rays are mandatory in all cases of GTN, as the lungs are the commonest site for metastases, and as a preparation for general anaesthesia. CT scans and MRI may be used judiciously in metastatic survey of other organs, especially the liver and brain.

Surgical management

Surgical management such as suction curettage or hysterectomy (if the patient has completed childbearing) is the mainstay of treatment; medical methods of evacuating the uterus (with oxytocin or cervical ripening agents like prostaglandins) or hysterotomy are no longer recommended.

The standard of care in the treatment of molar pregnancy is surgical evacuation of the uterus by suction curettage. This can be performed in any uterus, regardless of its size. It is advisable that the suction be performed with a concurrent oxytocin drip running in, to reduce the risks of haemorrhage, perforation and trophoblastic embolisation. A rare complication associated with evacuation of large uteri is onset of acute respiratory distress syndrome, thought to be due to the embolisation of trophoblasts into the circulation. Immediate ventilator support can be life-saving in these situations.[3]

A hysterectomy can be performed by an abdominal or vaginal route. All surgical specimens obtained should be sent for histological examination.

Postoperative care and surveillance

Fortunately, most of the accompanying symptoms of a complete molar pregnancy will resolve spontaneously after the molar tissue is evacuated.

After evacuation of the uterus, all patients should be followed up with weekly serum HCG until they become negative; then, monthly for six months. In the vast majority of patients, the HCG levels become negative by 8–12 weeks. Subsequent HCG measurements are required under the following circumstances: irregular vaginal bleeding, amenorrhoea or evidence of metastatic disease. In the serial monitoring of HCG, three patterns that raise suspicion of malignant GTN include: (1) persistent rise in the values; (2) plateauing of the values; and (3) a secondary rise after an initial fall.

Reliable contraception should be advised after evacuation of the mole, mainly to avoid the confusion that a new pregnancy can cause in the serial monitoring of HCG. Whilst barrier contraception may be the safest, they are also the least reliable. Intrauterine devices or implantable hormone devices may cause irregular vaginal bleeding, which might be mistaken for persistent GTN. Oral contraceptives are the preferred option.

The prognosis for future pregnancy is good, however the patient should be informed of the slightly increased risk of a recurrence of molar pregnancy. An early booking visit is advised for confirmation of a viable intrauterine pregnancy; and six weeks post-delivery, a serum HCG should be done to ensure that it is negative, in case of occurrence of a GTN. A phenomenon known as phantom HCG may be encountered, in which a persistent low level of HCG may be present due to circulating heterophilic antibodies. This can be overcome by sending both urine and serum samples to a reference HCG laboratory.

Placental Site Trophoblastic Tumour

This is a rare entity, characterised histologically by presence of intermediate trophoblastic cells. Levels of HCG are not as elevated compared to the other forms of GTN, and they tend to be indolent, slow-growing and metastasizing only very late in the course of progress. They are generally not chemosensitive and the main modality of treatment is hysterectomy.

Invasive Mole (IM)/Choriocarcinoma (CC)

This diagnosis can be made from a few situations: most commonly following evacuation of a complete mole, with plateauing or rising HCG levels noted on follow–up; or abnormal bleeding following a pregnancy event such as pregnancy loss, termination of pregnancy or a normal pregnancy. It is also known to present in a bizarre manner, for example sudden onset of neurological deficits in a lady remote from any pregnancy events. In these cases, the diagnosis is clinched by the markedly raised levels of HCG and absence of an intrauterine or extrauterine pregnancy sac. Radiological imaging is done, depending on the symptoms of the patient, as well as a full body metastatic survey once the diagnosis of invasive mole or choriocarcinoma is made, so that treatment can be administered.

A diagnosis of IM is seldom made clinically, without surgery. Most of the non-metastatic (low risk) GTN following a molar pregnancy is believed to be IM. The presence of a vascular nodule in the myometrium, following evacuation of a mole and persistent high levels or rising levels of HCG may be suggestive of an IM.

Chemotherapy, usually with a single agent, methotrexate (MTX) or actinomycin D (ACT-D) is the treatment of choice. In chemoresistant cases, resection of the nodule or hysterectomy may be indicated.

CC develops in about 3% to 5% of the patients with CHM. Of all CC, 50% are preceded by a hydatidiform mole, 25% by an abortion, and the other 25% by a full term pregnancy. A clinical diagnosis of CC is rare. Most of the metastatic (high risk) GTN, especially those outside the lungs, are believed to be CC. Chemotherapy with multiple agents (see below) is the treatment of choice.

Surgery has an important role in selected cases (see below).

GTN

A diagnosis of persistent GTN is made when any of the following criteria are fulfilled:

(a) There is a rise of HCG on three consecutive weekly measurements.
(b) There is plateauing of the HCG levels for three or more weeks.
(c) HCG levels remain elevated for six months or more.
(d) There is radiologic evidence of metastatic disease in the presence of positive HCG.
(e) There is histologic diagnosis of CC.

FIGO (2000) staging of GTN:

(I) Disease confined to the uterine corpus
(II) GTN extends to outside the uterus, but is limited to the genital structures (adnexae, vagina, broad ligament)

(III) GTN extends to the lungs, with or without genital tract involvement
(IV) All other metastatic sites

The mainstay of treatment for invasive mole or choriocarcinoma is chemotherapy. Hysterectomy has a role in reducing tumour burden in cases where disease is limited to the uterus, there is inadequate response to single-agent chemotherapy and/or the patient has already completed her family.

In general, the cases are stratified into low risk (score <7) or high risk categories (score 7 or higher), according to the presence of various factors in the FIGO scoring system.

TABLE 19.2   Factors Determining Risk for Choriocarcinoma

	Scores			
	0	1	2	4
Age of patient	<40	>=40	—	—
Antecedent pregnancy	Mole	Abortion	Term	—
Interval months from interval pregnancy	<4 months	4–<7 months	7–<13 months	>=13 months
Pre-treatment HCG levels	<1,000	1,000–10,000	10,000–100,000	>100,000
Largest tumour size	—	3–<5 cm	>=5 cm	—
Site of metastases	Lung	Kidney/Spleen	Gastrointestinal/Liver	Brain
Number of metastases	—	1–4	5–8	>8
Previous failed chemotherapy	—	—	Single drug	>2 drugs

For low risk cases, single-agent chemotherapy is used, such as methotrexate (intravenous or intramuscular), with or without folinic acid rescue. D-actinomycin can be used as well. HCG levels are monitored regularly. If the levels are falling adequately, the chemotherapy agent is continued until at least one course has been administered after the first normal HCG level is obtained. If there is an inadequate response, as demonstrated by slow decrease, plateauing or increase in HCG levels/detection of new metastases, the chemotherapy agent can be changed or a hysterectomy considered in suitable situations.

For high risk cases, or those refractory to single-agent therapy, multi-agent chemotherapy is recommended. The first-line used in Singapore is usually EMA-CO or EMA (preferred at National University Hospital), comprising etoposide, methotrexate, D-actinomycin, leucovorin, cyclophosphamide and vincristine. During the course of treatment, HCG is trended and this regimen is repeated until the normalisation of HCG, then continued for an additional two cycles. This chemotherapy regimen is generally well tolerated; side effects include alopecia, haematologic toxicity e.g. neutropenia, thrombocytopenia, and gastrointestinal symptoms like vomiting and diarrhoea. For patients with brain metastases, recurrent or resistant GTN, surgical options can be considered. Whole brain irradiation is also a treatment modality for those with metastases to the central nervous system.

The traditional role of surgery in GTN has been in a salvage setting, where despite multiple cycles of chemotherapy, resistant tumour foci exist. However, primary chemotherapy is not without danger in certain sites, especially the brain, where chemotherapy can cause necrosis and haemorrhage of the tumour which can have serious or even fatal consequences. Therefore, there has been a recent trend to do primary surgery in selected patients, to avoid prolonged chemotherapy and its complications. Examples of such surgery would include hysterectomy in low risk, non-metastatic disease; thoracotomy to remove large, solitary lung metastasis; and craniotomy in solitary brain metastasis at accessible sites.

Surgery may also be used when complications occur; for example, hysterectomy for a perforating invasive mole or choriocarcinoma with uncontrolled bleeding. Craniotomy may be necessary to stem cerebral haemorrhage from metastases.

With the availability of effective chemotherapy, radiation always had a limited role in the treatment of GTN. It has been employed most frequently to treat patients with brain or liver metastases, in an effort to minimise haemorrhagic complications from disease at these sites.

Response rate to chemotherapy is extremely good. Cure rates for non-metastatic/low-risk GTN approaches that of 100%; for high risk GTN it is now in the region of 80–90%, and even in the presence of metastases, the five year survival rates are more than 50%. The chemotherapy regimens used are not known to affect fertility or induce teratogenicity in future pregnancies. However, contraception use for a year following completion of chemotherapy is recommended to allow accurate disease monitoring with HCG and to minimise any remnant effects of chemotherapy on the ovary. Should a patient get pregnant, the same advice applies as that dispensed to the patient who has had a previous molar pregnancy.[4,5]

References

1. Ilancheran A. (1998) Optimal management of gestational trophoblastic disease: a review. *Ann Acad Med* **27**:698–704.
2. Altieri A, Franceschi S, Ferlay J, *et al.* (2003) Epidemiology and aetiology of gestational trophoblastic diseases. *Lancet Oncol* **4**(11):670–678.
3. RCOG Greentop guideline No. 38: *Gestational Trophoblastic Disease*. Published 4/3/2010.
4. Lurain JR. (2011) Gestational Trophoblastic Disease II: Classification and management of gestational trophoblastic neoploasia. *AJOG* **Jan 2011**:11–18.
5. Hancock BW, Newland ES and Benkowitz RS. (1998) *Gestational Trophoblastic Disease*.

20

PRENATAL SCREENING AND DIAGNOSIS

Citra Mattar

Introduction

The concept of screening or testing for chromosomal and genetic disease is best understood as a risk assessment of the foetus in the current pregnancy. Maternal risk assessment will be discussed elsewhere. The significance of chromosomal/genetic screening is that Down syndrome (Trisomy 21) is the most common chromosomal anomaly among live births, and thus the most prevalent cause of intellectual disability. Additional congenital structural anomalies may affect the child. Trisomy 18 and 13 are even more uncommon and are associated with severe structural and neurological anomalies, and intrauterine demise. The prevalence of the autosomal trisomies increases with increasing maternal age in the population. The prevalence of trisomies naturally decreases as gestational age increases due to the spontaneous pregnancy loss, and elective termination for women who wish to prevent the birth of an affected infant. For families who wish to carry on with an affected pregnancy, prenatal confirmation of the genetic diagnosis will allow time to prepare for life after birth, meeting with the paediatrician and communicating with Down syndrome and related associations. Certain single gene diseases cause pathology in utero (alpha thalassaemia major) while others manifest after birth, yet impose significant medical and socio-economic burden on affected families. For these reasons, prenatal screening is offered for Trisomies 21, 18 and 13 and the common single-gene disorders in the population. The information generated from such screening tests are important factors influencing the management of the affected pregnancy.

What is Prenatal Screening?

Prenatal screening is the process of assessing the risk of the foetus in the current pregnancy being affected by Trisomy 21, 18 or 13, and/or a single gene disease with non-invasive investigations. Examples of the latter commonly screened for are thalassaemia major (α- or β-) and other haemoglobinopathies, cystic fibrosis and DiGeorge syndrome. Targeted screening for foetal structural anomalies can be performed with an early gestation ultrasound scan from 11 to 14 weeks gestation.

Who are Candidates for Prenatal Screening?

Though maternal age is the main risk factor, prenatal screening should be offered to all pregnant women at the appropriate gestations, regardless of age if the mother understands the aims and limitations. Many women are willing to accept the small false negative risk in order to avoid the risk of pregnancy loss, such as women who have had recurrent miscarriages or fertility-assisted therapy. As non-invasive prenatal screening (NIPT) is currently more expensive than first trimester screening (FTS) and demands a longer processing time, it can be recommended as a second-line screening tool for women with intermediate to high risk FTS results. Increasingly, due to its uniquely high detection rate, NIPT is being offered as a first-line screen.

Women who would be anxious about the limitations of screening tests, who would prefer a confirmatory test straight away or who are considered high risk already may not be appropriate candidates for screening, and should be considered candidates for diagnostic testing as first-line.

Methods of Screening and Interpretation of Risk

Combined first trimester screening (FTS) and non-invasive prenatal testing by cell-free foetal DNA (NIPT) are available. These are screening tests for chromosomal and genetic conditions. An early gestation ultrasound at 11 to 14 weeks can be performed on its own in patients who decline the full FTS, for the purpose of early surveillance for structural defects.

First trimester screening (FTS)

FTS is a combination of maternal serum screening for biochemical markers (pregnancy-associated plasma protein-A, PAPP-A, and total β-human chorionic gonadotrophin, HCG) that are interpreted in the context of maternal age and ethnicity, the nuchal thickness (NT) measured by transabdominal US when the crown-rump length of the foetus ranges from 45–84 mm (or from a dated gestation of 11 weeks plus 3 days to 13 weeks plus 6 days), and the absence or presence of the nasal bone. The adjusted (aggregated) risk is often, but not always, lower that the risk associated with age alone.[1,2]

The concept of the risk threshold must be understood. By consensus opinion, the risk threshold for FTS is 1 in 250, i.e. a result of ≥1 in 250 should be investigated further. A risk <1 in 250 is considered a negative screen, and routine screening can resume throughout the pregnancy.

However, it is possible to further improve risk assessment by stratification into low, intermediate and high risk. Low risk results (≤1 in 1,000) require no further testing and routine foetal monitoring can resume. A high risk of ≥1 in 50 should be confirmed by an invasive test, due to the false positive rate (usually 5%), and the Odds of being Affected given a Positive Result (OAPR) of 3–5%, which means that the majority of high risk screening tests come from unaffected pregnancies. Intermediate risk patients (>1 in 1,000 but <1 in 50) may be considered for contingent testing, which varies by maternal-foetal units.

Non-invasive prenatal testing

NIPT with cffDNA in maternal blood is currently offered by several companies who use a variety of molecular analytical methods, including various forms of polymerase chain reaction (PCR) and high throughput shotgun sequencing. cffDNA is currently used to identify autosomal trisomies and sex chromosomal aneuploidies. Foetal sex (for X-linked genetic diseases), Rhesus factor and certain single-gene disease (β-thalassaemia and sickle cell disease, cystic fibrosis, haemophilia, Duchenne muscular dystrophy, spinal muscular atrophy, fragile-X syndrome) are possible. Depending on the molecular technology used, detection rate and false positive/negative rates differ between tests. Currently, we offer NIPT as the second-line or contingent test for intermediate risk patients. Additionally, high risk patients keen to avoid pregnancy loss who understand the limitations of NIPT may be offered this test.

NIPT detects >99% of pregnancies (detection rate) affected by aneuploidies overall, but the individual detection rate varies between the trisomies depending on the molecular analysis performed. The false positive rate is <0.5%, and in <1–5% of pregnancies there may not be sufficient cffDNA to make a diagnosis (uninformative rate). NIPT thus improves the stringency of selecting patients who would benefit from invasive testing.

Although it is not a diagnostic test, the high detection rate, particularly for Down syndrome, may allow some patients sufficient assurance in the quality of the test that pregnancy management may be based on these results alone, although this is not yet standard practice.

Early gestation ultrasound (11–14 weeks)

Use of the combined FTS which incorporates an ultrasound assessment at 11–14 weeks adds the value of being able to screen for certain structural anomalies during this gestational period. Even if the patient declines a formal combined FTS, she may be encouraged to have an early gestation ultrasound scan (at 11–14 weeks), for surveillance of the nuchal translucency, nasal bone, contiguity of the skull and limbs, and the abdominal wall. Evidence from this scan may be used to identify foetuses suspected to have cleft lip or palate, open abdominal wall or neural tube defects, cardiovascular anomalies or aneuploidies other than the trisomies, such as monosomy X, particularly if there is limited access to biochemical or molecular screening.[3,4]

When is Prenatal Screening Used in Clinical Practice?

FTS or NIPT can be used to screen for aneuploidies. FTS is beneficial to women who value early screening and discretion, as the test is conducted between 11 weeks and 13 weeks 6 days, allowing for chorionic villus sampling to be carried out by the end of the first or beginning of the second trimester. Once the diagnosis is confirmed, a woman may elect to terminate the affected pregnancy at a stage before she becomes visibly gravid. The FTS, due to the US component, also enables early screening for gross anatomical anomalies, such as open neural tube defects. FTS however is not designed to screen for single gene disorders (e.g. thalassaemia, cystic fibrosis). Currently, FTS is offered to all pregnant women regardless of maternal age.

NIPT may in some settings be offered as a first line screening test particularly if maternal age ≥35 years, or used as a second line test for high or intermediate risk results on FTS for patients who desire to avoid invasive testing. Due to its high detection rate, NIPT may also be offered to women who have had a previous pregnancy with aneuploidy, US findings associated with aneuploidy, or parental balanced Robertsonian translocation increasing the risk of foetal Trisomy 21 or 13. NIPT can be done as early as 10 weeks of gestation, although there may be some benefit in deferring the test to the early second trimester, when the risk of spontaneous miscarriage decreases and to coincide with the early gestation ultrasound scan at 11–14 weeks.

Every patient should be encouraged to have the early gestation ultrasound scan even if they decline FTS or NIPT for aneuploidies for the reasons described above.

Limitations of Prenatal Screening

Screening tests do not confirm the presence or absence of aneuploidy or genetic disease. The statistical limits are set to maximise the detection rate while minimising the incidence of false positive cases (that would put these pregnancies at risk of invasive procedure-related miscarriage). FTS detects approximately 90% of affected foetuses (when the false positive rate is 5%), and thus 10% of affected foetuses will be missed (false negative cases). Therefore, the patient must be instructed that "low risk does not mean no risk". If the screening US at 20–22 weeks detects a significant anomaly, invasive testing will still be recommended.

The limitations of NIPT currently are the variation in detection rate for trisomies 21 and 18, and 13 which is lower. The efficacy for sex chromosome aneuploidy is low. False negative results are still possible, and mosaicism is not reliably detected. NIPT is not yet validated for multiple pregnancies, and in cases of "vanishing twin" results may be inaccurate. Women with high body mass index are at higher risk of inaccurate or inconclusive results. Women carrying a foetus with significant risk of microdeletion syndrome and other single-gene diseases will still benefit from invasive testing.

Structural defects may be too subtle to detect on early gestation ultrasound; this should always be followed by second trimester structural screening, typically done between 18–22 weeks, which is more sensitive for structural anomalies.

Consequences of Screening: Low and High Risk Screening Test Results

All possible outcomes and related consequences should be considered. An intermediate or high risk screening test result could lead to adverse psychological effect including fear and anxiety. However it should be emphasised to the affected couple, before they undertake the test, that the majority of pregnancies (95–97%) with a positive result are ultimately normal (odds of being affected after a positive result, OAPR).

What is Prenatal Diagnosis?

Candidates for Prenatal Diagnosis

The use of the maternal age of 35 years as a "threshold" age at which to offer prenatal diagnosis has been reached by consensus, and chosen because the risk of

Down syndrome at this age approximates the risk of procedure-related pregnancy loss. However with other important factors to consider (e.g. the avoidance of pregnancy loss) this is no longer a stringent cut-off for offering screening tests. Consensus opinion is that all women should be offered FTS regardless of maternal age, and that all women should have the option of invasive testing, again regardless of maternal age.

Thus, invasive diagnostic testing should be considered in women with other high risk factors, such as a previous pregnancy complicated by trisomy, single or several structural abnormalities in the current pregnancy that are highly suggestive of trisomy, chromosomal translocation, inversion or aneuploidy in the mother or partner highly transmissible to the foetus, or a strong family history of single gene disorder in which the index mutation is known.[5]

Methods of Testing Including Rapid Tests

Diagnostic tests are available at different gestations when appropriate. Chorionic villus sampling (CVS) is performed between 11 and 13 weeks of gestation although it can be performed earlier under special circumstances. The transabdominal route is associated with better outcomes than the transcervical route. Chorionic villi are collected under US guidance, and the cultured cells are used for karyotype and genotype analyses. There is a 0.5–1% risk of pregnancy loss (approaching the incidence of amniocentesis-associated miscarriage in centres that perform a sufficiently high number of both procedures). Other risks include placental haematoma, amniotic fluid leakage and limb reduction sequence in CVS done earlier than recommended. 1–2% of pregnancies have placental mosaicism which does not reflect the chromosomal composition of the foetus, and maternal cell contamination is possible. Thus an abnormal karyotype on CVS should be confirmed by amniocentesis.

Amniocentesis is performed at 16–20 weeks of gestation, transabdominally and under US guidance. Around 20 mL of amniotic fluid is collected avoiding the placenta. Foetal cells (amniocytes) are cultured and used for karyotype/genotype studies. In addition to aneuploidies, and other chromosomal and genetic anomalies, amniotic fluid may be analysed for α-fetoprotein (neural tube defects) and surfactant for determination of lung maturity. In Rhesus alloimmunisation, bilirubin levels in amniotic fluid was previously assessed to determine the severity of foetal haemolysis; now this has been replaced by measurement of the peak systolic velocity of blood flow within the middle cerebral artery. Complications may include pregnancy loss (1 in 200 pregnancies, or 0.5%), amniotic fluid leak/membrane rupture, foetal trauma, chorioamnionitis, and preterm labour/delivery.

Foetal blood sampling, also known as cordocentesis or percutaneous umbilical blood sampling (PUBS), is performed from 20 weeks onwards and the aim is to collect foetal blood from the umbilical vein (under US guidance) to provide a means of rapid chromosome analysis. It is useful in situations where a CVS or amniocentesis were not performed or can no longer be performed due to gestational age. Done under US guidance, blood is collected from the placental or foetal attachment of the umbilical cord, with the foetus transiently paralysed using pancuronium if necessary. This test carries significant pregnancy loss risk of 1–2% and should be reserved for pregnancies determined to be at high risk for genetic disease. Other risks include haemorrhage at the puncture site, cord haematoma, fetomaternal haemorrhage, foetal bradycardia, and vertical transmission of communicable infections, such as HIV.

While the gold standard chromosomal analysis is by cell culture and karyotype, rapid diagnosis is possible by PCR or fluorescence *in situ* hybridisation (FISH) using locus-specific probes on uncultured amniocytes or other foetal cells, where data is available in 24 h or less. Commercial kits are available for this purpose.

Screening for Structural Anomalies

Methods of Screening

Structural anomalies are best visualised by US scan. An early 12 week scan at the time of FTS can identify major defects such as aneuploidy. If there is a suspicion of increased risk of structural or chromosomal/genetic defects, US screening for structural anomalies can be done at 16–18 weeks gestation to detect gross anomalies which affect 1–2% of pregnancies. Early detection can allow the necessary time for further investigations (e.g. karyotype) and sufficient time to consider the option of termination versus continuing the pregnancy. A full screening scan at 22 weeks is still recommended as subtle changes in complex structures, such as the heart, will be better visualised in a larger foetus.[6]

Foetal MRI can be performed for abnormalities on US not clearly defined, where additional information is important for management decisions involving prognostication, foetal therapy or delivery. Examples of defects detected on US in which the patient benefits from foetal MRI include anomalies of the cerebellar vermis in Arnold–Chiari malformations, lung volume in congenital diaphragmatic hernia (CDH), abnormal foetal eyes.

Gestational Age Makes a Difference

Screening for structural defects must be performed at a suitable gestational age such that the anatomy is clearly visualised, so that there is sufficient time for additional molecular confirmatory investigations (invasive testing) which may only yield results after 7–10 days, and time to consider and perform pregnancy termination, bearing in mind the gestational limit in effect (usually 24 weeks).

Communication

How to Counsel a Pregnant Woman on Prenatal Screening

Basic information on prenatal screening should be given to the mother a few weeks prior to the prescribed time of screening (11–13^{+6} weeks for combined first trimester screening, 10–20 weeks for NIPT). Counselling should include the rationale for screening, the procedure(s) involved, possible outcomes of screening, implications of positive screening results and subsequent confirmatory tests. Distinction between screening and diagnostic tests should be made while an explanation of detection rate and false positive/negative results must be included. Ideally, counselling should be provided by a dedicated nurse clinician well versed in counselling techniques. Written information should be provided to the mother to ensure she has a clear understanding of the available tests and their accuracy.

How to Counsel a Mother about a Positive Screening Test

Once a positive result is obtained, the mother should be counselled about the low odds of the pregnancy actually being affected. The option of diagnostic testing is to be discussed, with the appropriate procedures and associated risks discussed. The implications of having a child with Down syndrome or other anomalies, and options of continuing or terminating the pregnancy should be included.

What are the Options for a Foetus Diagnosed with a Molecular or Structural Anomaly?

Lethal Anomaly

Continue with the pregnancy with provision of emotional support to prepare for intrauterine or postnatal demise, or elective termination of pregnancy, if diagnosed at <24 weeks gestation, to avoid maternal emotional complications or if this is the patient's choice.

Non-Lethal Anomalies

In utero therapy

This has been described for selective foetal congenital diseases such as thalassaemia, osteogenesis imperfecta (intrauterine transplantation of haemopoietic or mesenchymal stem cells respectively), CDH (foetal endoscopic tracheal occlusion, FETO), twin–twin transfusion syndrome (fetoscopic laser ablation of placental anastomoses) and amniotic band syndrome (fetoscopic ablation/release of constriction bands).

Postnatal therapy

Where available, for selective diseases e.g. haemoglobinopathies.

References

1. Peralta CF, Falcon O, Wegrzyn P, *et al.* (2005) Assessment of the gap between the fetal nasal bones at 11 to 13 + 6 weeks of gestation by three-dimensional ultrasound. *Ultrasound Obstet Gynecol* **25**(5):464–467.
2. Prefumo F, Izze C. (2014) Fetal abdominal wall defects. *Best Pract Res Clin Obstet Gynaecol* **28**(3):391–402.
3. Rayburn WF, Jolley JA, Simpson LL. (2015) Advances in ultrasound imaging for congenital malformations during early gestation. *Birth Defects Res A Clin Mol Teratol* **103**(4):260–268.
4. Wiechec M, Anna K, Nocun A, *et al.* (2015) How effective is ultrasound-based screening for trisomy 18 without the addition of biochemistry at the time of late first trimester? *J Perinat Med* (3):129–273.
5. Robson SJ, Hui L. (2015) National decline in invasive prenatal diagnostic procedures in association with uptake of combined first trimester and cell-free DNA aneuploidy screening. *Aust N Z J Obstet Gynaecol* **55**(5):507–510.
6. Wiechec M, Knafel A, Nocun A, *et al.* (2015) How Effective Is First-Trimester Screening for Trisomy 21 Based on Ultrasound Only? *Fetal Diagn Ther* 1–45.

Part V

PREGNANCY CARE

Introduction

Pregnancy is accompanied by a multitude of normal physiological changes, affecting every system of the human body. These changes enable the woman to physically accommodate the "foreign" and enlarging foetus whilst ensuring the dynamic nutritive and developmental needs of the foetus are met at each stage of pregnancy. These adaptations, including cardiovascular, respiratory, metabolic, renal and haematological changes, albeit normal, can also be regarded as a "stress test" for the mother. As a clinician, it is important to understand these normal adaptations so one can distinguish them from pathological conditions, hence avoiding unnecessary intervention in normal pregnancy whilst recognising complications requiring active management. Although the majority of pregnancies are uncomplicated with good maternal and neonatal outcomes, pregnancy does impose increased maternal health risks. Risks are even greater for women who already have a health condition prior to conception.

Due to societal lifestyle changes and advances in assisted reproductive technology, increasing number of obese and older women are becoming pregnant. Furthermore, successes in medical management of congenital, childhood and young adult disorders have led to a substantial number of women entering pregnancy with a pre-existing medical condition. There has been an exponential increase in pharmacological and surgical interventions employed in young women with unknown safety profiles for pregnancy and on the foetus. All of these women are at greater risk of complications in pregnancy and would benefit from specialist advice and care before, during and after pregnancy.

The essence of optimum antenatal, intrapartum and postpartum care is to risk stratify, anticipate potential complications, then to seek to prevent, monitor for, identify and treat these complications in a timely and safe manner. Since pregnancy and foetoplacental development is a progressive and dynamic state, there are gestational windows for effective management, which if missed, may not be successfully addressed later in pregnancy. The importance of preconception and antenatal care is further emphasised by the DOHaD (Developmental Origins of Health and Disease) concept that the course of pregnancy can influence the long-term health trajectory for both the mother and baby, and even that of the subsequent generation.

The series of chapters here will address the key issues for various medical and pregnancy-related conditions with regard to antenatal care, intrapartum care and postpartum management, discussing both the impact on the mother as well as the implications for the foetus and neonate.

21

OBSTETRICS HISTORY TAKING AND EXAMINATION

Wong Yee Chee

Introduction

History and physical examination form the fundamental basis of obstetric management. A good history and a thorough examination allow the clinician to have a clear picture of the clinical scenario, and to formulate investigations and management that are appropriate for the mother and foetus to achieve the optimal outcomes.

Obstetric History

Unlike other medical disciplines, obstetric history is not incidence-based, i.e. not limited to the episode of presenting complaints. The main part of the history should contain details of the progress of the current pregnancy, highlighting risk factors and complications that unfold, as well as problems from previous pregnancies, which may significantly affect management of the current pregnancy.

- Confirm the gestational age of the foetus — through menstrual regularity and objective evidence from first trimester
- Identify High Risk Problems of mother and foetus — through details of her present pregnancy, previous pregnancies, medical and surgical history
- Evaluate the adequacy of obstetric care she has received — is it in keeping with current standard of antenatal care?
- Assess attitude of mother and partner towards the pregnancy

Components of Obstetric History

- Menstrual history and last menstrual period
- Antenatal progress
- History of past pregnancies
- Medical and surgical history
- Family history
- Social and dietary history

Menstrual history and last menstrual period

- With a known Last Menstrual Period (LMP), the Expected Delivery Date (EDD) is calculated by Neglee's Rule (EDD = LMP + 9 months and 7 days). The calculation assumes the menstrual cycle to be 28 days, with ovulation taking place on Day 14.

  However, this assumption may not hold true even in women with regular 28 days menstrual cycles, as 10–15% of this group have been shown to have ovulated earlier or later during the month of conception.

  This method of calculation of gestational age using menstrual cycles becomes even more unreliable in women with irregular menstrual cycles.

  In general, true gestational age of the foetus does not concur with menstrual age in some 30% of all pregnancies. The working motto in determination of gestational age should be "the calculated gestational age based on menses should be assumed to be inaccurate unless otherwise validated by objective methods."

- Check with mother the results of routine confirmation of gestational age by reliable objective means e.g. vaginal examination or dating ultrasound (US) scans at first trimester. In general, the first trimester US-verified EDD is regarded as the most accurate, and is used for subsequent calculation of gestational age.

  Accurate gestational age is vital for interpretation of antenatal foetal age-related tests, for foetal monitoring and for obstetric intervention.

History of antenatal progress

- The progress of pregnancy, including minor ailments, from first to third trimesters is tracked chronologically.
- Results of investigations, done as a routine or under specified circumstances, are to be known and interpreted.
- If pregnancy complications develop, the severity of the disease process, its effect on the patient and pregnancy, the treatment received and outcomes of treatment are to be documented and commented.

- To assess attitude of mother and partner towards the pregnancy, giving a good insight into their ability to cope with the stress of pregnancy and complications.
- The status of the foetus needs to be known, whether any foetal defect was detected. Know the pattern of maternal weight gain over the trimesters, and whether the foetus was noted to be growing normally, especially during the last trimester.

History of past pregnancies

Significant events in previous pregnancies need to be recorded in chronological order:

- Date of delivery and delivery gestation
- Antenatal problems/complications
- Length of labour; spontaneous/induced
- Type of delivery and complications e.g. normal vaginal delivery, caesarean section, assisted vaginal delivery, 3rd/4th degree perineal tears; postpartum haemorrhage
- Weight of baby in kg
- Any adverse neonatal complications e.g. cerebral palsy

Conditions affecting her previous pregnancies (like pre-eclampsia, intrauterine growth restriction, premature labour, abruptio placenta or prima postpartum haemorrhage) have an increased likelihood of recurring, thus affecting management of the current pregnancy.

Medical and surgical history

A survey of previous as well as current surgical and medical problems is carried out:

- Previous surgery on pelvic organs, hips or spine may pose special problems in pregnancy.
- Major pre-existing medical diseases that may impose adverse effects on mother and foetus during pregnancy include the following:
  - Diabetes mellitus — hypo-/hyperglycaemia, congenital anomalies, macrosomia, stillbirth
  - Hypertension — prematurity, intrauterine growth restriction, pre-eclampsia (superimposed)
  - Renal disease — hypertension, pre-eclampsia, urinary tract infection etc.
  - Thrombophilias — thrombosis, miscarriage, intrauterine death, venous thromboembolism
  - Connective tissue diseases — pre-eclampsia, intrauterine growth restriction, heart blocks

 o Epilepsy — congenital anomalies due to medications
 o Thyroid disease — foetal thyroid problems

Family history

- Diabetes in first-degree relatives is an indication to screen for gestational diabetes during pregnancy
- Anaemia affecting several family members should prompt the search for thalassemias in early pregnancy
- Congenital heart diseases (CHD) in mother and her siblings raise the risk of CHD in the foetus

Social and dietary history

- Good knowledge of patient social circumstances and financial status, including:
  - o Adequate dietary intake
  - o Accessibility to transport
  - o Access to help with caregiving when pregnancy complications develop

Presentation of Obstetric History

In the course of undergraduate studies, students will be required to present obstetric history in the following circumstances:

 i) Clinical case discussion/write-up
 ii) During ward round/hand-over round

Presenting obstetric history during clinical case discussion/write-up

- Introduce your patient by stating the patient's name, age, gravidity and parity, gestational age, followed by one to two sentences on the main issues of her pregnancy. This would give a preview of the contents of your forthcoming presentation.
- Start the pregnancy account by citing the LMP and the verified EDD. The historical account should be given in chronological order from first trimester to third trimester, describing any admission episodes at the appropriate time. Significant results or findings of routine tests would need to be highlighted; while for special investigations the reasons for ordering the tests is to be elaborated. Shortfalls in care received (versus the current standard of antenatal care) are to be highlighted. Whilst ensuring the flow of events is complete and

presented in coherent sequence, the presentation should be precise and preferably take no longer than 3–5 minutes.

It is important to conclude your presentation with a summary of the high risk factors (to mother/foetus/health personnel), including:

- Hepatitis B sAg carrier
- Pre-eclampsia since 30 weeks, with two previous admissions
- Mild intrauterine growth restriction noted since 32 weeks
- One previous lower segment caesarean section for foetal distress
- Postpartum haemorrhage after first delivery

The ability to completely list all of the problems encountered in the pregnancy reflects favourably on the clinical acuity of the presenter.

Presenting obstetric history during ward round/hand-over round

In these circumstances, detailed information on progress of the pregnancy is not normally required. Presentation should focus on the various problems detected to date, and to what extent they have been treated. Summarise the high risk factors at the end of the presentation (see above).

Management will be modified with specific investigations, and treatment targeted at these risk factors, to lower possible complications.

In conclusion, presentation of obstetric history should not just consist of US scan findings; it is the clinical problems encountered during pregnancy that should form the bulk of your presentation. US findings are only a small (though important) part of the whole clinical picture.

Obstetric Examination

General Physical Examination

At booking visit

- Body weight and height are taken and body mass index (BMI) calculated. Patients with low or high BMI are associated with increased pregnancy complications. Similarly, height of women generally correlates well with capacity of pelvis
- Nutritional status, including evidence of anaemia, is assessed
- Vital signs — blood pressure, pulse rate

- Check: Oral cavity for caries and gingivitis
- Neck for thyroid swellings
- Breasts for lumps and inverted nipples
- Lungs for air entry and adventitious sounds
- Cardiovascular examination to check for heart sounds and murmurs
- In women with severe hypertension and diabetes mellitus, fundoscopy of the eyes may be attempted to exclude associated vasculopathy

A pelvic examination is generally done during the booking visit in first trimester. Speculum examination is carried out to exclude infective vaginal discharges (where swab is taken for analysis) and abnormal appearance of cervix. A digital examination is then performed to ascertain that the size of the uterus is consistent with the gestational age of pregnancy, and also to exclude any pelvic masses.

Obstetric Examination of Gravid Abdomen

Ensure that the bladder is empty before the obstetric examination. Examination of the pregnant abdomen is carried out with the examiner standing to the right side of the mother and must be gentle and careful.

During antenatal visits in second and third trimesters, growth of the gravid uterus is monitored by serial measurement of symphysis fundus height (SFH), which is the distance between the symphysis pubis and the superior border of the fundus. Foetal heart sounds are determined by Doptone examination; the foetal heart sounds may also be heard with a stethoscope after 32 weeks.

Generally, foetal parts are not well felt until 28–30 weeks gestation. From 32 weeks onwards, systematic examination of the gravid abdomen is conducted at each review, to inspect the general appearance of the abdomen, and also to determine the uterine size, foetal parts by palpation, followed by auscultation of foetal heart sounds.[1-4]

Inspection of obstetric abdomen

The following observations on abdominal appearance in pregnancy are made (see photos):

- Degree of abdominal enlargement and shape
- Linea nigra
- Striae gravidarum (new/old)
- Appearance of umbilicus
- Presence of any surgical scars

- Presence of dilated veins
- Any Braxton Hicks contractions
- Any foetal movements

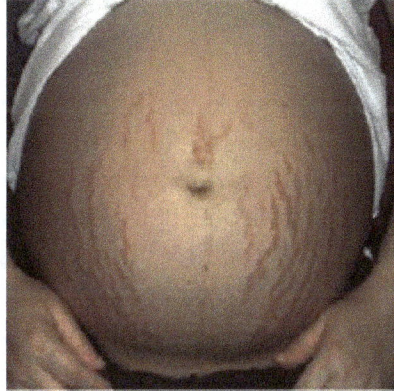

FIGURE 21.1 ■ Fresh striae gravidarum.

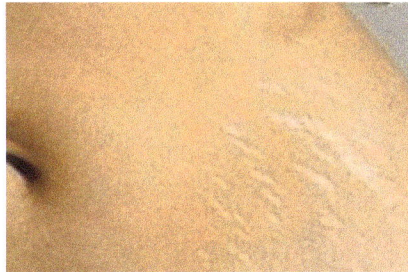

FIGURE 21.2 ■ Old striae gravidarum.

Palpation of gravid uterus (from 32 weeks onwards)

This is done in 4 steps (Modified Leopold and Sporlin's Manoeuvres) to ascertain the uterine size, foetal lie, foetal presentation, foetal back, foetal size, and liquor volume[5]:

- Step 1 Determination of uterine size (SFH)
  - (i) Ascertaining the highest point of uterine fundus
  - (ii) Measuring the symphysis fundal height

- Step 2 Palpation of presenting part and degree of engagement
- Step 3 Palpation of uterine fundus
- Step 4 Palpation of the sides of uterus

Step 1 Determination of uterine size and symphysis fundal height (SFH)

The uterine size is assessed by measuring the symphysis fundal height (SFH). The highest point of the uterine fundus in third trimester is usually situated over the right hypochodrium as a result of dextro-rotation of the gravid uterus. This is located by moving the left palm from the right coastal edge downwards until the radial border of the palm meets the first point of resistance, corresponding to the uppermost border of the uterine fundal wall (similar to movements in palpation of the liver edge), making sure not to reach the foetal parts which is lower than the uterine wall (Fig. 21.3).

The upper border of the symphysis pubis is next determined by feeling from

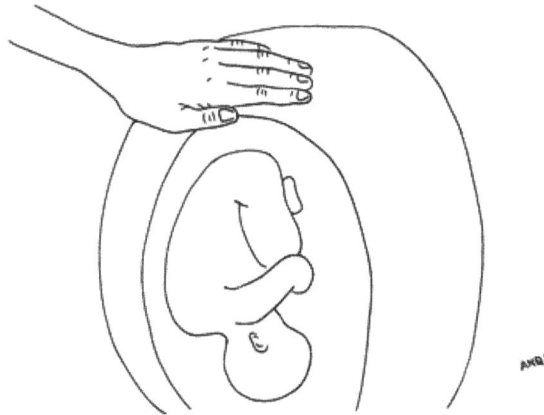

FIGURE 21.3 ■ Step 1 — Determination of uterine fundus.

the suprapubic area toward the pubic bone for the first bony prominence in the midline. The SFH is then measured by using a measuring tape from upper border of symphysis pubis to the uterine fundus (Fig. 21.4).

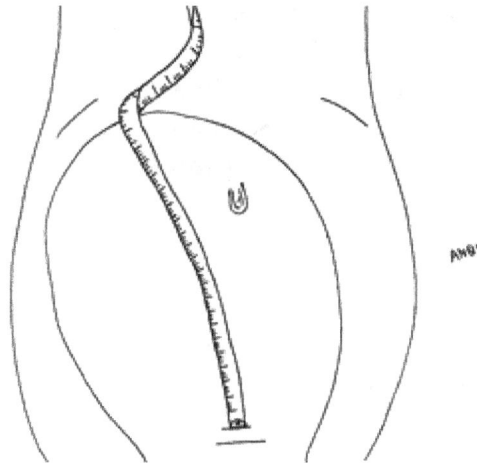

FIGURE 21.4 ■ Step 1 — Measurement of symphysis fundal height.

In general, from 16 to 36 weeks of gestation, the measured SFH in centimetres corresponds to gestational age ±2 cm (Table 20.1).

TABLE 21.1   Gestational Age Estimated from Symphysis Fundal Height

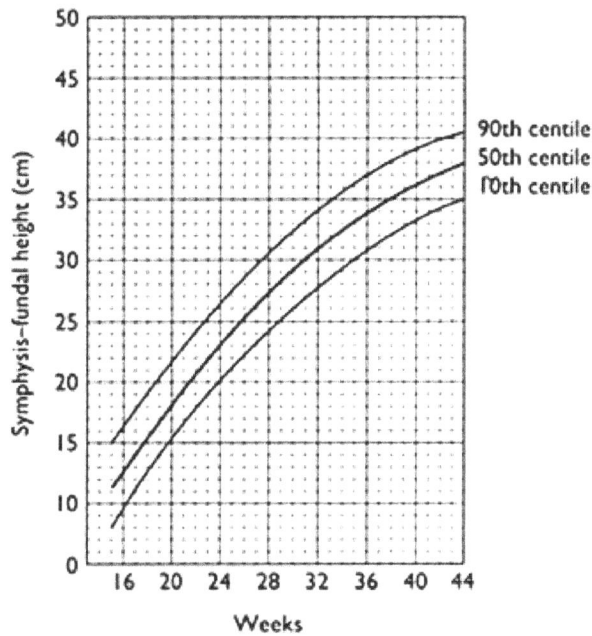

A measurement of SFH 2 cm more than expected for the given gestation can be suggestive of a macrosomic foetus, multiple pregnancy, polyhydramnios, maternal obesity, or an inaccurate estimated due date. Conversely, a measurement of 2 cm less than expected for gestation can be due to small for date foetus, oligohydramnios, foetus in oblique or transverse lie, or an inaccurate estimated due date.

Step 2 Palpation of presenting part and degree of engagement

This is done with the examiner facing the mother's feet, placing both hands on either side of the lower part of the uterus just above the symphysis pubis (with left hand on the patient's left side and right hand on the mother's right side) and pressing gently inwards to feel the presenting part between both palms. (Fig. 21.5)

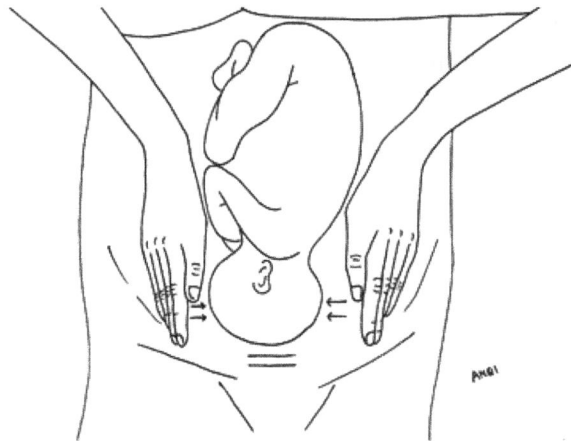

FIGURE 21.5 ■ Step 2 — Palpation of presenting part.

If the presenting part is the foetal head, the rounded structure can be balloted slightly from side to side by the fingers. Broad, irregular, firm foetal parts will indicate foetal buttocks, as seen in breech presentation.

The degree of engagement can then be assessed by moving the palms on both sides of the uterus towards the pelvic brim to ascertain the proportion of the presenting part felt above the brim.

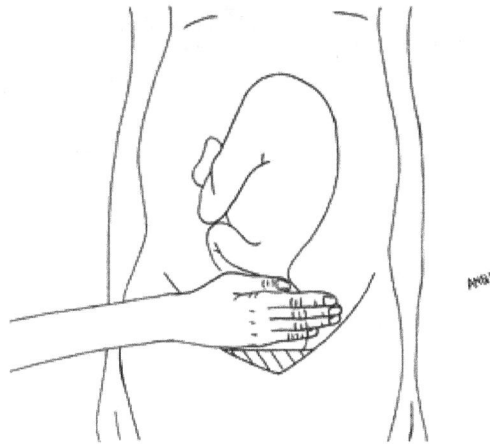

FIGURE 21.6 ■ Step 2 — Palpation of degree of engagement.

Alternatively, engagement of the presenting part may also be better assessed by putting the right palm centrally over the suprapubic area to feel the proportion of the foetal part above the brim (Fig. 21.6).

Degree of head engagement is quantified by arbitrarily dividing the foetal head into fifths — e.g. if only two-fifths or less of the head is palpable above the pelvic brim, the head is considered engaged into the pelvis i.e. the widest diameter of the head has descended into the pelvis. Serial assessment of foetal head engagement is an important part of monitoring the progression labour.

Pawlik's grip (using the thumb and index finger of the right hand, firmly grip the presenting foetal part between the fingers) for determination of presenting part and degree of engagement is strongly discouraged as it causes pain and discomfort to patient.

Step 3 Palpation of the uterine fundus

The fundal area is gently palpated with both palms, feeling for foetal parts at the upper pole, in an attempt to identify which pole of the foetus (head or breech) is occupying the fundus (Fig. 21.7).

Broad, irregular, firm foetal parts at the upper pole will indicate foetal buttocks, thus confirming cephalic presentation felt over the lower pole. With breech presentation, a ballotable rounded foetal head at the fundus will be found.

Step 4 Palpation of the sides of the uterus

Stabilising one side of the uterus with one palm, the examiner palpates the opposite side with the other palm and vice versa. Avoid palpating both sides of the uterus

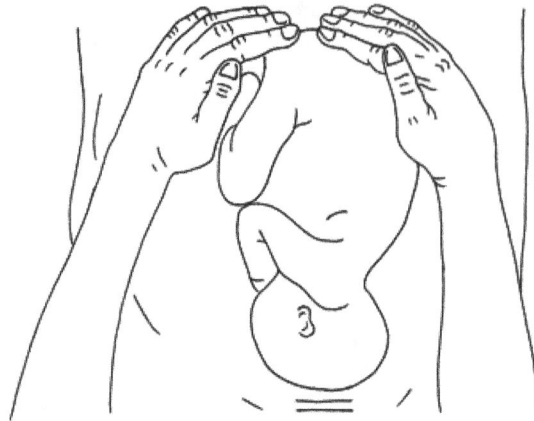

FIGURE 21.7 ■ Step 3 — Palpation of the uterine fundus.

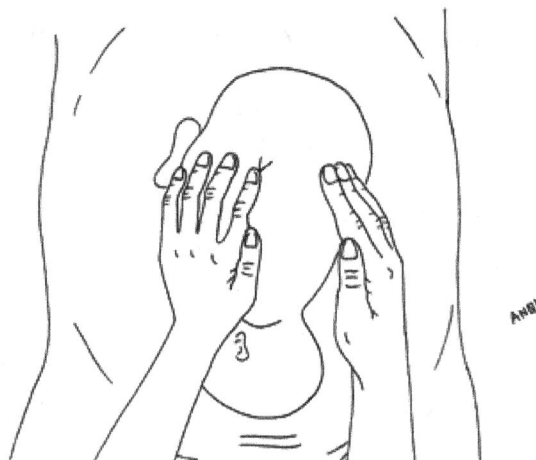

FIGURE 21.8 ■ Step 4 — Palpation of the sides of the uterus.

simultaneously as this may create uterine contractions and cause discomfort to patient (Fig. 21.8).

This step identifies on which side the smooth, firm back of the foetus or the knobbly limbs are, thus determining the foetal lie, the foetal back and approximate foetal size. It also allows the examiner to estimate the liquor volume by feeling for the liquor pockets surrounding the foetus, especially over the side of foetal limbs.

If there is an excessive amount of liquor (polyhydramnios), the uterus will be tense (with fluid thrills) and it will be quite difficult to feel for foetal parts. Conversely, if the liquor volume is reduced (oligohydramnios), the foetal outline and foetal parts are easily felt, with small fluid pockets felt between the foetal limbs.

Auscultation of foetal heart sound

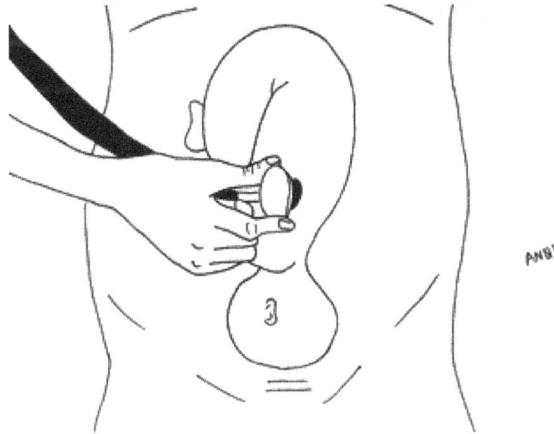

FIGURE 21.9 ■ Auscultation of foetal heart sound.

Foetal heart sound can be heard with Doptone (as gallop rhythms) from 12 weeks gestation and with stethoscope after 32 weeks. It is best heard over the anterior shoulder of the foetus (Fig. 21.9).

Foetal heart rate and regularity are recorded. Accelerations of heart rate associated with foetal movements are an indication of foetal health.

Presentation of Findings

Findings from palpation and auscultation of the abdomen are presented as follows:

- Symphysis fundal height (whether consistent with gestation)
- Number of foetuses
- Lie (longitudinal/transverse/oblique)
- Presentation (cephalic/breech/none)
- Degree of engagement
- Foetal back (maternal left/right)

- Foetal heart sound (location, regularity)
- Amount of liquor (normal/increased/decreased)
- Estimated foetal weight (kg)

References

1. Baker PN, Kenny Louise. (2011) *Obstetrics by Ten Teachers*, 19th edn.
2. Hanretty Kevin P. (2009) *Obstetrics Illustrated*, 7th edn.
3. Hacker NF, Gambore JC, Hobil CJ. (2010) *Essentials of Obstetrics and Gynaecology*, 5th edn.
4. Oats JN, Abraham S. (2010) *Llewellyn Jones Fundamentals of Obstetrics and Gynaecology*, 9th edn.
5. Leopold Sporlin. (1894) Conduct of normal births through external examination alone. *Arch Gynaekol* **45**:337.

22

ROUTINE ANTENATAL CARE

Chua Tsei Meng and Kuldip Singh

Introduction

The objective of antenatal care is to optimise obstetric outcomes for both the mother and the baby, i.e. the delivery of a healthy baby with minimal risk for the mother.

Regular antenatal care helps to identify and treat complications and to promote healthy behaviour. In addition to medical care, antenatal care includes counselling and education.[1-3]

First Antenatal Visit

History taking. to identify high risk factors. By identifying high risk pregnancies, it allows appropriate referral and co-management to achieve optimal obstetric outcomes.

The mother will be asked the following questions to identify risk factors:

- The date of the first day of her last period
- Her health
- Any previous illnesses and operations
- Any previous pregnancies and miscarriages
- Medication history and history of drug allergy
- Ethnic origins, to ascertain whether her baby is at risk of certain inherited conditions
- Her occupation

- Her emotional state
- Identify vulnerable situations that may require support, e.g. domestic abuse or violence

Look for past history of:

- Complications or infections in a previous pregnancy or delivery, such as pre-eclampsia or premature birth.
- Chronic disease, such as diabetes or high blood pressure.
- Family history of foetal abnormality, such as spina bifida.
- Family history of an inherited disease, such as sickle cell or cystic fibrosis.

Physical Examination

- Measurement of weight and body mass index:
  Maternal weight and height is measured at the booking appointment to calculate the woman's body mass index
- Check blood pressure
- Auscultate her heart and lungs
- Appropriate abdominal examination and pelvic examination

Ultrasound Scan for Dating

- Pregnant women are offered an early ultrasound scan in the first trimester to ensure that it is an intra-uterine pregnancy, check foetal viability, determine the gestational age and to detect multiple pregnancies.
- Ultrasound estimation of EDD is most accurate in the first trimester. The sonographically-derived EDD is used if it differs from that calculated using the LMP by more than five days in the first trimester of pregnancy.

Counselling

Pregnant mother will be provided with useful information on keeping healthy, to have a healthy pregnancy. She will be provided information about[4-5]:

Folic acid supplementation. Pregnant women will be informed that folic acid supplements, before conception and throughout the first 12 weeks, reduces the risk of having a baby with a neural tube defect. The recommended dose is 400 micrograms per day.

Lifestyle factors. that may affect her health or the health of her baby. Provide lifestyle advice, including smoking cessation, and the implications of recreational drug use and alcohol consumption in pregnancy.

Exercise advice. Pregnant women will be informed of the potential dangers of certain activities during pregnancy, for example: contact sports, high-impact sports and vigorous racquet sports that may involve the risk of abdominal trauma, falls or excessive joint stress, and scuba diving, which may result in foetal birth defects and foetal decompression disease.

Diet counselling. Provide information about nutrition, diet and food hygiene:

- Food hygiene, including how to reduce the risk of a food-acquired infection
- Pregnant women will be offered information on how to reduce the risk of **listeriosis** by:
  - Drinking only pasteurised milk
  - Avoiding eating ripened soft cheese such as Camembert, Brie and blue-veined cheese (there is no risk with hard cheeses, such as Cheddar, or cottage cheese and processed cheese)
  - Not eating pâté
  - Not eating uncooked or undercooked ready-prepared meals

Pregnant women should be offered information on how to reduce the risk of **salmonella** infection by:

- Avoiding raw or partially cooked eggs or food that may contain them (such as mayonnaise)
- Avoiding raw or partially cooked meat, especially poultry

Pregnant women will be informed of primary prevention measures to avoid **toxoplasmosis** infection, such as:

- Washing hands before handling food
- Thoroughly washing all fruit and vegetables, including ready-prepared salads, before eating
- Thoroughly cooking raw meats and ready-prepared chilled meals
- Wearing gloves and thoroughly washing hands after handling soil and gardening
- Avoid handling of cat faeces in cat litter or in soil

Prescribed medicines

- Few medicines have been established as safe to use in pregnancy.
- Prescription medicines should be used as little as possible during pregnancy and should be limited to circumstances in which the benefit outweighs the risk.

Over-the-counter medicines

- Pregnant women should be informed that few over-the-counter medicines have been established as being safe to take in pregnancy
- Over-the-counter medicines should be used as little as possible during pregnancy

Common symptoms of pregnancy

Inform patients of the possible common symptoms of pregnancy:

- Nausea and vomiting — occurs in 75–85% of pregnancies. It usually resolves spontaneously within 16–20 weeks. It is not usually associated with poor pregnancy outcome
- Heartburn — advise diet modification. Prescribe antacids if the symptom remains troublesome
- Constipation — diet modification
- Backache

Flu vaccination

During the flu season, pregnant mothers are recommended to receive flu vaccination as early as possible, regardless of the stage of pregnancy. Pregnant women are more likely to develop complications from flu, which can cause serious illness for both the mother and baby.

The flu vaccine will:

- Reduce her risk of serious complications, such as pneumonia, particularly in the later stages of pregnancy
- Reduce the risk of miscarriage or premature birth, stillbirth, or neonatal death
- Help protect the baby, which will continue to have some immunity to the flu during the first few months of its life

Screening Tests in Pregnancy

Screening tests are offered during pregnancy to identify any health problems that could affect the mother or her baby, such as infectious diseases, Down syndrome, or physical abnormalities.

Screening Tests Offered in Pregnancy

- Screening for haematological conditions
- Screening for infectious diseases (hepatitis B, HIV, syphilis, rubella)
- Screening for Down syndrome/chromosomal abnormalities
- Screening for abnormalities (foetal anomaly scan at 22 weeks)

Screening for haematological conditions

- *Full blood count*

Pregnant women are offered screening for anaemia. Screening should take place early in pregnancy when other blood screening tests are being performed. This allows enough time for treatment if anaemia is detected.

Haemoglobin levels outside the normal range for pregnancy (i.e. 11 g/100 ml at first contact) should be investigated and iron supplementation considered if indicated.

The **World Health Organization (WHO)** defines anaemia in pregnant women as haemoglobin <11 g/dL or hematocrit <6.83 mmol/L or 0.33 L/L (33%).

- *Blood grouping and red-cell alloantibodies*

Women are offered testing for blood group and rhesus D status early in pregnancy. Routine antenatal anti-D prophylaxis is offered to all non-sensitised pregnant women who are rhesus D-negative.

If a pregnant woman is rhesus D-negative, her partner is offered testing to determine whether the administration of anti-D prophylaxis is necessary.

<u>Blood group Rhesus negative mother</u>

Practice guidelines in the United States recommend administration of anti-D immune globulin to Rh(D)-negative pregnant women early in the third trimester, a single dose of 300 micrograms at 28 weeks of gestation. Other countries use a two dose regimen. For example, in the United Kingdom 100 micrograms of anti-D immune globulin are given at 28 and 34 weeks of gestation.

Women should be screened for atypical red-cell alloantibodies in early pregnancy and again at 28 weeks, regardless of their rhesus D status. Pregnant women with clinically significant atypical red-cell alloantibodies should be referred for further investigation and advice on subsequent antenatal management.

Screening for haemoglobinopathies

Screening for sickle cell diseases and thalassaemias is offered to all women as early as possible in pregnancy.

Screening for infectious disease

- *Hepatitis B virus*

Patient is offered serological screening for hepatitis B to allow effective postnatal interventions to decrease the risk of mother-to-child transmission.

- *HIV*

Pregnant women are offered screening for HIV infection early in antenatal care because appropriate antenatal interventions can reduce mother-to-child transmission of HIV infection.

Screening of HIV in pregnant women has proven substantially more effective than risk-based testing for detecting unsuspected maternal HIV infection and preventing perinatal transmission.

- *Rubella*

Rubella susceptibility screening is offered early to identify women who have not been immunised in childhood. This helps to identify women at risk of contracting rubella infection and to enable vaccination in the postnatal period for the protection of future pregnancies.

- *Syphilis*

Screening for syphilis is offered to all pregnant women at an early stage in antenatal care because treatment of syphilis is beneficial to the mother and baby.

T. pallidum crosses the placenta readily, resulting in foetal infection. Transplacental transmission can occur at any gestational age. The frequency of vertical transmission increases as gestation advances. But the severity of foetal infection decreases with infection as the pregnancy advances. Pregnancies complicated by untreated syphilis early in pregnancy are at increased risk of adverse outcomes: congenital infection and anomalies, intrauterine growth restriction, preterm birth, stillbirth and neonatal death.

Screening for Down syndrome and chromosomal abnormalities

- *Down syndrome*

A baby born with Down syndrome will have learning disability. The level of learning disability a baby has with Down syndrome can vary from mild to severe. Most cases of Down syndrome happen by chance. On rare occasions, it is inherited due to translocation.

Women of any age can have a baby with Down syndrome, although the chance of having a baby with the condition increases with age. The older a woman is, the more likely she is to have a baby with Down syndrome:

- A 20-year-old woman has a 1 in 1,500 chance of having a pregnancy affected by Down syndrome (this is a probability of 0.07%)
- A 30-year-old woman has a 1 in 900 chance of having a pregnancy affected by Down syndrome (a probability of 0.1%)
- A 40-year-old woman has a 1 in 100 chance of having a baby affected by Down syndrome (a probability of 1%)

These are background risks based on the woman's age alone.

- *Edwards' and Patau's syndromes*

Edwards' syndrome affects about 3 out of every 10,000 births.
Patau's syndrome affects about 2 out of every 10,000 births.

Anyone can have a baby with Edwards' or Patau's syndromes. The chance of having a baby with Edwards' or Patau's syndromes increases with age, so older mothers will have a higher chance of having a baby with these conditions.

All pregnant women are offered screening for Down syndrome, as well as tests for Edwards' and Patau's syndromes. It is their choice to embark on screening for Down syndrome.

For mothers younger than 35 years old, the "combined test" (nuchal translucency, beta-human chorionic gonadotrophin, pregnancy-associated plasma protein-A) is offered to screen for Down syndrome between 11 weeks 3 days and 13 weeks 6 days. The sensitivity of the test is 90% for Down syndrome with a false positive rate of 5%. (Refer to chapter on prenatal screening and diagnosis.)

Nuchal translucency (NT) measurement between 11 and 14 weeks gestation is a reliable marker for chromosomal abnormalities, including trisomy 21. Increased NT is associated with chromosomal anomalies and is a strong marker for adverse pregnancy outcomes such as miscarriage, intrauterine death, congenital heart defects and numerous other structural defects and genetic syndromes. (Refer to chapter on prenatal screening and diagnosis.)

- The result of the combined test is considered lower risk if the risk is less than 1 in 250.
- If the risk is between 1 in 250 and 1 in 1,000, it is considered intermediate risk, and the patient is offered non-invasive prenatal testing (NIPT).
- If the risk is 1 in 50 or higher, she is offered diagnostic tests of either amniocentesis or chorionic villous sampling.
- If the risk is between 1 in 50 and 1 in 250, she has the option of having NIPT or proceed with diagnostic test (amniocentesis or chorionic villous sampling).

For <u>mothers who are 35 years old or older</u>, the following options will be discussed with the mother:

Diagnostic tests: amniocentesis
Screening tests:

- First choice: **Non-invasive Prenatal Testing (NIPT) for Foetal Aneuploidy**
- Non-invasive prenatal testing uses cell-free foetal DNA from the plasma of pregnant women to screen for foetal aneuploidy. Cell-free foetal DNA allows the reliable non-invasive detection of trisomy 21 from maternal blood. (Refer to chapter on prenatal screening and diagnosis.)

Patients should be counselled with regards to the limitations of cell-free foetal DNA testing. They should be aware that:

- Cell-free foetal DNA testing should be an informed patient choice after pre-test counselling
- Patient has the option to choose no testing
- Cell-free foetal DNA test is a screening test with high sensitivity and specificity.
- The screening test provides information regarding only trisomy 21, trisomy 18 and trisomy 13. At the present time, it gives no other genetic information about the pregnancy
- It does not replace the precision obtained with diagnostic tests, such as chorionic villus sampling or amniocentesis, which remains an option for women
- A patient with a positive test result should be referred for genetic counselling and offered invasive prenatal diagnosis for confirmation of test results
- A negative cell-free foetal DNA test does not ensure an unaffected pregnancy. False-negative test results can occur as well
- A family history should be obtained before the use of this test to determine if the patient should be offered other forms of screening or prenatal diagnosis for familial genetic disease

Foetal anomaly scan

- *Ultrasound screening for foetal anomalies* is offered between 20–22 weeks.

  Patients should be informed of the limitations of routine ultrasound screening and that detection rates vary by the type of foetal anomaly.

- *Uterine artery* — Meta-analyses show that uterine artery Doppler analysis can predict women at increased risk of pre-eclampsia and intrauterine growth restriction. If the uterine arcuate resistance index is above 0.62, patient will be commenced on aspirin 100 mg daily until 35 weeks of gestation, if she has no known allergy to aspirin and no gastric problem.

Additional tests if indicated

- *Cervical length* — Patients with past history of preterm labour will be offered trans-vaginal measurement of cervical length. A shortened cervical length between 16 and 28 weeks of gestation is associated with an increased risk of spontaneous preterm birth <35 weeks. Cervical length can be measured when the patient undergoes ultrasound examination for foetal anomalies.
- Interventions with treatment of women with a short cervix with vaginal progesterone have reduced the rate of subsequent preterm birth. In some patients with a short cervix, cerclage or a cervical pessary may be effective.

Subsequent Antenatal Visits

The frequency of antenatal visits depends whether it is a low- or high-risk pregnancy. If the pregnancy is uncomplicated and the mother is in good health, the patient may not be seen as often as someone who needs to be more closely monitored.

In these antenatal visits:

- Urine test and blood pressure and weight measurement
- Check foetal growth by measuring symphyseal-fundal height
- Abdominal palpation to check the foetal lie and presentation
- Auscultation of the foetal heart
- Foetal movement counting: patient is advised to monitor foetal movement. If the foetal movements become reduced, they are advised to contact the hospital.
- All pregnant women will be provided with opportunity to discuss issues and ask questions.

Foetal Growth Scan at 32 weeks of Gestation

- To assess foetal growth and development
- To check amniotic fluid volume, foetal presentation and placental location

Monitor foetal growth in high risk pregnancy

- Ultrasound assessment of foetal growth is indicated in the third trimester in pregnancies at increased risk of foetal growth restriction
- If IUGR, offer close monitoring of foetal well-being
- Early identification of growth-restricted foetuses allows for closer surveillance and earlier intervention

Patient Education in Preparation for Labour and Delivery

Patient will be provided with the following information:

- The process of labour
- Pain relief in labour
- Recognition of active labour
- Breastfeeding
- Screening tests for newborn babies

Antenatal classes or parental craft classes can help to prepare the woman for delivery and learn how to look after and feed her baby. They help her to stay healthy during pregnancy, provide information and give her confidence.

Screening for Gestational Diabetes Mellitus (GDM)

- Screening for gestational diabetes is recommended at 24 to 28 weeks of gestation in patients with risk factors for GDM. First trimester screening is offered to patients with significant risk factors (e.g. body mass index >30 kg/m^2, gestational diabetes or baby >3,500 g in a prior pregnancy, family history of diabetes in a first-degree relative).
- At the booking appointment, the following risk factors for gestational diabetes should be determined. Women with any one of these risk factors should be offered testing for gestational diabetes:
  - Body mass index above 30 kg/m^2
  - Previous macrosomic baby weighing 3.5 kg or above

- Past history of gestational diabetes
- Family history of diabetes (first-degree relative with diabetes)
- Family origin with a high prevalence of diabetes: South Asian specifically women whose country of family origin is India, Pakistan or Bangladesh, black Caribbean, Middle Eastern

In order to allow a pregnant woman to make an informed decision about screening and testing for gestational diabetes, she will be informed that:

- 85% of women with gestational diabetes will respond to changes in diet and exercise
- 15% of them will need oral hypoglycaemic agents or insulin therapy if diet and exercise are not effective in controlling gestational diabetes
- If gestational diabetes is not detected and controlled there is an increased risk of birth complications, such as shoulder dystocia

Screening for Pre-eclampsia

- Blood pressure measurement and urinalysis for protein is carried out at each antenatal visit to screen for pre-eclampsia.
- At the booking appointment, the following risk factors for pre-eclampsia should be determined:
  - Age 40 years or older
  - Nulliparity
  - Family history of pre-eclampsia
  - Previous history of pre-eclampsia
  - Body mass index 30 kg/m^2 or above
  - Pre-existing vascular disease, such as hypertension
  - Pre-existing renal disease
  - Multiple pregnancy
- Pregnant women with any of the above risk factors will require more frequent blood pressure monitoring. They will be started on oral aspirin to reduce the risk of pre-eclampsia
- Women with significant hypertension and/or proteinuria will require increased surveillance
- Pregnant women should be made aware of the need to seek immediate advice if they experience symptoms of pre-eclampsia. Symptoms include:
  - Severe headache
  - Problems with vision, such as blurring or flashing before the eyes
  - Severe pain just below the ribs
  - Vomiting
  - Sudden swelling of the face, hands or feet

Group B Beta-Haemolytic Streptococcus Testing

- All pregnant women are offered screening for group B beta-haemolytic strepto-coccus (GBS) colonisation at 35 to 37 weeks with high vaginal swab.
- Intra-partum chemoprophylaxis of colonised women has been proven to reduce the incidence of early-onset neonatal GBS
- Patients who had GBS bacteriuria earlier in the current pregnancy or those who gave birth to a previous infant with invasive GBS disease are excluded from screening and they will receive intra-partum antibiotic prophylaxis regardless of the colonisation status.

37 to 42 Weeks of Gestation

- Weekly antenatal visits
- Foetal presentation is assessed by abdominal palpation because the presenta-tion will affect the mode of delivery
- From 40 weeks, women are offered antenatal foetal monitoring consisting of cardiotocography and ultrasound assessment of amniotic fluid index and Doppler blood flow studies

Women with uncomplicated pregnancies are offered induction of labour at 41 weeks plus 3 days of gestation.

References

1. National Collaborating Centre for Women's and Children's Health. (2014) *Antenatal Care: Routine Antenatal Care for the Healthy Pregnant Woman*. United Kingdom.
2. Hanretty KP. (2009) *Obstetrics Illustrated*, 7th edn.
3. Baker PN, Kenny L. (2011) *Obstetrics by Ten Teachers*, 19th edn.
4. Chamberlain G, Bowen Simpkins P. (2000) *A Practice of Obstetrics and Gynaecology: A Textbook for General Practice and DRCOG*.
5. Howell M. (2009) *Effective Birth Preparation Your Journey Guide to Better Birth*.

23

HYPERTENSIVE DISORDERS OF PREGNANCY

Pradip Dashraath and Claudia Chi

Introduction

Hypertensive disorders of pregnancy affect approximately 10% of all pregnant women worldwide. Whilst the latest report on Confidential Enquiries into Maternal Deaths in the UK concludes that mortality from pre-eclampsia and eclampsia is now at its lowest (at 0.49 per 100,000), it remains one of the leading causes of maternal and perinatal morbidity and mortality in much of Asia, Latin America and the African subcontinent.[1]

In Singapore, the incidence of pre-eclampsia is approximately 3.6% and has remained relatively static over the last half century. Conversely, the incidence of eclampsia has steadily declined and is attributable, in part, to the provision of evidence-based maternity care.[2]

How are Hypertensive Disorders of Pregnancy Classified?

The International Society for the Study of Hypertension in Pregnancy (ISSHP) and the National Institute of Clinical Excellence (NICE) Guidelines broadly stratify pregnant women with hypertension into the following categories[3]:

TABLE 23.1   Classification of Hypertensive Disorder of Pregnancy

(A) **Chronic hypertension**. Refers to hypertension present before 20 weeks' gestation and may be primary or secondary in aetiology.

(B) **Gestational hypertension**. Refers to onset of hypertension after 20 weeks' gestation *without* significant proteinuria. Also known as pregnancy-induced hypertension (PIH)

(C) **Pre-eclampsia**. Refers to onset of hypertension after 20 weeks' gestation *with* significant proteinuria (24-hour urine total protein >0.3 g/day or a spot urine protein:creatinine ratio >30 mg/mmol).

  • **Severe pre-eclampsia** is pre-eclampsia with severe hypertension with/without symptoms of impending eclampsia, haematological or biochemical impairment.

(D) **Chronic hypertension with superimposed pre-eclampsia**.

(E) **Eclampsia**. Refers to seizures associated with pre-eclampsia.

TABLE 23.2   Classification of Hypertension Severity in Pregnancy

Category	Systolic BP (mmHg)	Diastolic BP (mmHg)
Mild hypertension	140–149	90–99
Moderate hypertension	150–159	100–109
Severe hypertension	>160	>110

Why is gestational hypertension and pre-eclampsia only diagnosed after 20 weeks' gestation?

This is because the second wave of cytotrophoblastic invasion occurs between 16–20 weeks' gestation (see "Pathophysiology" below)

Pathophysiology

Pre-eclampsia is fundamentally mediated by placental anti-angiogenic factors (hence the older term, toxemia of pregnancy).

In normal pregnancy, cytotrophoblast invasion into spiral arteries in the placenta causes remodelling of the latter into high calibre, low resistance vessels. This allows for an optimal uteroplacental circulation. Soluble *pro-angiogenic* factors (VEGF, PLGF, TGF-β1) then maintain patency of these vessels.

In pre-eclampsia, cytotrophoblast invasion is shallow and placental vessels remain small calibre and high resistance resulting in placental ischemia. The ischemic placenta releases *anti-angiogenic* factors (sFLT-1 and sEng) which inhibit the activity of pro-angiogenic growth factors. These anti-angiogenic factors enter the systemic circulation and cause widespread endothelial dysfunction, accounting for the clinical features of pre-eclampsia.

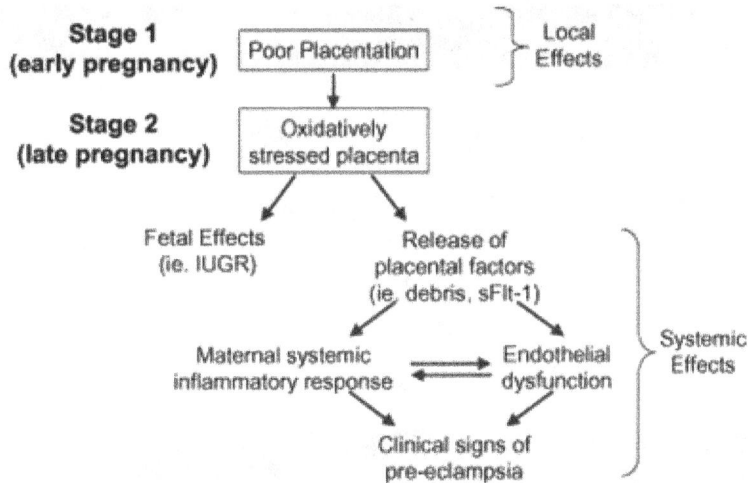

FIGURE 23.1 ■ Pathophysiology of pre-eclampsia.

Risk Factors

Risk factors for developing pre-eclampsia may be based on (i) Clinical history or (ii) Radiological findings.

Clinical Risk Factors

Risk Factor	Increased Risk of Pre-eclampsia
Age	>40 years of age
Family History	If mother or sister had pre-eclampsia
Body Mass Index (BMI)	BMI >35
Medical Co-morbidities	Increased risk in the presence of the following: (i) Pre-existing hypertension (ii) Pre-existing and gestational diabetes mellitus (iii) Connective tissue disease e.g., SLE
Obstetric factors	Primiparity Multiple pregnancy Previous pre-eclampsia

Radiological Risk Factors

Abnormal uterine artery Doppler (raised resistance with notching) is associated with increased risk of developing pre-eclampsia as it serves as a sonographic marker of poor placental perfusion which is fundamental in the pathophysiology of the disease.

Clinical Features of Disease

(1) **Weight gain**. Sudden and excessive weight gain may be the first sign of pre-eclampsia and is attributed to fluid retention.
(2) **Blood pressure**. Rise in the blood pressure is the most significant sign of pre-eclampsia with a persistent diastolic pressure of >90 mmHg.
(3) **Proteinuria**. Proteinuria of >2+ on a urine dipstick when coupled with high blood pressure is a red flag and behooves exclusion of pre-eclampsia.
(4) **Deep tendon reflexes**. Hyper-reflexia.

Investigations

The diagnostic workup in pre-eclampsia is targeted at (i) assessing the degree of proteinuria; and (ii) evaluating for complications of severe disease.

(A) Assessment of Proteinuria

24-hour urine total protein	>0.3 gm/day is diagnostic
Spot urine protein: creatinine ratio	>30 mg/mmol is diagnostic

(B) Evaluation for Complications

Full blood count	(i) Anaemia and thrombocytopenia — HELLP syndrome
	(ii) Raised haematocrit — hypovolemia
Liver function test	(i) Transaminitis — HELLP syndrome
	(ii) Raised LDH — haemolytic anaemia in HELLP
	(iii) Unconjugated hyperbilirubinemia — as above
Coagulation profile	(i) Raised PT/PTT/INR — DIVC
Renal panel	(i) Decreased renal function — worsening disease
Serum uric acid level	(i) Raised uric acid — reduced renal clearance
Foetal ultrasound	(i) Intra-uterine growth restriction
	(ii) Oligohydramnios ⎤ Signs of uteroplacental insufficiency
	(iii) Abnormal Dopplers ⎦

Clinical Consequences

The underlying pathological changes in pre-eclampsia affect both mother and foetus resulting in maternal and perinatal morbidity. The clinically significant complications of severe pre-eclampsia and their pathophysiological correlations are considered below:

(A) Maternal Complications

(1) Neurological
The patient may develop

- **eclampsia** as a result of hypertensive encephalopathy causing cerebral oedema and consequently, grand-mal seizures;
- **intra-cerebral haemorrhage** (ICH) as a result of hypertensive encephalopathy (ICH accounts for the most common cause of death in pre-eclampsia) and
- **temporary blindness (amaurosis)** as a result of focal oedema in the occipital lobe causing cortical blindness (posterior reversible encephalopathy syndrome).

(2) Cardiopulmonary
The patient may develop

- **acute pulmonary oedema** as a result of decreased plasma oncotic pressure (from hypoalbuminemia) and increased hydrostatic pressure and
- **hypertensive cardiomyopathy** as a result of diastolic dysfunction.

(3) Renal
The patient may develop

- **acute renal failure** as a result of intravascular volume depletion (pre-renal azotemia) and/or intrinsic renal failure secondary to glomerular capillary damage (glomerulocapillary endotheliosis).

(4) Hematological
The patient may develop

- **disseminated intravascular coagulopathy** (DIVC) as a result of fibrin activation and decreased fibrinolysis.

(5) Biochemical
The patient may develop

- the syndrome of **hemolytic anemia, low platelets and elevated liver enzymes** (HELLP) as a result of microangiopathy and hepatic ischemia secondary to vasospasm and fibrin deposition from endothelial dysfunction.

(B) Fetoplacental Complications

(1) **Hypoxia**

Vasoconstriction results in **uteroplacental insufficiency** which may be (a) acute, leading to foetal distress and in-utero foetal demise or (b) chronic, leading to intrauterine growth restriction (IUGR).

(2) **Placental abruption**

Vasoconstriction results in placental ischemia which predisposes to premature separation of the placenta (placental abruption).

Management of Pre-eclampsia

The aim in the management of pre-eclampsia is to balance the needs of both foetus and mother with a view to optimize the outcome for each.[4,5] The principles are as follows:

(A) Management of Maternal Condition

(1) **Blood pressure control**
   - Start anti-hypertensive medications in the presence of severe hypertension (BP >160/100 mmHg or MAP >125 mmHg). Various institution specific protocols exist.
   - Oral labetolol is generally regarded as first-line, with recourse to parenteral agents if uncontrolled. The medications used for blood pressure control are shown in Table 23.3.

(2) **Monitor for signs of severe disease**
   - Obtain a baseline assessment of biochemical and haematological parameters on admission.
   - Trend these investigations at least twice weekly with a view to delivery should severe disease (e.g. HELLP syndrome) develop.

(3) **Evaluate the need for magnesium sulphate**
   - $MgSO_4$ is used in the prophylaxis against eclamptic seizures and is started in women with evidence of severe disease (Table 23.4). Once initiated however, attention should be directed towards delivery within the next 24 hours.

TABLE 23.3 Anti-Hypertensive Medications used in the Management of Gestational Hypertension and Pre-Eclampsia

Medication	Mechanism of Action	Effects on Cardiac Output	Side Effects
Labetolol	α and β adrenergic blocker	Unchanged	Flushing and headache. Contraindicated in asthma or heart failure
Nifedipine	Calcium channel blocker	Unchanged	Orthostatic hypotension and headache
Hydralazine	Direct peripheral vasodilator	Increased	Flushing and headache. Contraindicated in severe mitral regurgitation or left ventricular outflow tract obstruction
Methyldopa	False neurotransmission	Unchanged	Fever, lethargy, transaminitis and haemolytic anaemia

(B) Management of Foetal Condition

(1) **Corticosteroids for lung maturity.** Pre-eclampsia is one of the leading causes of iatrogenic prematurity. If delivery is considered likely within 7-days in women between 24–34 weeks gestation, a two-dose regime of intramuscular (IM) dexamethasone 12 mg 12-hours apart is given to promote foetal lung maturity and reduce the risk of respiratory distress syndrome at birth.

(2) **Foetal monitoring**
   - Consideration are made for serial assessment of amniotic fluid index and umbilical artery Doppler velocimetry weekly and foetal growth every 3-weekly.
   - When in labour, continuous foetal monitoring via cardiotocography (CTG) is recommended.

TABLE 23.4 Features of Severe Pre-eclampsia

Signs and symptoms	(i) Headache (ii) Blurred vision, scintillating scotoma or amaurosis (iii) Epigastric tenderness (iv) Hyper-reflexia and clonus (>3 beats) (v) Treatment recalcitrant severe hypertension
Investigations	(i) HELLP syndrome (ii) Worsening thrombocytopenia (platelet $<100 \times 10^9/\text{L}$) (iii) Worsening transaminitis (ALT or AST >70 IU/L)

Labour and Delivery

The following are pertinent considerations regarding delivery in a patient with pre-eclampsia:

  (i) **Timing of delivery.** Patients with severe pre-eclampsia must be delivered as soon as possible and preferably after completion of corticosteroids if between 24–34 weeks' gestation. Patients without severe features of disease are delivered from 37 weeks' gestation.
 (ii) **Mode of delivery.** Vaginal delivery is not contraindicated and caesarean section is reserved for the usual obstetric indications.
(iii) **Use of regional anesthesia.** Epidural and spinal analgesia are relatively contraindicated if maternal platelet counts are $<75 \times 10^9$/L due to the risk of neuraxial haematoma and paralysis.
(iv) **Postpartum haemorrhage prophylaxis.** Ergometrine is contraindicated as it may precipitate a hypertensive crisis.

Future Pregnancy Implications

  (i) **Risk of recurrence.** Women should be counseled that their risk of developing hypertensive disorders in the subsequent pregnancy is as follows:

Category	Future risk of gestational hypertension	Future risk of pre-eclampsia
Gestational hypertension	50%	5%
Pre-eclampsia	50%	15%
Severe pre-eclampsia <34 weeks GA	—	25%
Severe pre-eclampsia <28 weeks GA	—	55%

 (ii) **Role of aspirin.** Low-dose aspirin (75 mg/day) started before 16 weeks gestation until birth is recommended for women with history of pre-eclampsia in subsequent pregnancies as this has been shown to reduce the risk of recurrent disease.

Eclampsia

Eclampsia is a serious complication of pre-eclampsia and is an obstetric emergency with high maternal and perinatal morbidity and mortality.

It presents as a generalsied tonic-clonic seizure as a result of ischemic cerebral hypoxia from oedema and intense vasospasm. There is no urinary or bowel incontinence.

When seizures occur, attention must be given to:

- Protecting the maternal airway, breathing and circulation by way of supplemental oxygen and turning the patient to the left lateral position.
- The seizure must then be aborted with magnesium sulphate using the Collaborative Eclampsia Trial regimen with a loading dose of 4 g given intravenously over 5 minutes, followed by an infusion of 1 g/hour maintained for 24 hours. Recurrent seizures should be treated with a further dose of 2–4 g given over 5 minutes. If the foetus is still *in utero*, delivery must be expedited.
- Other anticonvulsants, such as diazepam and phenytoin, are rarely used as they are not as effective and have potential adverse effects on the foetus.
- All women on magnesium sulphate should be catheterised for strict monitoring of urine output (as it is renally excreted) and
- Examined frequently for signs of magnesium toxicity. Therapeutic levels of $MgSO_4$ are 4 to 6 mg/dL with toxic concentrations having predictable consequences (Table 23.5).

TABLE 23.5   Features of Magnesium Sulphate Toxicity

Serum Concentration (mg/dL)	Clinical Manifestation
1.5–3	Normal concentration
4–6	Therapeutic concentration
5–10	ECG changes: Increased PR and QT intervals
8–12	Hyporeflexia, flushing, somnolence and slurred speech
15–17	Muscle paralysis and desaturation
30	Cardiac arrest

Magnesium sulphate toxicity is reversed with 10 ml of 10% calcium gluconate administered as a slow intravenous bolus over 10 minutes, alongside supplemental oxygen and cardiorespiratory support if required.

- Control of blood pressure using oral or parenteral medication as shown in Table 23.3.
- Terminate the pregnancy at any gestation by the most suitable method in the interest of the mother.

Chronic Hypertension

Chronic hypertension in pregnancy is defined as the presence of hypertension before 20 weeks gestation or hypertension present before pregnancy, which may either be primary (essential hypertension) or secondary.

The main concern with chronic hypertension is the high risk of developing superimposed pre-eclampsia or eclampsia as the pregnancy progresses.

TABLE 23.6   Secondary Causes of Chronic Hypertension

Organ system	Aetiology
Cardiovascular	(i) Coarctation of the aorta — unequal pulses
Renal	(i) Renal artery stenosis — abdominal bruit
Endocrine	(i) Cushing's syndrome — central adiposity and hirsutism
	(ii) Hyperthyroidism — goiter, tachycardia and weight loss
	(iii) Hyperaldosteronism — muscle weakness
	(iv) Phaeochromocytoma — flushing and diaphoresis

The principles of management of chronic hypertension in pregnancy therefore involve close monitoring of maternal blood pressure and proteinuria for acute worsening and monitoring of the foetus for appropriate growth.

Maternal

- Stop ACE-I, ARB and hydrochlorothiazide preconception as these are teratogenic.
- Advise home BP monitoring with an appropriately sized cuff.
- Start antihypertensive therapy if BP persistently >150/100 mmHg. Options include methyldopa, labetolol or nifedipine.
- Measure serum creatinine and obtain 24-hour urine collection at booking for baseline assessment of renal function and proteinuria.
- Start aspirin prior to 16 weeks gestation to reduce the risk of superimposed pre-eclampsia.

- Assess blood pressure and urine dipstick for proteinuria at every antenatal visit; superimposed pre-eclampsia is diagnosed when there is an acute worsening of BP and degree of proteinuria.

Foetal

- Obtain serial ultrasound assessments of foetal growth, amniotic fluid index and Dopplers as IUGR, oligohydramnios and raised uterine artery resistance indices are surrogate markers of uteroplacental insufficiency in the setting of chronic hypertension.

Labour and Delivery

- **Timing of delivery**
  Consider Delivery from 37 weeks of gestation unless superimposed pre-eclampsia warrants earlier delivery.
- **Mode of delivery**
  Vaginal delivery is not contraindicated and caesarean section is reserved for the usual obstetric indication.

References

1. Knight M, Tuffnell D, Kenyon S, *et al.* (eds.) on behalf of MBRRACE-UK. (2015) Saving lives, improving mothers' care — Surveillance of maternal deaths in the UK 2011–13 and lessons learned to inform maternity care from the UK and Ireland. Confidential Enquiries into Maternal Deaths and Morbidity 2009–13. Oxford: National Perinatal Epidemiology Unit, University of Oxford.
2. Kwek K, Yeo GS. (2006) Epidemiology of pre-eclampsia and eclampsia at the KK Women's and Children's Hospital, Singapore. *Singapore Med J* **47**(1): 48–53.
3. National Institute for Health and Care Excellence (NICE) Guideline 107. (2010) Hypertension in pregnancy: The management of hypertensive disorders in pregnancy.
4. American College of Obstetricians and Gynecologists. (2002) Diagnosis and management of preeclampsia and eclampsia. ACOG Practice Bulletin No. 33. *Obstet Gynecol* **99**(1):159–167.
5. World Health Organization (WHO). (2011) WHO recommendation for prevention and treatment of pre-eclampsia and eclampsia. Available from http://apps.who.int/iris/bitstream/10665/44703/1/9789241548335_eng.pdf.

24

DIABETES IN PREGNANCY

Pradip Dashraath and Claudia Chi

Introduction

Diabetes mellitus is the most commonly encountered medical condition in pregnancy. It may be present either before pregnancy (pre-existing diabetes mellitus) or develops during the course of pregnancy (gestational diabetes mellitus GDM).[1,2]

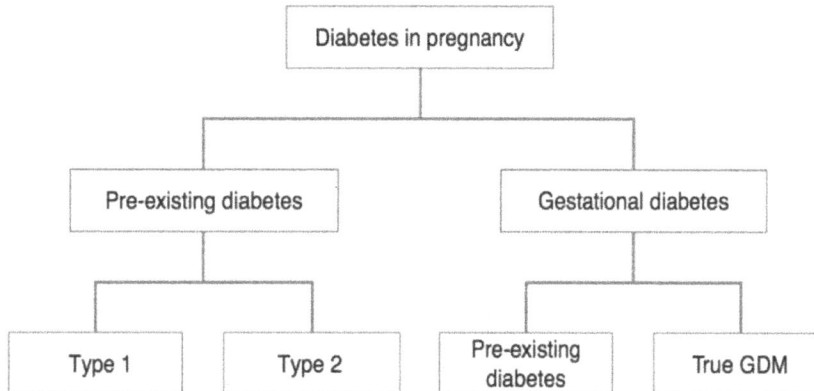

```
                    Diabetes in pregnancy
                            |
          +-----------------+-----------------+
          |                                   |
  Pre-existing diabetes             Gestational diabetes
          |                                   |
    +-----+-----+                      +-------+-------+
    |           |                      |               |
  Type 1      Type 2            Pre-existing        True GDM
                                 diabetes
```

The fundamental principle in the management of diabetes in pregnancy is to achieve euglycaemia, so as to attenuate the maternal and foetal complications associated with hyperglycaemia[3] (Tables 24.1 and 24.2). Appropriate management with diet modification accompanied by appropriate regular exercise and in certain cases, the addition of insulin therapy, can help to lower the risk of developing perinatal complications.

TABLE 24.1   Maternal Complications of Diabetes Mellitus

Effect of diabetes on pregnancy	(i) Increased risk of pre-eclampsia
	(ii) Increased risk of infection such as urinary tract infections, pyelonephritis and vulvovaginal candidiasis
	(iii) Increased risk of operative delivery/Caesarean section
Effect of pregnancy on diabetes	(i) Increased risk of progression of diabetic retinopathy
	(ii) Worsening proteinuria and oedema; deterioration of pre-existing diabetic nephropathy
	(iii) Worsening of glycaemic control and increased insulin requirements due to antagonistic effect of human placental lactogen, glucagon and cortisol (all of which are increased in pregnancy)
	(iv) Increased risk of ketoacidosis in the presence of hyperemesis, infection, corticosteroid therapy
	(v) Paradoxical predisposition to hypoglycaemia as a result of both intensified glycaemic control and hypoglycaemia unawareness from autonomic neuropathy

TABLE 24.2   Foetal and Neonatal Complications of Diabetes Mellitus

	Effect of Hyperglycaemia
First trimester (i) Miscarriage (ii) Organogenesis	(i) Increased risk of miscarriage: (ii) Increased risk of congenital abnormalities
Second and third trimester (i) Foetal growth	(i) Increased risk of accelerated foetal growth and macrosomia as hyperglycaemia stimulates secondary foetal hyperinsulinaemia, which promotes fat disposition including intra-abdominal fat
	(ii) Increased risk of polyhydramnios predisposing to preterm delivery
(ii) Lung maturation	(i) Hyperinsulinaemia delays lung maturation by inhibiting surfactant proteins, increasing the risk of distress syndrome in the newborn
(iii) Stillbirth	(i) Increased risk of chronic foetal hypoxia and of sudden unexplained intrauterine death
Delivery (i) Birth trauma	(i) Foetal macrosomia increases the risk of shoulder dystocia, birth trauma and asphyxia
Neonate (i) Hypoglycaemia	(i) Foetal hyperinsulinaemia predisposes to neonatal hypoglycaemia

(*Continued*)

TABLE 24.2 (*Continued*)

	Effect of Hyperglycaemia
(ii) Polycythaemia	(ii) Foetal hyperinsulinaemia promotes antepartum extramedullary haematopoiesis. Polycythaemia in turn increases the risk of neonatal jaundice
Adolescence/ adulthood	
(i) Obesity and type 2 diabetes mellitus	(i) Intrauterine exposure may predispose to metabolic syndrome and type 2 diabetes mellitus later in life independent of genetic susceptibility by way of metabolic programming (Barker hypothesis)

Management of Pre-Existing Diabetes in Pregnancy

The structured, multidisciplinary approach to the management of pre-existing diabetes in pregnancy is discussed below.

Pre-Conception Counselling

Physicians caring for women with diabetes who are contemplating pregnancy should refer these patients to a High Risk Pregnancy Clinic for pre-conception counselling. This is to allow for optimisation of glycaemic control prior to conception, as well as assessment for the presence and severity of antecedent diabetic complications. It is also an opportunity to discuss the potential complications in pregnancy associated with diabetes in pregnancy and the ways to reduce these complications.

(A) *Glycaemic control*

Women should be counselled that good glycaemic control and lower HbA1c levels reduce the risk of congenital anomalies in the foetus and the risk of pre-eclampsia, and are associated with improved perinatal outcomes. It is recommended that HbA1c should be less than 6.1% at the time of conception if this can be achieved safely. The frequency of home blood glucose monitoring will need to be increased to achieve better glycaemic control.

(B) *Review medications*

It is recommended for all women with pre-existing diabetes mellitus to take peri-conception folic acid (5 mg/day) for the prevention of neural tube defects.

In general, women on oral hypoglycaemic agents are switched to insulin during pregnancy for tighter glycaemic control; however, the latest evidence supports the use of metformin as an adjunct or alternative to insulin.

Women on angiotensin-converting enzyme inhibitors (ACE-I) and angiotensin-receptor blockers (ARBs) should have these medications stopped and changed to suitable alternatives due to the potential for teratogenicity.

(C) *Screen for diabetic complications*

The risk of diabetic micro- and macrovascular complications increases with the duration of the disease and, as outlined previously, may be exacerbated by pregnancy.

All women with pre-existing diabetes should have:

- A baseline ophthalmological assessment for diabetic retinopathy if their annual assessment was more than 6 months ago; this is repeated at 28 weeks' gestational age (GA) if the first assessment is normal, or at 16–20 weeks' GA if there is evidence of antecedent retinopathy.
- Baseline assessment of renal function — serum urea and creatinine, degree of proteinuria (spot urine protein:creatinine ratio or 24-hour urine total protein collection). NICE Guidelines recommend referral to a nephrologist if serum creatinine is >120 µg/L or proteinuria >2 g/day. The risk of pre-eclampsia is increased in the presence of microalbuminuria (30–300 mg/day), albeit to a lesser degree compared to frank nephrotic syndrome (>300 mg/day).[4]
- A baseline assessment of diabetic autonomic neuropathy.

(D) *Screen for non-diabetic complications*

Women with type 2 diabetes are more likely to harbour features of the metabolic syndrome including obesity, hypertension and hyperlipidaemia. Obesity in itself is a risk factor for late stillbirth, birth trauma and maternal complications postpartum such as postpartum haemorrhage. Weight reduction and optimisation of body mass index in obese women prior to pregnancy would reduce the risks of these complications.

Antepartum Management

Multidisciplinary management of women with diabetes in pregnancy is recommended and should involve the obstetrician, endocrinologist, diabetic nurse and dietician.

(A) *Early dating ultrasound*

Women with diabetes should receive a dating scan in the first trimester to assess the viability of the pregnancy and obtain an accurate gestational age. Ultrasonography performed later in a diabetic pregnancy is less accurate as feotal growth restriction or acceleration may be present.

(B) *Prevention of pre-eclampsia*

Women with pre-existing diabetes should be advised to take daily low-dose (75 mg) aspirin from 12 weeks gestation to reduce the risk of developing pre-eclampsia during pregnancy.

(C) *Screening for congenital abnormalities*

Women with pre-existing diabetes should receive an early foetal anomaly scan between 18–20 weeks' gestation to assess for major congenital abnormalities, particularly of the spine, kidneys and heart. This is repeated between 21–24 weeks' gestation, paying close attention to the four-chamber view of the heart and ventricular outflow tracts.

(D) *Assessment of foetal growth*

An assessment of foetal growth and liquor volume at the end of the second trimester and thereafter every 4 weeks is recommended for women with pre-existing diabetes. Diabetic pregnancies are predisposed to macrosomia and polyhydramnios as a result of foetal hyperinsuli-naemia.

Growth restriction in the setting of a diabetic pregnancy, however, is a red-flag and implicates: (i) intervening pre-eclampsia, (ii) hyperglycaemia-induced toxic placental senescence, (iii) diabetic macrovascular disease of the placenta, or a combination of these factors. Regardless of the aetiology, growth restriction serves as a harbinger of uteroplacental insufficiency with its attendant risk of in-utero foetal demise.

(E) *Optimisation of glycaemic control*

It is an important clinical point to note that in pregnancy, excess maternal glucose is preferentially transferred across the placenta rather than being peripherally metabolised. It is recommended to optimise glycaemic control in pregnancy by aiming to achieve the glucose limits as shown in Table 24.2 in order to minimise the associated complications.

Pre-prandial target	3.5–5.5 mmol/L
Post-prandial target	5.5–6.6 mmol/L

Women with diabetes are instructed to record a 7-point blood glucose profile (pre- and postprandial and once before bedtime) for at least two days of the week (preferably a weekday and a weekend as dietary patterns may vary) throughout the antenatal period more frequent monitoring would usually be recommended for those on insulin.

Women with diabetes are monitored closely throughout pregnancy (usually at 1- to 2-weekly intervals), and titration of insulin doses is made on the basis of the home blood glucose profile. One should be cognizant of the fact that insulin requirements are likely to increase as the pregnancy advances, as a result of the physiological rise in the production of human placental lactogen (hPL) which antagonises the effect of insulin.

Equally important is the recognition and remediation of hypoglycaemia symptoms, the risk of which is increased with tight glycaemic control.

(F) *Clinical assessment for maternal well-being*

It is recommended for blood pressure and urinalysis to be performed at every antenatal visit as diabetic pregnancies are associated with an increased risk of pre-eclampsia. New-onset hypertension > 140/90 mmHg with proteinuria 2+ or greater in any woman beyond 20 weeks' gestation mandates exclusion of pre-eclampsia.

Enquire about foetal movements from the appropriate gestation as diabetic pregnancies are associated with an increased risk of stillbirth. Bedside Doptone assessment of the foetal heartbeat is reassuring for both patient and practitioner and should be performed at every antenatal visit if available.

(G) *Timing and mode of delivery*

The risk of late stillbirth among women with diabetes is approximately four-fold higher than for the non-diabetic population and it is for this reason that guidelines recommend delivery around 38 and 39 weeks of gestation for women on insulin.

Diabetic pregnancy in itself is not a contraindication to vaginal delivery and Caesarean section should be reserved for the usual obstetric indications. The issue of mode of delivery for large for gestational age (LGA) foetuses is multifactorial; the decision must be individualised, taking into consideration the patient's parity, previous obstetric history, her own BMI and personal preference.

Intrapartum Management

(A) *Principle of insulin therapy during labour*

The goal of intrapartum insulin therapy is strict glucose control, regardless of whether the woman is induced or arrives in spontaneous labour. Once the woman is in active labour, a sliding scale of intravenous short acting insulin infusion and dextrose (5% or 10%) is commenced. The capillary blood glucose is checked hourly and the insulin infusion rate is altered according to a sliding scale determined by the individual daily insulin requirements. The usual dose range is between 2–6 U/hr. The target glucose level during labour and delivery is between 4–7 mmol/L. Insulin drives extracellular potassium into the cells hence it is important to monitor and replace potassium in the intravenous dextrose to avoid hypokalaemia.

(B) *Postpartum haemorrhage (PPH) prophylaxis*

Due consideration should be given to the active management of the 3rd stage of labour and PPH prophylaxis with an intravenous infusion of a uterotonic agent, as maternal obesity, foetal macrosomia and polyhydramnios all increase the risk of uterine atony.

Postpartum Management

Insulin requirements fall to pre-pregnancy levels with delivery of the placenta. As such, in women with pre-existing diabetes, insulin is generally resumed at 50% of the pre-pregnant dose once she is tolerating a normal diet. The dose can then be titrated over the following weeks until optimal.

Neither insulin nor metformin are contraindications to breastfeeding, and mothers should be fully encouraged to exclusively breastfeed their infants.

Gestational Diabetes Mellitus

Gestational diabetes mellitus (GDM) is defined as "diabetes first diagnosed in the second or third trimester that is clearly not pre-existing".[1] It used to be defined as "carbohydrate intolerance with onset or first recognition during pregnancy" but it is becoming more acceptable to use the former definition to distinguish true GDM from pre-existing but undiagnosed diabetes.

Worldwide, GDM affects approximately 5–12% of pregnancies with the highest prevalence in women of Southeast Asian origin. Singapore has one of the hightest GDM rates, affecting approximately 1 in 5 pregnancies (20%). High prevalence of obesity and advanced maternal age have contributed to the increase in GDM.

The pathophysiology relates to changes in maternal carbohydrate metabolism and decreased insulin sensitivity, driven primarily by human placental lactogen which antagonises the action of endogenous insulin.

Diagnosing GDM

In Singapore, GDM is diagnosed by performing a 75-g oral glucose tolerance test (OGTT) between 24–28 weeks of pregnancy — this period coincides with an increase in gestational insulin resistance. The diagnosis of GDM is based on The International Association of Diabetes and Pregnancy Study Group (IADPSG) 3-point diagnostic criteria (Table 24.3), which has replaced the 1999 WHO criteria used in the past.

Table 24.3.   GDM Diagnostic Criteria

Plasma Glucose Levels	Previous Criteria (WHO 1999)	Currect Criteria (IADPSG)
Fasting	≥7.0 mmol/L	≥5.1 mmol/L
1-hour post OGTT	NA	≥10.0 mmol/L
2-hour post OGTT	≥7.8 mmol/L	≥8.5 mmol/L

HbA1c should be avoided for both the screening and diagnosis of GDM as it is neither validated in GDM diagnosis nor sensitive in detecting postprandial hyperglycaemia. Additionally, HbA1c values are generally lower during pregnancy as a result of increased red cell turnover and may therefore be spuriously reassuring.

It is important to note that for women not known to have pre-existing diabetes but have high risk factors for diabetes (such as BMI more than 30 kg/m^2, history of GDM, 40 years and older, and history of pre-diabetes), considerations should be given to screen for pre-existing diabetes as early as possible in pregnancy to allow appropriate management to reduce complications associated with diabetes.

Screening for GDM — Risk Based or Universal?

Currently in Singapore, universal screening is recommended over risk-based screening because Asians have a higher prevalence of GDM.[1] Apart from detecting more GDM cases, universal screening is associated with improved maternal and foetal outcomes.

Management of GDM

The management of GDM is similar to that of pre-existing diabetes mellitus.

Medical Treatment

The aim is also to achieve optimal glycaemic control in pregnancy. The mainstay of treatment is diet modification and appropriate regular exercise. It is recommended that all women with GDM be referred to a dietician. The pre-prandial glucose target is less than 5.5 mmol/L and post-prandial target less than 6.6 mmol/L.

Women with GDM are instructed to record a 7-point blood glucose profile (pre- and post-prandial and once before bedtime) for at least two days of the week (preferably a weekday and a weekend as dietary patterns may vary) throughout the antenatal period. They are monitored closely throughout pregnancy (usually at 1–2 week intervals). If the pre- and post-prandial target cannot be achieved by diet modification and exercise, insulin treatment would be introduced.

Insulin, if required, is given as fast-acting insulin analogues before meals as with pre-existing diabetes; however, it may only be needed before certain meals depending on the post-prandial glucose readings. Intermediate-acting insulin may be required at bedtime and/or before breakfast for fasting hyperglycaemia. The insulin regime is adjusted according to the pre- and post-prandial glucose readings.

Obstetric Management

GDM is associated with an increased risk of pre-eclampsia, hence women should have regular checks of blood pressure and urinalysis.

As GDM develops in the second half of the pregnancy, it is not associated with increased risk of foetal congenital abnormalities as opposed to pre-existing diabetes. However, regular foetal growth scan is recommended as women with GDM have a higher incidence of macrosomia. In addition, the growth of the foetus may influence the timing and mode of delivery, as well as the decision to start insulin treatment.

Elective birth by induction of labour or caesarean section (if indicated at 40–41 weeks' gestation) is offered to women with uncomplicated, well controlled GDM, on diet modification alone. Elective birth at 38–39 weeks' gestation should be considered for women with GDM on insulin or with poor glycaemic control.

Intrapartum Management

Intrapartum target blood glucose levels of 4–7 mmol/L are the same as pre-existing diabetes. The majority of women with GDM do not require insulin during labour. However, those on larger doses of insulin (>20 U/day) are managed as women with pre-existing diabetes, with insulin sliding scale. Following delivery, the insulin treatment would be discontinued.

Postnatal Management

Plasma glucose levels usually revert to pre-pregnancy levels 6-weeks after delivery. It is therefore recommended that women have a 2-point 75 g OGTT performed between 6–12 weeks after delivery to reassess glycaemic status using non-pregnancy thresholds.

Women with GDM have a seven-fold increased risk of developing type 2 diabetes in their lifetimes. In Singapore, an estimated 4 in 10 women with GDM develop pre-diabetes or diabetes in the 5-years following their delivery. Sustained lifestyle modifications have been shown to reduce this risk of progression by 35% over 10 years.[5]

References

1. Ministry of Health Singapore. (2018) Gestational diabetes mellitus An update on screening, diagnosis, and follow up. MOH Appropriate Care Guide. 28 May 2018. Available from www.ace-hta.gov.sg
2. World Health Organisation (WHO) (2013) Diagnostic Criteria and Classification of Hyperglycaemia first detected in Pregnancy. WHO/NMH/MND/13.2. WHO 2013. Available from http://www.who.int/diabetes/publications/Hyperglycaemia_In_Pregnancy/en/
3. HAPO Study Cooperative Research Group (2008) Hyperglycaemia and adverse pregnancy outcomes. *N Engl J Med* **358**:1991–2002.
4. National Institute of Health and Clinical Excellence (NICE) (2015) Diabetes in pregnancy: management of diabetes and its complication from pre-conception to the postnatal period. Feb 2015. Available from http://www.nice.org.uk
5. Aroda VR *et al.* (2015) The effect of lifestyle intervention and metformin on preventing or delaying diabetes among women with and without gestational diabetes: the Diabetes Prevention Program outcomes study 10-year follow-up. *J Clin Endocrinol Metab.*

25

ANAEMIA IN PREGNANCY

Vanaja Kalaichelvan and Kuldip Singh

Introduction

Anaemia is a common medical disorder in pregancy. The incidence varies in different populations and in local studies it is between 3–10 present of all pregnant mother. It is defined as a Haemoglobin level of less than 11.0gm%.

Pathophysisology

- During pregnancy: Blood volume increased by 40%
  Cardiac output increased by 40%
  Plasma volume increased by 40%
  Red cell mass increased by 18–20%

- Due to a greater increase in blood volume than the rise in red cell mass, haemodilution develops, especially in the third trimester of pregnancy
- Daily absorption of iron from gut increases from 10% to 20% because of increased Beta-globulin in pregnancy, including transferrin

- There is net increased requirement of iron in pregnancy as shown below

Debit	Credit
(a) Foetus 400 mg	(a) Red blood cells in puerperium 500 mg
(b) Placenta 100 mg	(b) Pregnancy amenorrhoea 150 mg
(c) Red blood cells 500 mg	
(d) Blood loss during delivery 150 mg	
(e) Lactation requirements 150 mg	
Total Debit 1300 mg	Total Credit 650 mg

*The net requirement in pregnancy is 650 mg.

Classification of Anaemia in Pregnancy

- Iron Deficiency — 85% to 90% of cases
- Megaloblastic
  - (a) Folic acid deficiency
  - (b) Vit B_{12} deficiency
- Haemolytic

(a)	Congenital	(b)	Acquired
	— Sickle cell anaemia		— Infection
	— Thalassaemia		— Physical/chemical agents
	— Hereditary spherocytosis		— Drugs
			— Autoimmune

- Refractory Anaemia or Anaemia of Jolly
  - — A form of mild bone marrow suppression occurring only during pregnancy, reverting to normal after pregnancy. It is refractory to current known normal treatment.

Causes of Anaemia

Decreased Intake or Absorption

- Poor diet
- Nausea, vomiting in pregnancy
- Fasting
- Food fads
- Drugs decreasing iron absorption e.g. magnesium trislicate, phenytoin, alcohol
- Gut disease
- Gut surgery e.g. peptic ulcer
- Worm infestation

Decreased Production

- Bone marrow suppression — drugs
  — chemicals
  — irradiation
  — malignancy
- Haemoglobinopathies
- Chronic systemic illnesses

Increased Destruction/Increased Loss

- Heavy menstruation
- Analgesics
- Gastritis
- Piles
- Antepartum haemorrhage, threatened abortion
- Postpartum haemorrhage in previous pregnancy
- Haemolytic diseases — including Rhesus incompatibility

4. Increased Demand

- Repeated pregnancy — especially closely spaced
- Multiple pregnancy

Effect of Anaemia on Mother and Foetus

Mother	Foetus
(1) Circulatory changes — High output congestive cardiac failure	(1) Foetal hypoxia leading to intra-uterine growth retardation
(2) More prone to (a) infection (b) puerperal sepsis	(2) Increased incidence of preterm labour
(3) Increased risk of postpartum haemorrhage	(3) Increased incidence of low birth weight infants
(4) Less able to withstand blood loss during complicated labour	(4) Foetal distress in labour

Clinical Presentation

Asymptomatic — anaemia found on peripheral examination or routine investigation[2-4]

Symptomatic — unusual

History

Menstrual history — heavy flow, number of pads, clots

Present obstetric history

- Dating of the pregnancy
- At what stage of gestation now?
- Is this a multiple pregnancy?
- When was diagnosis of anaemia made?
- Any antepartum haemorrhage in this pregnancy?
- General — lassitude, malaise, weakness
  - breathlessness, especially on exertion
  - chest pains, palpitation
  - dizziness, tinnitus
- Treatment — transfusion
  - injections
  - infusions
  - oral haematemics
- Complications of treatment — constipation, nausea, vomiting

Past obstetric history

- No. of children
- Lactating?
- Any abortions/stillbirths
- Birthweight of all babies
- Any anaemia in previous pregnancies
- Antepartum and postpartum haemorrhage

Past medical/surgical history

- Gastritis, gastric ulcer, duodenal ulcer
- Haemorrhoids
- Gastrointestinal surgery

Family history of "blood related disorders"

- Anaemia
- Haemoglobinopathies
- Haemolysis
- Gallstones at an early age
- Transfusion

Dietary history

- What composition, quantity?
- How much money spent on food?
- Any food fad?
- Fasting (especially in Malays)
- Alcohol
- Family income, socioeconomic status
- Cooking method; Indians tend to overcook their vegetables

Drug and toxin exposures

- Analgesics, anticonvulsants, chloramphenicol, sulphonamides
- Irradiation
- Chemical exposure

Physical Examination

General

- Patient's well-being, propped up, stature, nutritional status
- Pallor — conjunctival, oral mucosa, palmar creases, retina
  - Jaundice in haemolytic anaemia

- Stigmata of nutritional deficiency — glossitis
  - angular stomatitis
  - koilonychias

- Vital signs
- Cardiovascular system — tachycardia, showing increased heart rate
  - cardiac murmurs due to hyperkinetic circulation

- Respiratory system — evidence of congestive cardiac failure
- Splenomegaly — difficult to palpate unless early pregnancy

Abdomen and perineum

- Operation scar — evidence of past surgery
- Lax abdomen
- No. of foetuses, multiple pregnancy
- Foetal size
- Any placenta praevia with malpresentation
- Foetal movement, foetal heart
- Amount of liquor
- Haemorrhoids

Investigations

- **Full Blood Count** — Haemoglobin — <11 gm%
  - Haematocrit — <35%
  - Total White and Platelet Count
  - Reticulocyte Count

- Peripheral Blood Film
  - Hypochromic, microcytic — Iron deficiency anaemia
  - Macrocytes, megaloblast — Folate deficiency anaemia
  - Target cells — Suggestive of Beta Thalassaemia
  - Hbh bodies — Suggestive of Alpha Thalassaemia

- Howell-Jolly bodies
- Spherocytes
- Fragmented cells

- Red Blood Cell Indices
  - Mean Corpuscular Volume — decreased when less than 85 f litre
  - Mean Corpuscular Haemoglobin — decreased when less than 27 pico grams
  - Mean Corpuscular Haemoglobin Concentration — decreased when less than 32%

- Iron Metabolism
  Serum Iron of <600 µgm% suggests iron deficiency
  - Total Iron Binding Capacity → an increase (>450 µg%) suggestive of iron deficiency
  - Ferritin → decrease (<8 µg%) suggestive of iron deficiency

Management

Mode of Treatment Depends On
- Severity of anaemia
- Underlying cause
- Urgency of treatment — gestational age
- Response to treatment — symptoms
  — haemoglobin
  — reticulocyte count

- Tolerance of side effects

Modalities of Treatment for Iron Deficiency Anaemia

Oral iron preparations
- first line
- organic preparations e.g. fumerate, gluconate preferred as less side effects. Dose of 200 mg tds with folic acid and vitamin C
- newer preparations available such as Iberet Folate with less side effects
- other prophylactic preparations are not effective for therapeutic treatment
- administered 30–45 min before meals to enable maximal absorption
- reticulocyte count increased within 48 hours
- side effects include gastritis, nausea, vomiting, diarrhoea, constipation

Parenteral iron preparation

- Indicated if:
  - non-compliance with oral therapy
  - rapid restoration e.g. close to term
  - gastrointestinal tract intolerance to oral forms
  - decreased gastrointestinal tract absorption
  - no response to oral treatment

- Efficiency is shown to be much better than oral therapy, but it should not be the first line of therapy unless the mother is in advanced pregnancy and close to term.[5]
- Dose of parenteral iron is calculated on the basis of basic bodyweight, haemoglobin deficiency and pregnancy requirements.
- Intramuscular — 2 to 4 mL given at one time into buttocks
  (Ferrosig 200 mg/2 mL) — repeated 2–3 times/week until total dose is given
    — 'z' technique of injection to minimise staining of site of injection
    — rarely used in current practice

- Intravenous
  - Iron III carboxymaltose (Ferrinject) or Iron III hydroxide in sucrose (Venofer) allow for controlled delivery of iron within the reticuloendothelial system (bone marrow primarily) and subsequent delivery to the iron binding proteins ferritin and transferrin. It is administered intravenously as a single dose of 1000 mg over 15 minutes (maximum 15 mg/kg by injection or 20 mg/kg by infusion) if the requirements for iron is greater than >1,000 mg.

Side effects are rare:

Mild

 (i) light headedness
 (ii) headache (mild)
(iii) flushing

Moderate

 (i) nausea/vomiting
 (ii) diarrhoea

Severe

 (i) dyspnoea
 (ii) tachycardia
(iii) sweating
(iv) shock

Blood transfusion

- Indications:
    - (i) Antepartum Haemorrhage
    - (ii) Haemolytic Crisis
    - (iii) Severe anaemia with impending cardiac failure

- Complications of Blood Transfusion

Immediate	Late
(i) Allergic reaction	(i) Isosensitisation esp. Rhesus
(ii) Febrile reaction	(ii) Disease transmission h. e.g. Hepatitis, Autoimmune deficiency syndrome, HIV
(iii) Circulatory overload	(iii) Transfusion of siderosis
(iv) Haemolysis	(iv) Development of circulatory anticoagulants e.g. AHG, Ab
(v) Thrombophlebitis	
(vi) Air embolism	

- Complications of Massive Transfusion:
    - (i) Hypothermia
    - (ii) Circulatory overload
    - (iii) Citrate intoxication
    - (iv) Hyperkalaemia
    - (v) Acidosis
    - (vi) Coagulation defect
    - (vii) Pulmonary complications
    - (viii) Decreased platelets

We need to treat anaemia in pregnancy early because:

- To prevent complications to mother and foetus
- To ensure that the mother can withstand the hypovolaemic shock of postpartum haemorrhage, if it occurs
- Treatment of Anaemia induced Cardiac Failure:
    - (i) Prop patient up
    - (ii) Give oxygen if necessary
    - (iii) Diuretics
    - (iv) Digitalise
    - (v) When cardiac failure is under control, slow transfusion of packed cells
    - (vi) Careful monitoring of mother and foetus
    - (vii) Avoid postpartum haemorrhage by control of cord traction and the use of intravenous oxytocics

Megaloblastic Anaemia

Incidence

5% in Singapore and is generally due to folic acid deficiency

Pathophysiology

- Folic acid stored largely in the liver and is normally sufficient for six weeks
- Necessary for nucleic acid synthesis which increases during pregnancy
- Steps in development
  (i) Diminished folate stores
  (ii) Low serum folate (three weeks)
  (iii) Hypersegmentation of marrow neutrophils (five weeks)
  (iv) Low red blood cells folate (16 weeks)
  (v) Megaloblastic anaemia (19 weeks)
- Daily requirement of folate
  (i) Non pregnant 50 μg
  (ii) Pregnant 150–300 μg for positive folate balance as
  (i) Decreased folate absorption in gastrointestinal tract
  (j) Increased maternal requirements
  (k) Foetal parasitism

Effects

Suggested (not proven), especially if it occurs in early pregnancy:

- Spontaneous abortion
- Foetal malformations
- Premature delivery
- Abruptio placentae

Investigation

- Buffy coats smear
  (i) Megaloblasts
  (ii) Hypersegmented Neutrophils: 75% of folate deficient patients have 4% or more neutrophils with >= 5 lobes i.e. lobe counts of 4%

(iii) Macropolycytes: giant neutrophils with very numerous lobes
(iv) Orthochromatic macrocytes (>12 mm in longest diameter)

- Peripheral blood film
  (i) Howell-Jolly bodies in red blood cells
  (ii) Normoblasts showing premature haemoglobinisation

- Low serum folate
- Low red blood cell folate
- Bone marrow biopsy (rarely)

Prevention

- Proper diet
- Small amounts of folic acid with supplemental iron given routinely. Recommended dosage of 300–500 µg

Treatment

- Folic acid 15–20 mg/day

Thalassaemia in Pregnancy

Incidence

- Incidence of gestational thalassaemia is 0.8%
- Gene frequency in population is 4% for alpha, and 2% for beta thalassaemia

Definition

Thalassaemia is a genetic defect in which there is a partial or complete suppression of synthesis of either the alpha or Beta globulin chain, resulting in reduced haemoglobin context in the red blood cells.

HbA   = 2 alpha 2 beta
HbA2 = 2 alpha 2 delta
HbF   = 2 alpha 2 gamma

Types

Alpha Thalassaemia

Bart's (4 gamma) — Intrauterine death
                    Bart's Foetalis

HbH disease (4 Beta) — not lethal
                     — born alive
                     — anaemia under stressful conditions
                       e.g. pregnancy
                     — HbH inclusion bodies seen on peripheral blood film
                       with cresyl blue

Beta Thalassaemia

Major — does not normally reach childbearing age
       — increased foetal haemoglobin (Hbf)

Minor   — not lethal
           — anaemia under stressful conditions e.g. pregnancy
           — HbA2 increased, 2 × normal
           — HbF increased
           — HbA decreased

Diagnosis

- Hb electrophoresis at pH 8.6

   Normal Hb electrophoresis

   HbA > 95%
   HbF < 1%
   HbA2 up to 2–3%

   At pH 8.6: HbF and HbE travel slower than HbA
              HbH and Bart's Hb travel faster than HbA

Treatment

- Folic acid, vitamin C supplement
- No iron supplements unless concomitant
  Iron deficiency anaemia present
- Blood transfusion if severe
- Partner should be screened to determine if he is a carrier, and if so the couple
  should be counselled for prenatal screening and diagnosis

Refractory Anaemia or Anaemia of Holly

- a form of mild bone marrow suppression occurring only during pregnancy, reverting to normal after pregnancy
- it is refractory to current known normal treatment

References

1. Singh K, Fong YF, Arulkumaran S. (1998) Anaemia in Pregnancy — a cross-sectional study in Singapore. *Eur J Clin Nutr* **52**:65–70. (United Kingdom).
2. Symonds I, Baker P, Kean L. (2002) *Problem Orientated Obstetrics and Gynaecology*.
3. Powrie RO, Greene MF, Camann W. (2010) *F de Sweit's Medical Disorders in Obstetric Practice*, 5th edn.
4. James D, Steer PI, Weiner CP, Gonik B. (2011) *High Risk Pregnancy Management Options*, 4th edn.
5. Singh K, Fong YF, Kuperan P. (1998) A comparison between intravenous iron polymatose complex (Ferrum Hausmann®) and oral ferrous fumarate in the treatment of iron deficiency anaemia in pregnancy. *Euro J Haematol* **60**:119–124.

26

AUTOIMMUNE DISEASES IN PREGNANCY

Anita Kale

Introduction

The body's immune system helps against invasion by foreign pathogens. It is able to distinguish biologic self from non-self. Loss of this distinction leads to autoimmune diseases. These are characterised by typical clinical signs and symptoms and serologic evidence of autoantibodies. For many autoimmune conditions, these autoantibodies play a role in tissue damage.

Autoimmune diseases are more prevalent in women of reproductive age group. More than 70% of patients are women of reproductive age. Pregnancy associated fluctuations in sex hormones substantially affect the disease activity. Diseases with cellular pathology, such as rheumatoid arthritis (RA) and multiple sclerosis (MS) are associated with remission during pregnancy; whereas diseases characterised by autoantibody production, such as systemic lupus erythematosus (SLE) and Grave's disease tend towards increased severity in pregnancy.[1-3]

In the scope of the undergraduate curriculum, this chapter will cover two common conditions, namely SLE and anti-phospholipid syndrome (APS).

Systemic Lupus Erythematosus

SLE is an idiopathic chronic multisystem disorder that may affect skin, joints, kidneys, lungs, serous membranes and other organs in the body. The most common complaint is extreme fatigue, the others being fever, weight loss, myalgia and arthralgia. There is a possible genetic predilection, as approximately 10% of patients with SLE have an affected relative.[4]

Diagnosis

To be classified as having SLE, an individual must have 4 out of 11 clinical and laboratory criteria, at one time or serially.

TABLE 26.1   Revised American College of Rheumatology Classification Criteria for SLE[5]

Criterion	Definition
(1) Malar rash	Fixed erythema, flat or raised, over the malar eminences, tending to spare the nasolabial folds
(2) Discoid rash	Erythematous raised patches with adherent keratotic scaling and follicular plugging; atrophic scarring possible in older lesions
(3) Photosensitivity	Skin rash as a result of unusual reaction to sunlight, by patient history or physician observation
(4) Oral ulcers	Oral or nasopharyngeal ulceration, usually painless
(5) Arthritis	Nonerosive arthritis involving two or more peripheral joints, characterised by tenderness, swelling or effusion
(6) Serositis	(a) Pleuritis — convincing history of pleuritic pain or rubbing heard by a physician, or evidence of pleural effusion (b) Pericarditis — documented by ECG or rub or evidence of effusion
(7) Renal	(a) Persistent proteinuria >0.5 g/day or >3+ if quantitation not performed (b) Cellular casts — red cell, haemoglobin, granular, tubular or mixed
(8) Neurologic	(a) Seizures — in the absence of offending drugs or known metabolic derangements (e.g. uraemia, ketoacidosis or electrolyte imbalance) (b) Psychosis — in the absence of drugs or metabolic derangements
(9) Haematologic	(a) Haemolytic anaemia — with reticulocytosis (b) Leukopenia — <4,000/μL on 2 or more occasions (c) Lymphopenia — <1,500/μL on 2 or more occasions (d) Thrombocytopenia — <100,000/μL in absence of drugs
(10) Immunologic	(a) Anti-DNA — antibody to native DNA in abnormal titre (b) Anti-SM — presence of antibody to Sm nuclear antigen (c) Positive finding of antiphospholipid antibodies used based on (1) an abnormal serum level of IgG or IgM anticardiolipin antibodies (2) a positive test result for lupus anticoagulant using a standard method, or (3) a false-positive serologic test for syphilis for six months
(11) Antinuclear Antibody	An abnormal ANA titre by immunofluorescence or an equivalent assay at any time and in the absence of drugs known to be associated with "drug-induced lupus syndrome"

In pregnancy, anti-dsDNA antibodies correlate with disease flare and preterm delivery. Anti-Ro/SS-A and anti-La/SS-B antibodies found in both SLE and Sjogren's syndrome patients are associated with neonatal lupus.

Effects of Pregnancy on SLE

Women with SLE are advised to try for pregnancy when the disease is in remission. Flares are more common in the second half of pregnancy. Active disease at the time of conception increases the risk of flare during pregnancy. Disease flare during pregnancy may pose diagnostic difficulty as many features such as fatigue, oedema, erythema and musculoskeletal pain also occur in normal pregnancy. Distinction between pre-eclampsia and SLE flare is also difficult. The distinguishing features of SLE flare are rising anti-dsDNA titres, fall in complement levels and presence of casts on urine microscopy; whereas pre-eclampsia will cause elevation in transaminases.

Effects of SLE on Pregnancy

SLE is associated with increased risk of spontaneous early as well as late miscarriage, foetal death, intrauterine growth restriction, pre-eclampsia, and preterm delivery. Risks are increased if there is active disease at the time of conception. Pregnancy outcome is particularly affected by the presence of renal disease and anti-cardiolipin antibodies.

Management

Ideally, this should begin with pre-conception counselling. Knowledge of anti-Ro, anti-La, antiphospholipid, renal and blood pressure status allows prediction of the risks to the woman and her baby. Outlook is better if conception occurs during remission. Pregnancy care requires a multidisciplinary approach. Regular monitoring is required for disease activity as well as for foetal growth. Hydroxychloroquine, prednisolone, sulphasalazine and azathioprine can be safely used during pregnancy. Patients on prednisolone should be screened for gestational diabetes.

Neonatal Manifestations

In the presence of anti-Ro/SS-A and anti-La/SS-B antibodies there is a 5% risk of neonatal cutaneous lupus and 2–3% risk of congenital heart block (CHB). The risk of neonatal lupus increases up to 25% if there is a history of previously affected foetus.

Cutaneous lupus appears in form of a skin rash, usually on the face and scalp. The rash disappears spontaneously by six months of life. Residual pigmentation may persist up to two years, but permanent scarring is unusual.

In contrast to cutaneous lupus, CHB appears in utero, is permanent and may be fatal. The majority of those who survive need pacemakers in early infancy.

Anti Phospholipid Syndrome (APS)

Antiphospholipid antibodies (aPL) are a family of autoantibodies that bind to negatively charged phospholipids or phospholipid-binding proteins. Anti-cardiolipin antibodies (aCL) and lupus anticoagulant (LA) are overlapping subsets of aPL antibodies. The link between aPL antibodies and pregnancy was established around mid-1970s.

Diagnosis

APS is diagnosed when a woman has one from each of the clinical and laboratory criteria listed in the table below (as per the Sydney revised classification criteria, 2006).[6]

Clinical criteria:

(1) Thrombosis (venous/arterial)
(2) Pregnancy complication (recurrent pregnancy loss, unexplained foetal death beyond 10 weeks' gestation, premature birth because of severe pre-eclampsia or intrauterine growth restriction)

Laboratory criteria: All lab criteria should be present on two or more occasions, at least 12 weeks apart

(1) Presence of lupus anticoagulant
(2) Presence of aCL antibody, IgG or IgM
(3) Anti-beta 2 glycoprotein antibody, IgG or IgM

Risks of APS and Pregnancy

Thrombotic complications

Numerous retrospective studies have confirmed the link between APS and venous or arterial thrombosis. Over half the cases of thromboembolism in women with APS occur in relation to pregnancy or the use of combined oral contraceptive.

In the two largest series of prospectively followed APS pregnancies, the rates of thrombosis and stroke were 5% and 12% respectively.

Obstetric complications of APS

In the original description of APS, the sole obstetric criterion for diagnosis was foetal loss (at gestation more than 10 weeks). More recently, it has been extended to include women with recurrent early pregnancy losses. 10–20% of women with recurrent pregnancy losses have positive serology for APS.

The median rate of gestational hypertension/pre-eclampsia in pregnancies complicated by APS is 32%. Pre-eclampsia may develop as early as 15–17 weeks' gestation.

The risk of intrauterine growth restriction (IUGR) is also high, in the range of 30%. Hypercoagulability causing defective uteroplacental circulation is supposed to be responsible for these late pregnancy complications.

Management

Patients with APS require close monitoring due to increased risk of maternal as well as foetal complications. Serial ultrasound assessment of foetal growth should be performed. Combined use of low molecular weight heparin (LMWH) and low dose aspirin has been shown to be beneficial in terms of reducing the risk of thrombosis, as well as improved pregnancy outcome. The LMWH is discontinued before labour and delivery, to allow use of regional anaesthesia and to reduce the risk of excessive blood loss at the time of delivery. Aspirin should be discontinued at around 36 weeks or 8–10 days prior to delivery. The treatment is restarted post-delivery and is continued for six weeks post-partum.

References

1. Beeson PB. (1994) Age and sex association of 40 autoimmune diseases. *Am J Med* **96**:457–462.
2. Nelson-Piercy C. (2010) *Handbook of Obstetric Medicine*, 4th edn.
3. Hacker NF, Gambore JC, Hobil CJ. (2010) *Essential of Obstetrics and Gynaecology*, 5th edn.
4. Tan EM, Cohen AS, Fries JF, *et al*. (1982) The 1982 revised criteria for the classification of systemic lupus erythematosus, *Arthritis Rheum* **25**:1271–1277.
5. Hochberg MC. (1997) Updating the American College of Rheumatology revised criteria for the classification of systemic lupus erythematosus. *Arthritis Rheum* **40**:1725.
6. James DK, Steer PJ, Weiner CP, Gonik B. (2010) *High Risk Pregnancy Management Options*, 4th edn.

27

THYROID DISORDERS IN PREGNANCY

Chan Shiao-Yng

Introduction

Recommendations for the management of thyroid disease pre-conceptually and during pregnancy are being refined as new evidence emerges. Several controversies remain unresolved whilst awaiting the conclusion of ongoing clinical trials. These include issues of screening for thyroid disease in pregnancy, thresholds at which treatment should be started and whether to treat euthyroid Thyroid Peroxidase antibody positive women. Hence, there are differences in the specific strategies employed by various units, but the basic principles are generally similar. Of note is that reference ranges for thyroid function tests vary according to the laboratory assay, geographical population, ethnicity and gestational age. Thyroid hormone levels are particularly critical in the first trimester of pregnancy in determining pregnancy outcome. Treatment of thyroid disorders should be optimised prior to conception, with clear management plans in place for when pregnancy is confirmed. Adequate treatment and control of both hypothyroid and hyperthyroid disease in pregnancy is associated with good obstetric outcome.

Normal Physiological Changes

Placental human chorionic gonadotrophin (HCG) peaks at around 10 weeks of gestation and increases maternal oestrogen levels, which stimulates the hepatic production of thyroxine binding globulin (TBG), and subsequently the binding of free thyroid hormones in the circulation. HCG, which has weak thyrotrophic activity, can also directly stimulate the maternal thyroid gland to produce thyroid hormones. The placenta, which is rich in deiodinase type 3 enzymes, metabolises maternal thyroid hormones. Despite this, the foetus receives physiologically important amounts of maternal thyroid hormones by transplacental supply from five weeks of gestation onwards. This is particularly critical for foetal neurodevelopment prior to the onset of endogenous foetal thyroid hormone production, at around 16–18 weeks of gestation in humans. In addition, renal iodide clearance is increased and the requirement for iodine, an essential constituent of thyroid hormones, rises. As a result, any iodine deficiency or thyroid insufficiency can be exacerbated in pregnancy as the thyroid struggles to increase thyroid hormone production to compensate for normal physiological changes. On the other hand, thyrotoxicosis is more likely to occur, particular under specific pregnancy circumstances.[1,2]

Gestational Transient Thyrotoxicosis

Biochemical hyperthyroidism (suppressed TSH with elevated free T4) is found in about 3% of normal pregnancies, usually in association with hyperemesis gravidarum in the first and early second trimesters, with spontaneous reversion to euthyroidism by late second trimester. This is attributable to the thyrotropic effect of HCG, thus molar pregnancies and multiple pregnancies, which have increased placental mass, may be particularly affected. Severe hyperemesis gravidarum has been associated with increased risk of small for gestational age neonates but whether transient thyrotoxicosis mediates this risk is unclear. There is no evidence that treatment of thyrotoxicosis *per se* is beneficial in such cases. Only symptomatic support is indicated if required.

Hyperthyroidism

In women of reproductive age, pre-pregnancy hyperthyroidism is secondary to Graves' disease in over 90% of cases. New presentation of Graves' disease during pregnancy is much rarer than gestational transient thyrotoxicosis. They can be distinguished as Graves' disease is often associated with symptom-onset predating pregnancy (e.g. significant weight loss, heat intolerance, palpitations, etc.), a positive family history of thyroid disease, a diffuse goitre and the presence of TSH receptor autoantibodies (TRAb). TRAb stimulate the thyroid gland resulting in elevated circulating free T4 and free T3 concentrations, which suppress TSH production by the pituitary gland. Uncontrolled maternal thyrotoxicosis is associated with many complications in pregnancy (Table 27.1) and must be treated. The transplacental passage of TRAb may cause foetal/neonatal hyperthyroidism in 1% of cases, whilst overtreatment with anti-thyroid drugs can induce foetal hypothyroidism.

TABLE 27.1 Complications Associated with Uncontrolled Maternal Graves' Disease

• Thyroid storm (1st and 2nd trimester)	• Foetal growth restriction
• Congestive cardiac failure	• Foetal thyrotoxicosis
• Pre-eclampsia	• Foetal hypothyroidism
• Placental abruption	• Stillbirth
• Preterm delivery	• Perinatal death

The anti-thyroid drugs carbimazole/methimazole and propylthiouracil (PTU) show no significant differences in their potential to induce foetal hypothyroidism, and no differences in childhood neurodevelopmental assessments compared to unexposed siblings. Both drugs are potentially teratogenic, with the former slightly more so than the latter. Overall, the incidence of birth defects is in the region of 1.5 times the background risk for both. There has been an unproven causal link between carbimazole/methimazole and the rare benign scalp condition of aplasia cutis, as well as choanal/oesophageal atresia and dysmorphic facial features in the foetus; whilst PTU has been associated with face, neck and urinary tract defects. However, the risks to the pregnancy of uncontrolled hyperthyroidism far outweighs the risk of teratogenicity, thus treatment is still recommended. PTU is currently favoured over carbimazole/methimazole in women planning a pregnancy, given its more favourable teratogenic profile. Since PTU is associated with the rare side effect of severe liver impairment in 1 in 10,000 cases, some have advocated converting treatment back to carbimazole/methimazole in the second and third trimesters once organogenesis is complete.

The natural history of Graves' disease is improvement with advancement of pregnancy. Under the careful monitoring of an endocrinologist, anti-thyroid drugs could be gradually reduced and often stopped, since Graves' disease commonly enters remission in the second half of pregnancy. Thyroid function tests should be performed about four weeks after each dose change, and in some cases fortnightly monitoring is required in the first half of gestation when rapid physiological changes occur. The aim is to maintain the free T4 level in the upper third of the normal range on as low a dose of the anti-thyroid drug as possible, to protect the foetus from hypothyroidism. It is common to find that TSH concentrations remain low or fully suppressed and is thus not a good indicator of disease control.

In addition to regular assessments of maternal blood pressure and urine as screening tests for pre-eclampsia, foetal growth should be monitored with regular ultrasound scans during the third trimester. Levels of TRAb should be quantified to help predict the risk of foetal/neonatal thyrotoxicosis. Left untreated, foetal thyrotoxicosis is associated with intrauterine growth restriction, foetal goitre, foetal hydrops, preterm delivery and foetal death. Thus, any suspicion of this diagnosis through the detection of persistent foetal tachycardia on auscultation warrants urgent ultrasound scanning of the foetus and treatment in a specialist Foetal Medicine centre.

There is a 60–80% chance that Graves' disease will flare postpartum, and thyroid function tests should be performed over the course of the following 6 to 9 months. Breast-feeding is safe with low doses of carbimazole/methimazole and PTU administered in divided daily doses post-feeds. Monthly thyroid function tests in the baby should be considered on higher dose regimens.[3,4]

Hypothyroidism

Worldwide iodine deficiency remains the leading cause of hypothyroidism, and in affected countries the WHO has recommended routine iodine supplementation to ensure a daily iodine intake of 250 μg during pregnancy and lactation.

In iodine-replete countries, the incidence of hypothyroidism diagnosed before pregnancy is about 1%, the commonest cause being primary thyroidal failure due to autoimmune thyroiditis. In addition, approximately 2.5–5% of pregnant women have subclinical hypothyroidism, defined by a mildly elevated serum TSH concentration but normal free T4 and free T3 concentrations. This can be indicative of the early stages of thyroid insufficiency or inadequate thyroxine replacement in previously diagnosed overt hypothyroidism.

The risks of untreated overt hypothyroidism in pregnancy are well documented (Table 27.2). Maternal thyroid hormones are believed to be crucial for the normal development of the placenta and the foetus, particularly the central nervous system, especially in the first trimester of pregnancy. Adequate treatment of overt hypothyroidism from the very start of pregnancy is associated with good obstetric outcomes.

TABLE 27.2   Obstetric Complications Associated with Untreated Overt Maternal Hypothyroidism

• Miscarriage (1st and 2nd trimester)	• Preterm birth
	• Placental abruption
• Gestational hypertension	• Low birthweight
• Pre-eclampsia	• Stillbirth
• Anaemia	• Perinatal death
• Postpartum haemorrhage	

Several studies have now also associated subclinical hypothyroidism during the first half of pregnancy with an increased risk of miscarriage, preterm delivery, and neuropsychological deficiencies in the offspring. However, one large clinical trial (CATS study) has reported that screening for and treatment of subclinical hypothyroidism is of no benefit to offspring neurodevelopment, whilst a meta-analysis of several small studies suggests a reduction in miscarriage risk if levo-thyroxine is commenced early in the first trimester, particularly in TPO (thyroid peroxidase) antibody positive women. The treatment of subclinical hypothyroid-ism in pregnancy remains controversial.

Clinical practice guidelines, largely based on the consensus opinion of experts, have recommended that in women with pre-existing hypothyroidism, the TSH level should be kept below 2.5 mU/L before embarking on a pregnancy. When pregnant, levothyroxine doses should be empirically increased by 4–6 weeks of gestation and by an increment of 30–50% of the existing dose. The aim should be to replicate normal physiology, anticipate increased dose requirements and pre-vent (rather than react to) abnormalities in thyroid function test results during pregnancy. Since there has been no evidence that subclinical hyperthyroidism (suppressed TSH with normal free T4) is associated with adverse outcomes, the balance of risk is in favour of thyroxine dose increases in maternal hypothyroid-ism. Thyroid function should be checked four weeks after every dose change and dose change recommendations should be made promptly. Results should be interpreted using trimester-specific reference ranges where available, otherwise TSH concentrations should be kept between 0.1–2.5 mU/L, 0.2–3.0 mU/L and 0.3–3.0 mU/L in the first, second and third trimesters respectively. Thyroid func-tion should ideally be tested pre-conception, at the diagnosis of pregnancy, at antenatal booking and monthly until 20 weeks' gestation, then at least once in the third trimester of pregnancy. (See Table 27.3)

TABLE 27.3 Recommendations for Thyroid Function Monitoring in Pregnancy in the Absence of Trimester-Specific Reference Ranges

	TSH Target (mU/L)	Thyroxine Adjustments	Thyroid Function Test Monitoring
Pre-conception	0.4–2.5	Adjust by 25–50 mcg at a time.	4–6 weeks after each dose change
1st trimester	0.1–2.5	Increase thyroxine by 30–50% when pregnancy test is positive.	Every 4 weeks
2nd trimester	0.2–3.0	Adjust by 25 mcg at a time.	Every 4 weeks, or 4 weeks after dose change
3rd trimester	0.3–3.0	Adjust by 25 mcg at a time.	4 weeks after dose change. If stable, at least once.
Postpartum	Non-pregnant range	Reduce thyroxine back to pre-pregnancy dose.	6 weeks postpartum

Euthyroid Thyroid Peroxidase (TPO) Antibody Positivity

TPO antibodies are associated with thyroid autoimmune disorders but the vast majority of TPO antibody positive women are euthyroid. TPO antibody positivity is highly prevalent, affecting around 10–20% of reproductive-aged women, with higher prevalence reported in those with recurrent miscarriages and infertility compared to the unselected population. Approximately 15–20% of TPO antibody positive women who are euthyroid outside pregnancy will develop hypothyroidism or subclinical hypothyroidism by the third trimester of pregnancy. This may indicate a subtle reduction in thyroid reserve, which is unable to adapt to the physiological changes of pregnancy. Thus, in untreated TPO antibody positive women, thyroid function monitoring is warranted in each trimester of pregnancy.[5]

TPO antibody positivity is associated with increased risks of miscarriage and preterm delivery independent of thyroid dysfunction. It is also associated with subfertility and a significantly increased risk of postpartum thyroiditis. Two small clinical studies demonstrated a reduction in miscarriages with levothyroxine treatment and one also reported a reduction in preterm birth rate. Two large randomised controlled trials are currently underway to confirm these findings (TABLET trial and T4life trial).

Goitre

The normal thyroid gland increases in size by at least 10% during pregnancy. Therefore, pre-existing goitres may enlarge further and can present with or without thyroid dysfunction.

Women with goitre should be assessed for:

- Thyroid dysfunction (due to autoimmune hypothyroidism or hyperthyroidism, functioning nodule(s), iodine deficiency)
- Tracheoesophageal compression (assessed by a flow volume loop spirometry investigation, especially if the goitre is large or if symptoms of dysphagia, dysphonia, snoring, breathing difficulty are present)
- Malignancy (ultrasound scan plus fine needle aspiration if there is a highly suspicious lesion).

Failure of intubation is higher in pregnant women anyway. Should a pregnant woman with a goitre require a general anaesthetic in an emergency, the risk of a failed intubation may be further elevated. Anaesthesiologists should be involved in antenatal assessment in the third trimester of pregnancy, prior to labour onset, in preparation for the possibility of an emergency operative delivery.

Postpartum Thyroiditis

Postpartum thyroiditis can occur not only after the delivery of a full term pregnancy but also after an early pregnancy loss. This condition affects around 10% of women, with around a four-fold higher incidence in TPO antibody positive women.

Postpartum thyroiditis is a transient inflammation of the thyroid gland, which typically develops between 2–6 months after the end of a pregnancy. Most women will have a short period of thyrotoxicosis for a few weeks or months, followed by a short period of hypothyroidism for the next few months, although the pattern of changes can vary and some will only experience one of the phases without the other. Symptoms can be variable and are mostly non-specific and vague such as tiredness. Some women may not experience any symptoms at all, even when the thyroid function tests are abnormal. Treatment is only indicated if symptoms are present.

Thyrotoxicosis is due to the excessive release of previously synthesised thyroid hormones from thyroid tissue destruction (i.e. not due to increased thyroid hormone production, thus drugs which suppress thyroid hormone synthesis would not be an effective treatment). Treatment of thyrotoxicosis with a short course of beta-blockers is only required for symptom control. Similarly, levothyroxine treatment is only indicated if there are significant symptoms or if there is no spontaneous resolution to euthyroidism.

Women who develop postpartum thyroiditis have about a 10% chance of remaining permanently hypothyroid and will therefore require lifelong levothyroxine replacement. In the rest, who spontaneously recover in the short term, there is then a 30–50% chance of developing overt hypothyroidism in the next five years. Thus, annual thyroid function testing is recommended in these women. They should also be checked when planning for their next pregnancy.

References

1. Glineor D. (1997). The regulation of thyroid function in pregnancy: pathways of endocrine adaptation from physiology to pathology. *Endoc Rev* **18**:404–433.

2. Krassas GE, Poppe K, Glinoer D. (2010) Thyroid function and human reproductive health. *Endocr Rev* **31**(5):702–755.

3. Stagnaro-Green A, Abalovich M, Alexander E, *et al.* (2011) Guidelines of the American Thyroid Association for the diagnosis and management of thyroid disease during pregnancy and postpartum. *Thyroid* **21**(10):1081–1125.

4. Mestman JH. (2004) Hyperthyroidism in pregnancy. *Best Pract Res Clin Endocrinol Metab* **18**(2):267–288.

5. Chan SY, Boelaert K. (2015) Optimal management of hypothyroidism, hypothyroxinaemia and euthyroid TPO antibody positivity preconception and in pregnancy. *Clin Endocrinol (Oxf)* **82**(3):313–326.

28

CARDIAC DISEASE IN PREGNANCY

Chan Shiao-Yng

Introduction

In the Western world, cardiac disease is now the leading cause of maternal mortality. With the success of the treatment of congenital heart disease (affected girls are living longer and healthier lives), with rising maternal age and prevalence of metabolic syndrome and hence ischaemic heart disease, the number of women entering pregnancy with a heart condition is on the rise. Rheumatic heart disease remains a dominant group of cardiac diseases in pregnant women originating from non-Western countries. Still, a significant proportion of cardiac deaths occur in women who were not known to have a cardiac disorder prior to labour, and who presented for the first time in the peripartum period. Hence, continued vigilance and awareness of cardiac disease remains key to minimising the risk of such tragic consequences. The specific management of each different cardiac disorder is beyond the scope of this chapter. Rather, general principles in the management of cardiac disease in pregnancy will be considered.[1-3]

Normal Physiological Changes in Pregnancy

Pregnancy induces significant haemodynamic changes from as early as five weeks of gestation, with cardiac output reaching an antenatal peak around 28 weeks of gestation (when most cardiac decompensation of pre-existing cardiac disease typically occurs), with further dynamic changes peripartum. The changes that occur in a normal pregnancy are summarised in Table 28.1.

TABLE 28.1   Normal Haemodynamic Changes in Pregnancy

Parameter	Changes in Normal Pregnancy
Blood volume	Increase by 40–50% from first trimester, reach a peak around 24 weeks. Declines post-partum by autodiuresis.
Systemic vascular resistance	Decrease from first trimester onwards until postpartum due to peripheral vasodilatation
Blood pressure	Decrease by approximately 10 mm Hg by second trimester and returns to pre-pregnancy levels towards term. In labour BP increases: systolic BP by 15–25%, diastolic BP by 10–15%
Stroke volume	Increase in first and second trimester (due to increased end-diastolic volume, muscle wall mass and contractility). Decline in the third trimester due to reduced venous return secondary to inferior vena caval compression by uterus
Heart rate	Increase by 10 to 15 beats per minute from mid-trimester and peaks at 32 weeks, stays elevated until a few days postpartum
Cardiac output	Increase by 20% at 8 weeks and 40–50% by 20–28 weeks, then plateau until labour. Increase further by 15% in early labour, 25% in first stage, 50% in active second stage due to autotransfusion from uterus during contraction (300 500 mls per contraction) and sympathetic stimulation from pain and anxiety. Increase by 80% in immediate postpartum due to autotransfusion from involuting uterus, relief of aortocaval compression and resorption of peripheral oedema
Heart size	Increase by up to 30%, partly due to dilatation
Haemostatic factors	Hypercoagulability antenatally and for several weeks postpartum due to increased coagulation factors, fibrinogen, platelet adhesiveness, decreased fibrinolysis, venous stasis secondary to venous compression by uterus

Aortocaval compression becomes significant after 20 weeks' gestation, so pregnant women should avoid lying supine. The left lateral position is preferred but a semi-recumbent position is also acceptable.

Given these significant cardiovascular changes, women with cardiac diseases are at significantly increased risk in pregnancy.

Pre-Pregnancy Risk Assessment and Counselling

Upon entering child-bearing age, women with cardiac disease should be counselled of the implications of pregnancy for their heart condition and the potential risks of adverse pregnancy outcome. Contraception appropriate for their medical condition should be prescribed, and advice given to seek specific pre-pregnancy counselling in specialist centres prior to stopping contraception. Given the risks associated with pregnancy, the occurrence of unwanted or unplanned pregnancies should be avoided.

The Modified WHO classification is one way of categorising maternal cardiovascular risk in pregnancy according to the underlying cardiac disease, current cardiovascular status and symptoms (Table 28.2, Adapted from ESC Guideline 2011).

TABLE 28.2 Categorising Maternal Cardiovascular Risk in Pregnancy[4]

WHO Risk Class	Risk Description	Examples of Cardiac Conditions
I	No increased risk of maternal mortality. No, or mild, increase in morbidity.	Uncomplicated and mild pulmonary stenosis, patent ductus arteriosus, mitral valve prolapse, successfully repaired septal defects, atrial or ventricular ectopic beats
II	Small increased risk of mortality or moderately increased morbidity.	A well patient with uncomplicated unoperated septal defect, repaired Tetralogy of Fallot, most arrythmias
II–III	Small increase in risk of mortality or moderately increased morbidity. (Consideration of individual factors required.)	Relatively asymptomatic patient with mild left ventricular impairment, hypertrophic cardiomyopathy, native or tissue valvular disease (except those in Class III and IV), Marfan syndrome without aortic dilatation, aorta <45 mm associated with bicuspid aortic valve, repaired coarctation.
III	Significantly increased risk of maternal mortality or severe morbidity. Intensive monitoring by a multidisciplinary team (Obstetricians, Cardiologists, Anaesthetists) in specialist centres throughout pregnancy and puerperium is recommended.	Mechanical heart valve, systemic right ventricle, Fontan circulation, unrepaired cyanotic heart disease, complex congenital heart disease, Marfan syndrome with aortic dilatation 40–45 mm, bicuspid aortic valve with aortic dilatation 45–50 mm.
IV	Extremely high risk of mortality or severe morbidity. Pregnancy contraindicated. Termination of pregnancy should be discussed. If decision is to continue with pregnancy, intensive multidisciplinary monitoring is essential.	Pulmonary arterial hypertension, severe systemic ventricular function (left ventricular ejection fraction <30%, New York Heart Association class III/IV), previous peripartum cardiomyopathy with residual left ventricular impairment, severe mitral stenosis, severe symptomatic aortic stenosis, native severe coarctation, Marfan syndrome with aortic dilatation >45 mm, aortic dilatation >50 mm with bicuspid aortic valve.

Foetal Risks

Apart from reviewing the risk of pregnancy to the woman, preconception counselling and early pregnancy care should also include the risks to the foetus. There are situations where the risk to the mother has to be weighed against the risk to the foetus, and individual management plans need to be made taking into consideration the wishes of the mother.

(1) Teratogenic implications of drugs: Where possible teratogenic drugs (e.g. ACE inhibitors, warfarin) should be stopped or switched to safer alternatives. In women with a mechanical prosthetic valve warfarin is better than heparin preparations in protecting the mother against thromboembolism. However, it is associated with the risk of teratogenesis in the first trimester (nasal bridge hypoplasia, congenital heart disease, agenesis of corpus callosum, ventriculomegaly, stippled epiphyses), miscarriage, stillbirth and foetal intracranial haemorrhage. A compromise approach may be to switch to LMWH in the first trimester, then back to warfarin from 13 weeks' gestation when organogenesis is complete, then again to LMWH two weeks prior to planned delivery. Management plans should be individualised and jointly decided by a multidisciplinary team and the woman.

(2) Increased risk of congenital heart defects (about 5% compared to a background population risk of 1%). Foetal echocardiogram should be performed at the mid-trimester anomaly scan.

(3) Inheritance of genetic conditions (e.g. autosomal dominant inheritance of Marfan syndrome). Many congenital heart defects have a polygenic inheritance with variable penetrance. Referral to a geneticist may be appropriate where there is evidence of a syndrome or where other family members are affected. Prenatal diagnosis (e.g. chorionic villous sampling) may be offered where the gene defect is known. In other cases, nuchal fold thickness could be measured at the end of the first trimester with increased thickness associated with increased risk of a cardiac defect (sensitivity 40%, specificity 99%).

(4) Risk of obstetric complications like pregnancy loss (miscarriages and perinatal loss), prematurity and foetal growth restriction (FGR) should be discussed. Prematurity may be spontaneous or iatrogenic due to a deterioration in maternal condition, development of pre-eclampsia or poor foetal growth. FGR is one of the unwanted effects of beta-blockers and may also be exacerbated by relative hypooxygenation of the uteroplacental circulation. Serial growth scans in the third trimester is appropriate.

(5) Breast-feeding is encouraged unless the women requires drugs which are absolutely contraindicated for breast-feeding. The safety profile of many drugs used to treat cardiovascular disease is not established and the relative benefits of breast-feeding need to be weighed against the risk to the neonate.

Antepartum management

History taking (personal and family history) and cardiovascular examination in early pregnancy is important in making a risk assessment and to anticipate potential complications. This is also relevant to those who are not known to have ongoing cardiac disease, who may have risk factors and need to be identified. If there is a positive history, signs or symptoms then appropriate baseline investigations such as BP, pulse, oxygen saturations, ECG and cardiac ECHO should be considered. Women identified to be at significant risk should be jointly managed by multidisciplinary teams experienced in the care of pregnant women with cardiac disease in specialist centres. Regular monitoring, preferably by the same healthcare professionals throughout gestation, is required.

Intrapartum and delivery management

A clearly documented multidisciplinary delivery plan should be made around 32–34 weeks of gestation. The aim is to minimise peripartum cardiovascular stress.

Vaginal birth is the preferred choice in most cases except in particular circumstances. Examples include:

- Warfarin therapy in mothers with mechanical heart valves, with inadequate time to stop treatment (about 10 days required) and convert to heparin (which does not cross placenta), to allow reversal of foetal anticoagulation which can result in the risk of foetal intracranial haemorrhage during a vaginal birth
- Women who are unable to mount the increased cardiac output required during labour such as those with severe aortic stenosis
- In extremely high risk cases with precarious cardiovascular status where very intensive monitoring and control is required, such as severe pulmonary hypertension
- Acute events, like acute heart failure and aortic dissection, where expediting delivery may be required.

In most cases of a planned vaginal birth, an early slow incremental epidural is advocated to reduce sympathetic activity from pain and minimise additional load on the heart, whilst taking care to minimise the risk of acute cardiovascular fluctuations (e.g. acute peripheral vasodilatation and hypotension). To avoid the detrimental effects of the Valsalva manoeuvre, active pushing in the second stage of labour should be minimised, or avoided by allowing passive foetal head descent to the perineum (promoted by uterine contractions) followed by an elective instrumental delivery.

Thromboprophylaxis with heparin or low molecular weight heparin is usually withheld peripartum. Particularly in those with a prosthetic mechanical valve, the period of stopping anticoagulation should be kept to the minimum. Optimising the timing of delivery in association with anticoagulation management requires the multidisciplinary expertise of Obstetricians, Cardiologists and Haematologists.

There has been a general shift in policy away from antibiotic use to prevent infective endocarditis in patients with valvular heart diseases, even outside of pregnancy. There is no evidence that vaginal delivery or caesarean section is associated with infective endocarditis. Hence, the need for intrapartum and immediate pre-caesarean antibiotic prophylaxis should only be considered in the highest risk patients, which include those with a prosthetic heart valve and a previous history of infective endocarditis. The specific antibiotics to be given should follow the latest local antimicrobial recommendations for high risk procedures (e.g. dental procedures), with checks that the recommended drugs are safe in pregnant and lactating women.[5]

Postpartum care

Prophylaxis against postpartum haemorrhage usually involves a slow low dose infusion of oxytocin, avoiding the usual bolus dose in order to prevent a sudden sharp rise in autotransfusion from the uterus. Accepting the potential oxytocin side-effects of peripheral vasodilation, tachycardia and fluid retention (hence pulmonary oedema) is arguably better than the acute consequences of a postpartum haemorrhage. Ergometrine and carboprost are contraindicated. In caesarean section cases, prophylactic uterine compression sutures should be considered.

High risk cases should be nursed in the high-dependency unit or intensive care unit in the immediate postpartum period, usually for at least 24–48 hours. This is the time when the risk of pulmonary oedema is greatest, following autotransfusion from the uterus and movement of extravascular fluid into the intravascular space. In unstable cardiac conditions a more prolonged stay in hospital may be required.

Contraception in the immediate postpartum period should be actively encouraged to avoid unwanted pregnancies. Non-user dependent progesterone-only preparations such as Depo-Provera and Implanon subcutaneous implants may be inserted within five days of delivery and are most commonly recommended.

Specific high risk cardiac conditions

Myocardial infarction

Pregnancy itself is a risk factor for acute myocardial infarctions. The incidence of myocardial infarctions in pregnancy and postpartum are increasing. Up to a third of these women will die. Most women have risk factors for ischaemic heart disease (smoking, diabetes, obesity, chronic hypertension, advance maternal age, renal transplant, family history). A high index of suspicion and early detection with the use of ECG and troponin 1 quantification is warranted.

Aortic dissection

The aorta is particularly vulnerable to systolic hypertension in pregnancy particularly in Marfan's syndrome and those with a dilated aortic root with bicuspid aortic valve. However, aortic dissection may also occur in pregnant women without these risk factors and usually presents in the latter part of pregnancy or immediately post-partum. A high index of suspicion in women presenting with chest pain is required. Diagnosis can be made by CT scan. To prevent aortic dissection in vulnerable women, systolic hypertension needs to be prevented or treated aggressively with beta blockers.

Valvular heart disease

Mitral stenosis, severe aortic stenosis and complicated mechanical heart valves present the greatest management challenges. Mitral and aortic stenosis prevent women from mounting adequate increases in cardiac output, so they are therefore at significant risk of pulmonary oedema. Sudden decreases in systemic vascular resistance must be avoided in severe aortic stenosis. Women may be unaware of their valve lesion (commonly secondary to rheumatic heart disease), particularly if they originate from less developed countries where there is limited healthcare. Echocardiograms should be arranged as soon as possible where there is a suspicion of an undiagnosed valvular condition. The challenges of thromboprophylaxis in women with mechanical heart valves are discussed above.

Pulmonary hypertension

Pregnancy in women with pulmonary hypertension, regardless of cause, has a 30–50% mortality risk. If termination of pregnancy is declined by the patient, very close monitoring and detailed delivery plans must be made by an experienced multidisciplinary team in specialist units.

Peripartum cardiomyopathy

This condition typically presents in late pregnancy or in the first few months post delivery. The cause is unknown and it has an incidence ranging from 1:300 to 1:4000 pregnancies, depending on the population. Mortality could be as high as

10–15% in some regions. Women usually present with dyspnoea exacerbated by lying flat. A quarter of these cases will also show hypertension. The diagnosis can be by chest X-ray and echocardiography. Approximately 50% of women will spontaneously recover over the first six months. The remainder will mostly have some residual impairment but the worse cases require cardiac transplantation. The recurrence risk in subsequent pregnancies is 30–50%.

References

1. Bowater SE, Thorne SA. (2010) Management of pregnancy in women with acquired and congenital heart disease. *Postgrad Med J* **86**:100–105.
2. Curry R, Swan I, Steer PJ. (2009) Cardiac disease in pregnancy. *Curr Opin Obstet Gynecol* **21**:508–513.
3. James DK, Steer PJ, Weiner CP, Gonik B. (2011) *High Risk Pregnancy Management Options*, 4th edn.
4. ESC Guidelines on the management of cardiovascular diseases during pregnancy. (2011). *Eur Heart J* **32**:3147–3197.
5. RCOG Good practice guidelines. (2011) Cardiac Disease and pregnancy (Good practice No. 13).

29

VENOUS THROMBOEMBOLISM (VTE) IN PREGNANCY

Jeslyn Wong and Claudia Chi

Introduction

Venous thromboembolism (VTE) is one of the most common causes of maternal death. Pregnancy is associated with a 6–10 fold increase in the risk of VTE compared to non-pregnant state. Many substantial changes in the coagulation and vascular systems occur during normal pregnancy, leading to a hypercoagulable state. For instance, there is a progressive increase in plasma concentration of several clotting factors, including factor VIII, factor X and fibrinogen levels and a reduction in the anticoagulant mechanisms including decreased protein S activity and increased resistance to activated protein C.[1]

Several studies have suggested that Asian populations have lower rates of VTE as compared to those of other racial groups. This may be attributed to low clinical suspicion in a perceived low-risk population, resulting in under-diagnosis of VTE.[2] In Singapore, Malays were found to have the highest incidence of VTE (70 per 100,000), followed by Indians (56 per 100, 000), and Chinese (51 per 100, 000) outside pregnancy.[3] Whereas the incidence of VTE among North Americans of European origin has been estimated to be between 103 and 149 per 1000,000.[4-6]

The consequences of VTE are important. It can be associated with significant maternal morbidity and mortality. Maternal hypoxia and circulatory failure resulting from pulmonary embolism poses significant maternal and foetal risk. Therapeutic measures for VTE also have potential maternal and foetal adverse effects.

This chapter aims to highlight the risk factors for VTE in pregnancy, and to discuss prevention and the acute management of VTE in a pregnant patient.

Risk Factors for Venous Thromboembolism in Pregnancy

The risk factors for VTE in pregnancy may be classified into pre-existing, obstetric and transient risks.

Prevention of VTE in Pregnancy (Antenatal)

Women with Previous VTE

In the group of women with previous VTE, it is important to differentiate them into 2 main groups: those who had a single previous episode of VTE and those with a history of recurrent VTE.

Many individuals with recurrent VTE are on long term warfarin. Warfarin crosses the placenta and is associated with an increased risk of congenital abnormalities including a characteristic warfarin embryopathy in about 5% of foetuses exposed between 6 and 12 weeks of gestation. Therefore once pregnancy is confirmed, warfarin should be stopped, and converted to low molecular weight heparin (LMWH). This should ideally be done before the 6th week of pregnancy. Women who are not on warfarin would be advised to start LMWH as soon as they have a positive pregnancy test.[6]

As for women with a previous single episode of VTE, it is useful to stratify them into the following groups:

- Unprovoked VTE
- Estrogen- provoked (estrogen-containing contraception or pregnancy) VTE
- Thombophilia or family history associated VTE
- Temporary risk factor (e.g. surgery, trauma) associated VTE

Women with recurrent VTE, unprovoked VTE, estrogen-provoked VTE, thrombophilia or family history (1st degree relative) associated VTE, are at high risk of VTE in the current pregnancy. Antenatal LMWH should therefore be considered in such women, and should be continued until 6 weeks post-partum.

Women with previous VTE provoked by a temporary risk factor that are no longer present are at intermediate risk, and do not generally require antenatal LMWH if no other risks factors. They should, however, be offered LMWH for 6 weeks postpartum.

TABLE 29.1   Risk Factors for Venous Thromboembolism in Pregnancy

Pre-existing	Obstetric	Transient

• Previous VTE
• Thrombophilia
  • Heritable
    • Antithrombin deficiency
    • Protein C/S deficiency
    • Factor V Leiden
    • Prothrombin gene G20210A
  • Acquired (antiphospholipid syndrome)
• Medical co-morbidities (e.g. heart/lung disease, systemic lupus erythematosus (SLE), cancer, nephotic syndrome, sickle cell disease, intravenous drug user (IVDU))
• Age >35 years
• BMI >30kg/m^2
• Parity ≥ 3
• Smoking
• Gross varicose veins
• Paraplegia
	• Multiple pregnancy, assisted reproductive therapy
	• Pre-eclampsia
	• Caesarean section
	• Post-partum haemorrhage > 1L requiring transfusion
		• Surgical procedures in pregnancy or puerperium
		• Hyperemesis/dehydration
		• Ovarian hyperstimulation syndrome (OHSS)
		• Admission or immobility
		• Systemic infection
		• Postpartum wound infection
		• Long- distance travel (>4 hours)

Women with Thrombophilia

Thrombophilia can be divided into heritable thrombophilia, and acquired thrombophilia. Examples of each group are included in Table 29.1 above, under "pre-existing" risk factors.

Women with thrombophilia and previous VTE and women with inherited thrombophilia associated with high risk of VTE (such as antithrombin deficiency, homozygous factor V Leiden or combined defects) are considered high risk and hence prophylactic LMWH during the antenatal period and for 6 weeks postpartum are recommended.

On the other hand, women with asymptomatic (no previous VTE) thrombophilia (except for women with antithrombin deficiency or homozygous or compound heterozygous defects) and no other risks factors, may potentially be managed without antenatal prophylactic LMWH; however, individualised care and expert opinion should be sought and postpartum LMWH be considered for at least 7 days postpartum.

In women with antiphospholipid syndrome (APS) and previous VTE, antenatal LMWH and post-partum LMWH for 6 weeks are recommended. Women with

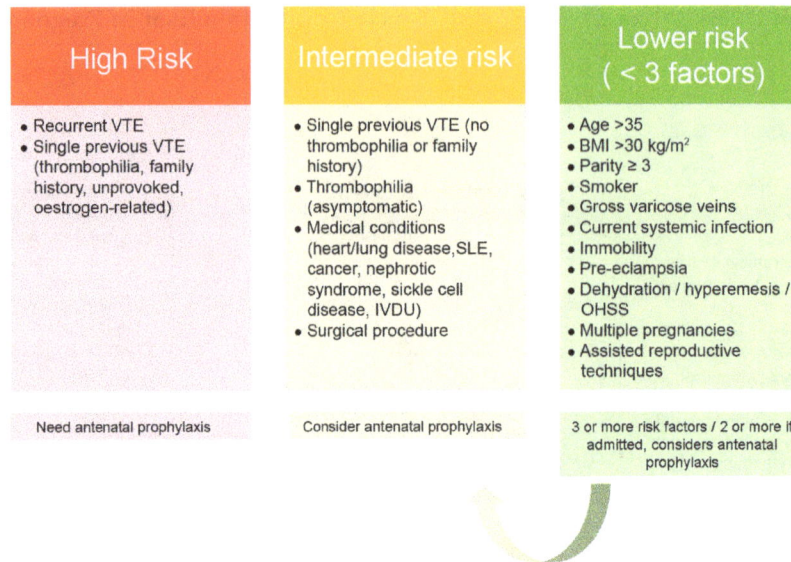

High Risk	Intermediate risk	Lower risk (< 3 factors)
• Recurrent VTE • Single previous VTE (thrombophilia, family history, unprovoked, oestrogen-related)	• Single previous VTE (no thrombophilia or family history) • Thrombophilia (asymptomatic) • Medical conditions (heart/lung disease, SLE, cancer, nephrotic syndrome, sickle cell disease, IVDU) • Surgical procedure	• Age >35 • BMI >30 kg/m^2 • Parity ≥ 3 • Smoker • Gross varicose veins • Current systemic infection • Immobility • Pre-eclampsia • Dehydration / hyperemesis / OHSS • Multiple pregnancies • Assisted reproductive techniques
Need antenatal prophylaxis	Consider antenatal prophylaxis	3 or more risk factors / 2 or more if admitted, considers antenatal prophylaxis

FIGURE 29.1 ■ Antenatal thromboprophylaxis risk assessment and management.[6]

APS with no previous VTE and no other risk factors or foetal indications for LMWH may potentially be managed without antenatal LMWH; but similarly, individualised care and expert opinion should be sought and postpartum LMWH be considered for at least 7 days postpartum.

Prevention of VTE in Pregnancy (Postnatal)

For patients at high risk of VTE, and who were on antenatal LMWH, LMWH should be continued for 6 weeks post-partum. For patients at intermediate risk, LMWH should be continued for 1 week post-partum.

Risk factors for VTE associated with delivery include:

- Caesarean section
- Post- partum haemorrhage >1L or blood transfusion
- Use of mid-cavity rotational forceps for delivery
- Prolonged labour

Other pre-existing conditions that increase the risk of VTE (Table 29.1) include obesity, smoking history, parity of 3 or more, pre-eclampsia, advanced maternal age, thrombophilias with or without previous VTE and other medical co-morbidities like nephrotic syndrome, heart disease, and systemic lupus erythematosus. The following

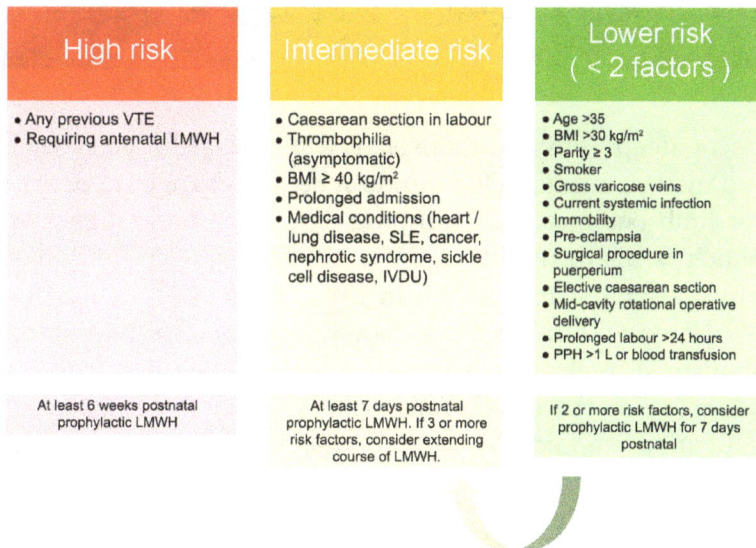

FIGURE 29.2 ■ Postnatal thromboprophylaxis risk assessment and management.[6]

flow chart (Fig. 29.2) summarises the thromboprophylaxis risk assessment and management during the postpartum period.

Contraindications to LMWH

- Active antenatal or post-partum haemorrhage
- High risk of bleeding e.g. placenta previa
- Bleeding diathesis
- Thrombocytopenia
- Acute stroke in last 4 weeks
- Severe renal disease (decreased excretion)
- Severe liver disease (with impaired coagulation profile)
- Uncontrolled hypertension (>200/120 mmHg)

Dosage of Prophylactic LMWH

The dosage of prophylactic dose of LMWH in the form of enoxaparin (Clexane®), is 0.6 mg/kg/day.

Suggested thromboprophylactic doses of enoxaparin:

<50 kg → 20 mg daily
50–90 kg → 40 mg daily
91–130 kg → 60 mg daily
131–170 kg → 80 mg daily

Diagnosis of VTE

The signs of deep vein thrombosis (DVT) and pulmonary embolism may be subtle, and may be mistaken for common benign changes in pregnancy. For example, lower limb oedema and cramping is a common benign symptom in pregnancy, which is also present in DVT, although lower limb swelling and pain almost always occurs unilaterally in DVT. Perception of dyspnea is also commonly associated with normal pregnancy, but may also be a symptom of pulmonary embolism. Therefore, it is important that a detailed history is taken, which includes identifying the risk factors for VTE in the patient. Physical examination and investigations should also be performed in order to confirm the diagnosis.

Signs and Symptoms of DVT Include:

- Lower limb swelling and pain (generally unilateral)
- Pain on compression of the calf or on deep palpation in the femoral triangle
- Dorsiflexion of the foot may elicit pain in the leg (Homan's sign)
- Leg swelling and pain may be preceded by low back pain
- Low grade fever

Signs and Symptoms of Pulmonary Embolism Include:

- Shortness of breath
- Pleuritic chest pain of acute onset
- Hemoptysis may occur
- Low grade fever
- Tachycardia
- Desaturation of the patient
- Increased jugular venous pressure (JVP)
- Hypotension, cyanosis and collapse and sudden death can occur

Any patient with high clinical suspicion of VTE should be promptly started on therapeutic doses of LMWH (unless any contraindication), and continued on the treatment until the diagnosis is excluded using objective testing.

Investigations

— DVT
  - Compression duplex ultrasound

- Pulmonary embolism
  - Electrocardiogram (ECG)
    - Look for "S1Q3T3", signs of right heart strain, RBBB
  - Arterial blood gas
  - Echocardiography
    - Regional wall motion abnormalities with sparing of the apex of the right ventricle (McConnell's sign) is suggestive of pulmonary embolism
  - Chest X ray (CXR) — with lead shielding of the foetus
  - If CXR and compression duplex ultrasound are negative, but clinical suspicion of pulmonary embolism is still high, consider ventilation-perfusion scan (V/Q scan) or CT pulmonary angiogram (CTPA).
    - V/Q scan increases the risk of childhood cancer (1 in 280,000, vs 1 in 1,000,000 in CTPA)
    - CTPA increases risk of maternal breast cancer (increased up to 13.6%, background risk of 1 in 200)
- Blood test
  - D-Dimer is not useful in diagnosing DVT/pulmonary embolism, as it raised even in normal pregnancy due to physiological changes in pregnancy.
  - Blood tests for full blood count, coagulation screen, renal and liver panel should be taken before starting treatment
    - Use of anticoagulation therapy is influenced by renal and liver function

Management of VTE

LMWH (such as enoxaparin, Clexane®) is given in 2 divided doses per day, with the dosage titrated according to the patient's weight.

For enoxaparin, the recommended therapeutic dosage is 1 mg/kg twice a day.

Therapeutic anticoagulation should be continued throughout pregnancy, suspended for delivery, and restarted for at least 6 weeks post-partum and until at least 3 months of treatment has been given in total. When a patient suspects that she is in labour, she should stop injecting LMWH. If the delivery is planned, LMWH should be withheld for 24 hours before planned delivery. LMWH can then be restarted postnatally when the risk of bleeding if deemed to be low.

Patients should be offered a choice between LMWH and warfarin once they have delivered. Both forms of anticoagulation are safe for use when breastfeeding. However, monitoring of warfarin would require regular blood tests especially in the first 10 days of initiating the drug, and should be started at least 3–5 days after delivery due to risk of haemorrhage.

Rarely, patients may present with acute cardiorespiratory collapse in a massive pulmonary embolism. Basic resuscitative measures should be administered by a multidisciplinary team, including both the medical team and obstetrical team. Once the patient is stabilised, intravenous unfractionated heparin is the anticoagulation of choice as it is more favourable in these circumstances due to its rapid effect. When the diagnosis is confirmed with echocardiography or CTPA, thrombolysis or surgical embolectomy by cardiothoracic surgeons should be considered.[7]

Implications of LMWH on Regional Anaesthesia during Labour and Delivery

It is recommended that regional anaesthesia should not be undertaken until at least 24 hours after the last therapeutic dose of LMWH (twice- daily regimen) and at least 12 hours after the last prophylactic dose of LMWH.[2] The epidural catheter should not be removed within 12 hours of the most recent LMWH injection. LMWH should not be given at least 4 hours after the epidural catheter has been removed.

References

1. James DK, Steer PJ, Weiner CP, Gonik B. (2010) *High Risk Pregnancy, Management Option,* 4th edn.
2. Zakai NA, McClure LA. (2011) Racial differences in venous thromboembolism. *J Thromb Haemost,* **9**: 1877–82.
3. Molina JA, Jiang ZG, Heng BH, Ong BK. (2009) Venous thromboembolism at the National Healthcare Group, Singapore. *Ann Acad Med Singapore* **38**:470–8.
4. White RH, Keenan CR. (2009) Effects of race and ethnicity on the incidence of venous thromboembolism. *Throm Res* **123**(Suppl 4):S11–7.
5. Silverstein MD, Heit JA, Mohr DN. Petterson TM, O'Fallon WM, Melton LJ III. (1998) Trends in the incidence of deep vein thrombosis and pulmonary embolism: a 25 years population-based study. *Arch Intern Med* **158**:585–93.
6. Thrombosis and embolism during pregnancy and the puerperium, reducing the risk. Royal College of Obstetrician and Gynaecology. Green-top Guideline no. 37a, 2015.
7. Thrombosis and embolism during pregnancy and the puerperium, the acute management of. Royal College of Obstetrician and Gynaecology. Green-top Guideline no. 37b, 2015.

30

ANTEPARTUM HAEMORRHAGE

Su Lin Lin

Introduction

Obstetrics haemorrhage (antepartum haemorrhage and postpartum haemorrhage) remains the leading cause of maternal morbidity and mortality in developing countries. In developed countries, the incidence of haemorrhage-related mortality is much lower, but it remains one of the predominant causes of maternal mortality which do not appear to decrease over the trienniums.

Antepartum haemorrhage (APH) is defined as bleeding from or into the genital tract, occurring from 24 + 0 weeks of pregnancy and prior to the birth of the baby. The two main causes of antepartum haemorrhage are placenta praevia and placental abruption. The other differential diagnosis is shown where the woman often presents with vaginal spotting or blood streaked through mucus.

Placenta Praevia

Definition. The implantation of placenta over the lower uterine segment. It is the leading cause of antepartum haemorrhage, affecting 0.4–0.5% of pregnancies.[1] The risk factors for placenta praevia are tabulated in Table 30.1 (Malden *et al.*).

Presentation

With the advances in and more routine use of ultrasonography, placenta praevia has increasingly become an incidental finding. Diagnosis is often made during

TABLE 30.1 Risk Factors for Placenta Praevia

Risk Factors	Odds Ratio
Previous caesarean sections	2.7
Maternal age (extremes of age)	9.1
Prior abortion	1.9
Parity ≥5	2.3
Parity 2–4	1.9

routine growth scan. Placental location is surveyed during the routine foetal anomaly scan. With the diagnosis of low-lying placenta at the gestation, no intervention is required as most of the placenta would not be low-lying at the later gestation as the lower uterine segment continued to form. However, advice would be given for admission with any antepartum haemorrhage, and also for avoidance of sexual intercourse.

The typical presentation is painless vaginal bleeding. This commonly occurs around 32 weeks of gestation, although the presentation can be in earlier gestation. Physical presentation reveals non-tender uterus. Malpresentation is another way placenta praevia presents in pregnancy, occurring in about 35% of cases of placenta praevia.[2] Vigilance should therefore be exercised regarding the placental location when the foetus is in a non-cephalic presentation.

Placenta Abruptio

Placenta abruptio is defined as the premature separation of the placenta from the decidual-placental interface prior to the delivery of the foetus. It complicates 0.4–1% of pregnancies[3] and is a significant cause of maternal and perinatal morbidity and mortality. Perinatal deaths can occur in utero as stillbirths or postnatally as neonatal deaths. In developed countries, approximately 10% of all preterm births and 10–20% of all perinatal deaths are caused by placental abruption.[3]

Risk Factors for Placental Abruption

The major risk factors for placental abruption are listed in Table 30.2. Smoking is one of the few modifiable risk factors for abruption. The combination of smoking and hypertension has a synergistic effect on the risk of placental abruption.[4] Sudden abdominal trauma or rapid uterine decompression have been postulated to cause shearing of the placenta, due to sudden stretching or contraction of the underlying uterine wall.

TABLE 30.2 Major Risk Factors for Placenta Abruptio

Previous history of placenta abruptio

Pregnancy-induced hypertension/pre-eclampsia

Polyhydramnios

Abdominal trauma

Smoking

Cocaine use

Presentation

Women with acute placental abruption typically present with an abrupt onset of acute abdominal pain and vaginal bleeding. This is known as "revealed" abruption. "Concealed" abruptio occurs in 10–20% of placental abruptions, where the women present with abdominal pain of varying degree in the absence of vaginal bleeding. All or most of the blood is trapped between the foetal membranes and decidua, rather than escaping though the cervix and vagina.[5] These cases may pose a diagnostic challenge and a delay in treatment.

Assessment of Women Presenting with Antepartum Haemorrhage

History Taking

Features elicited from history help to distinguish the cause of antepartum haemorrhage.

- Painless haemorrhage is suggestive of placenta praevia, vasa praevia or lower genital tract causes.
- Haemorrhage associated with constant abdominal pain is consistent with the diagnosis of placental abruption. However, the diagnosis of concealed abruption (which can present with painless bleeding or abdominal pain without bleeding) should always be borne in mind.

Identification of risk factors from history also aid in diagnosis.

Physical Examination

- Vital signs, especially blood pressure and pulse rate, are crucial as they determine the potential hypovolaemic state that the woman is in. They also determine the degree of resuscitation required for the woman.

- The woman should be assessed for tenderness or signs of an acute abdomen. The tense or "woody" feel to the uterus on abdominal palpation indicates a significant abruption.

Speculum Examination

- Not contraindicated in women who present with antepartum haemorrhage. A speculum examination can be useful to identify cervical dilatation or visualise a lower genital tract cause for the APH.

Digital Vaginal Examination

- If placenta praevia is a possible diagnosis (for example, a previous scan shows a low placenta, there is a high presenting part on abdominal examination or the bleed has been painless), digital vaginal examination should not be performed until an ultrasound has excluded placenta praevia. Digital vaginal examination can provide information on cervical dilatation if APH is associated with pain or uterine activity.

Investigations

Maternal Investigations

Blood tests

- Full blood count and determination of blood group including Rhesus should always be performed.
- Group and cross-match with at least four units of blood should be made available for major haemorrhage.
- Blood should also be dispatched to screen for disseminated intravascular coagulation which is invariably associated with massive abruption. One practical point is to order fresh frozen plasma during the time when packed cells are being requested.

Ultrasound

- Ultrasound to assess the location of the placenta is crucial unless prior information about the location of the placenta is available. However, placenta abruptio is a clinical diagnosis and ultrasound has limited sensitivity to detect the presence of a retroplacental clot. The absence of retroplacental haematoma does not exclude the possibility of severe abruption because blood may escape through the cervix and vagina instead of collecting behind the uterus. The sensitivity for detection of retroplacental haematoma is around 25%.[6] However, a positive finding is associated with worse neonatal outcome.[7]

Foetal Investigations

- An assessment of the foetal heart trace via cardiotocography should be performed as this helps decision making regarding the timing as well as the mode of delivery.

Management

- Women presenting with spotting who are no longer bleeding and where placenta praevia has been excluded can go home after a reassuring initial clinical assessment.
- All women with APH heavier than spotting and women with ongoing bleeding should remain in hospital at least until the bleeding has stopped. At present, there is no evidence to support recommendations regarding duration of inpatient management.
- The use of a course of corticosteroids to enhance foetal lung maturity should be considered for all pregnancies between 24 and 34 weeks of gestation. One exception is women who present with minor spotting, where preterm delivery is deemed unlikely. The other scenario in which corticosteroids will be of minimal benefit are women who require immediate delivery; for example, women with a clinical diagnosis of placental abruption associated with abnormalities on foetal cardiotocography.
- If foetal death is diagnosed, vaginal birth is the recommended mode of delivery for most women (provided maternal condition is satisfactory), but caesarean birth will need to be considered for some cases.
- If the foetus is compromised, a caesarean section is the appropriate method of delivery with concurrent resuscitation of the mother.
- Postpartum haemorrhage (PPH) should be anticipated in women who have experienced APH. Women with APH resulting from placental abruption or placenta praevia should be strongly advised to receive active management of the third stage of labour.

References

1. Faiz AS, Ananth CV. (2003) Etiology and risk factors for placenta praevia: an overview and meta-analysis of observational studies. *J Maternal-Foetal Neonatal Med* **13**(3): 175–190.
2. Cotton DB, Read JA, Paul RH, Quilligan EJ. (1980) The conservative aggressive management of placenta praevia. *Am J Obstet Gynaecol* **137**(6): 687–695.
3. Tikkanen M. (2011) Placental abruption: epidemiology, risk factors and consequences. *Acta Obstet Gynecol Scand* **90**(2): 140–149.
4. Ananth CV, Savitz DA, Bowes WA Jr, Luther ER. (1997) Influence of hypertensive disorders and cigarette smoking on placental abruption and uterine bleeding during pregnancy. *Br J Obstet Gynaecol* **104**(5): 572.
5. Oyelese Y, Ananth CV. (2006) Placental abruption. *Obstet Gynecol* **108**: 1005.
6. Sholl JS (1987). Abruptio placentae: clinical management in nonacute cases. *Am J Obstet Gynaecol* **156**: 40.
7. Glantz C, Purnell L. (2002) Clinical utility of sonography in the diagnosis and treatment of placental abruption. *J Ultrasound Med* **21**: 837.

31

FOETUS SMALLER THAN DATES

Biswas Arijit

Introduction

A small for gestational age (SGA) foetus is one whose estimated foetal weight or abdominal circumference is less than 10th percentile of that expected for that gestational age. The diagnosis can only be confidently made in accurately dated pregnancies. A SGA foetus could either be truly growth restricted (Foetal Growth Restriction, FGR) or constitutionally small. Seventy percent of SGA foetuses are constitutionally small. The incidence of true FGR is about 5% in general obstetric population.

It is important to identify the FGR foetus because there is an inverse relationship between the birth-weight percentile and adverse perinatal outcome. The greatest risk is when the weight is below the third percentile for gestational age. The constitutionally small baby also has a slightly increased risk of perinatal complications.

What are the Causes of FGR?

Extrinsic Factors. Factors that affect supply of nutrients and oxygen.

- Decreased utero-placental blood flow — Hypertensive diseases. Chronic renal disease. Collagen vascular disease

- Chronic hypoxaemia — Chronic pulmonary disease. Cyanotic heart disease. Living in high altitudes
- Chronic nutritional deficiency
- Autoimmune diseases
- Drugs & toxins — Substance abuse. Cigarette smoking. Drugs like anticonvulsants, antineoplastic agents
- Primary Placental problem — Idiopathic FGR
- Multiple pregnancy

Intrinsic Factors Factors that affect growth potential

- Chromosomal abnormalities
- Congenital syndromic abnormalities
- Intrauterine transplacental infections — Toxoplasma. Cytomegalovirus. Varicella-Zoster. Malaria. Rubella. Syphilis

What are the Types of FGR?

Based on the relative size of the head and the abdomen, FGR can be classified into 2 types

Symmetric FGR—All organs are proportionately small. Foetal Head Circumference (HC)/Abdominal Circumference (AC) ratio is within normal range. 20–30% of FGR are of this type. This is usually the type of FGR seen in those resulting from Intrinsic Factors. Constitutionally small foetuses are also usually symmetrically small.

Asymmetric FGR — This results from relatively greater decrease in abdomen size compared to head size. Abdomen is smaller because of a smaller liver volume compared to the relatively unaffected brain size. HC/AC ratio is higher than the expected range. This pattern of FGR is the commonest form resulting from Extrinsic factors affecting growth support. The asymmetry results from foetal adaptation to inadequate growth support by redistributing blood flow preferably to vital organs (brain and heart) at the expense of non-vital organs (kidneys, abdominal viscera)

Why is FGR Important?

FGR is one of the leading causes of perinatal morbidity and mortality. Foetuses with FGR due to intrinsic foetal causes generally have poorer prognosis because of the etiological factors like chromosomal abnormalities and intrauterine infection, which lead to poor "growth potential." FGR resulting from utero-placental insufficiency i.e. those resulting from poor "growth support," if unrecognized, may lead to intrauterine death or hypoxic neurological damage to the foetus. Hence, the aim of management is to deliver the baby before metabolic acidosis sets in from uncompensated hypoxia. The challenge is to continue conservative management until adequate foetal maturity is achieved. There is increasing evidence that FGR babies have increased risks of chronic diseases like diabetes and hypertension when they reach adulthood.[1–3]

How is the Diagnosis Made?

Clinical

- Clinical suspicion is important, especially in presence of one or more predisposing factors. Even in low risk pregnancies, clinical assessment is the important starting point. The most important pre-requisite is an accurate assessment of gestational age, because normal and abnormal foetal size is diagnosed on the basis of gestational age. Early establishment of gestational age through dating ultrasound scan early in pregnancy is imperative for all pregnancies.
- Symphysis-Fundal Height Measurements (SFH) — Measurement of the distance between the upper edge of the pubic symphysis and the top of the uterine fundus using a tape measure is a simple and inexpensive clinical tool. After 24 weeks the SFH in centimetres roughly corresponds to the gestational age. Discordance is suspected when it is more than 3 cm from that expected for the gestational age. This method performs best when the same clinician does all the serial measurements. While the sensitivity of SFH measurement is not particularly high in the detection of SGA foetus, it performs better than plain abdominal palpation alone.

Ultrasound Measurements of Foetal Growth—A routine screening ultrasound scan for foetal growth is usually performed at around 32 weeks in many centres around the world. No real evidence exists that supports the role of routine third trimester scans in the detection and improvement of outcome in SGA foetuses. Whenever clinical suspicion of FGR is present, ultrasound assessment of foetal growth is important. Prenatal diagnosis is wholly based on ultrasonographic detection of small foetal size. The most important ultrasound parameter is the foetal abdominal circumference (AC). Abdominal circumference is an indirect estimate of foetal liver size and glycogen storage. Foetal weight can be roughly estimated by using formulae that incorporate foetal AC, Head circumference (HC) and Femur length (FL). Ultrasound diagnosis of SGA foetus is made when either the Estimated Foetal Weight (EFW) or the foetal AC is less than 10th centile expected for that gestational age, which can be assessed by using available growth curves. Customised and individualised growth curves may improve diagnostic performance.

How Should We Manage?

Once a diagnosis of FGR is made, the most important issue is to distinguish the constitutionally small foetus from the growth-restricted foetus. A constitutionally small foetus achieves its normal growth potential and has a good prognosis, whereas the foetus whose growth potential is restricted is at increased risk of perinatal morbidity and mortality. FGR resulting from intrinsic foetal factors such as aneuploidy, congenital malformations and foetal infection carries a guarded prognosis that often cannot be improved by any intervention. FGR resulting from uteroplacental insufficiency has a better prognosis if delivered at an optimum gestation.

Initial Assessment, therefore, should be targeted to identify a cause:

- Detailed Foetal Anomaly scan — to look for structural abnormality. Approximately 10 % of severe FGR (EFW below 3%) are associated with structural abnormality.
- Karyotype — by amniocentesis or foetal blood sampling for cases of FGR with foetal abnormality or early onset severe symmetrical FGR or FGR with polyhydramnios.
- Infection screen — Maternal blood to check for seroconversion for cytomegalovirus (CMV), Toxoplasma and Rubella in cases of FGR with markers of infection like intracranial or intrahepatic calcification or increased echogenicity.

In absence of an identifiable cause and in presence of a predisposing factor like hypertensive disease, renal disease, autoimmune disease, thrombophilic disorders etc. the most likely cause for FGR is utero-placental insufficiency. In absence of such predisposing conditions, it is important to differentiate between constitutional small foetus and FGR due to idiopathic placental insufficiency. In these cases, effort should focus on identification of symptoms/signs associated with chronic foetal hypoxia. These are:

Clinical — Foetal movements assessed by Foetal Movement Charts. Decreased foetal movement may be associated with chronic foetal hypoxia.

Investigations

- Doppler Velocimetry —
  (i) Umbilical artery Doppler velocimetry to assess placental vascular resistance. An increase in umbilical artery resistance, leading to reduced end diastolic flow, is consistently seen when 30% of the villous vasculature ceases to function. As placental dysfunction worsens, umbilical artery blood flow resistance increases and transfer of substrates, oxygen, and foetal waste products becomes increasingly impaired. Normal end diastolic flow is infrequently associated with significant perinatal morbidity or mortality and is strong evidence of foetal well-being. Absent or reversed end-diastolic flow in the umbilical artery occurs when 60–70% of the villous vasculature is obliterated and is evidence of poor foetal condition and hence an indication to deliver the foetus.
  (ii) Middle Cerebral artery (MCA) Dopplers — Vasodilation and high diastolic flow in the middle cerebral artery reflect compensatory cerebral vasodilatation (brain-sparing effect) secondary to foetal hypoxia and result in a reduced pulsatility index (MCA-PI). In a term foetus, a relatively lower resistance index in MCA compared to the umbilical artery (Reversed Cerebro-Placental Ratio) is an indication to deliver the foetus.
- Assessment of Amniotic Fluid Volume — Amniotic fluid is semi-quantitatively assessed by ultrasound by measuring the Amniotic Fluid Index (AFI). Chronic foetal hypoxia from placental dysfunction in the FGR foetus results in redistribution of blood flow in the foetus away from non-vital organs like kidney, liver or intestines to the brain and heart. This results in decreased foetal urine production and decreased amniotic fluid. AFI less than five is considered as severe oligohydramnios and this is one of the indications to deliver a FGR foetus.
- Cardiotocography (CTG) — Abnormal CTG in the form of poor baseline variability, absence of accelerations and presence of spontaneous decelerations is

usually a late sign of foetal hypoxia in a FGR foetus. An abnormal CTG would indicate urgent delivery.

Frequency of foetal assessment — Once FGR is diagnosed by clinical and ultrasound examination, foetal growth should be assessed by foetal biometry every 2 to 3 weeks. Foetal well-being should be assessed by Daily Foetal Movement chart and weekly/twice weekly AFI, Doppler velocimetry and CTG. The frequency of assessment depends on the severity of FGR.

When and How to Deliver?

The essence of management of the FGR foetus is optimum timing of delivery, before the foetus develops metabolic acidosis. The mode of delivery is determined by usual obstetric considerations and the degree of urgency of delivery. Antenatal corticosteroids for enhancing lung maturity should be administered for FGR foetuses who might need delivery prior to 34 weeks.[4,5]

The following are a few important guidelines, which might help to time delivery:

- In presence of normal foetal assessment parameters, the FGR foetus or constitutionally small foetus should be delivered once it reaches 37–38 weeks.
- Between 34–37 weeks, elevated umbilical artery RI or S/D ratio, especially in presence of oligohydramnios is an indication to deliver.
- In FGR foetuses remote from term (<34 weeks of gestation), evidence of normal umbilical artery flow by Doppler velocimetry is reassuring with regard to immediate foetal outcome. Prolongation of pregnancy to gain further foetal maturity is reasonable in these cases.
- For pregnancies beyond 34 weeks, absent EDF in umbilical artery is an indication to deliver.
- For pregnancies beyond 28 weeks, reversed EDF in umbilical artery or an abnormal CTG is an indication to deliver.
- Prior to 28 weeks, the decision to deliver should be taken with due consideration of neonatal intensive care facilities and after carefully discussing the options with the couple. Normal venous Dopplers might allow continuation of pregnancy for a few days even when umbilical artery Dopplers show absent or reversed EDF. Between 26 and 29 weeks of gestation, each day in utero has been estimated to improve survival by 1–2%.

Salient Points

- True FGR is an important cause of perinatal mortality and morbidity.
- Diagnosis is suspected clinically either because of the presence of a predisposing condition in the mother and/or smaller symphysis fundal height.
- Diagnosis is confirmed on ultrasound scan. Foetal AC and EFW are the two most important measurements on ultrasound for diagnosis.
- Accurate early dating is essential to make the diagnosis confidently.
- It may be difficult to isolate the true FGR foetus from the constitutionally small foetus.
- True FGR foetus is at risk of chronic hypoxia, foetal neurological damage and even death.
- Close monitoring of foetal growth and well-being with the use of foetal movement chart, ultrasound Doppler velocimetry, AFI and CTG are important.
- The aim of management is to deliver a reasonably mature foetus before it develops metabolic acidosis.

References

1. James DK, Steer PJ, Weiner CP, Gonik B. (2010) *High Risk Pregnancy Management Options*, 4th edn.
2. Baskett TF, Calder AA, Sabaratnam A. (2014) *Munro Kerr's Operative Obstetrics*, 12th edn.
3. Hacker NF, Gambore JC, Hobil CJ. (2010) *Essential of Obstetrics and Gynaecology*, 5th edn.
4. SOGC Clinical Practical Guidelines No. 295. (2013) *Intrauterine Growth Restriction: Screening, Diagnosis, and Management*. Society of Obstetrics and Gynaecology, Canada.
5. Royal College of Obstetricians and Gynaecologists Green-top Guidelines No. 31. (2013) *Small-for-Gestational-Age Fetus, Investigation and Management*.

32

MULTIPLE PREGNANCY

Harvard Lin, Biswas Arijit and Kuldip Singh

Introduction

Multiple pregnancy is the presence of more than one foetus in the uterus during pregnancy, the commonest being twin pregnancy.

The incidence of multiple pregnancy is 3% of live births

Frequency calculated using Hellin's rule is

Twins	1 in 80 pregnancies
Triplets	1 in 80^2 pregnancies
Quadruplets	1 in 80^3 pregnancies

However, over the past few decades, there has been a 40% increase in twinning rates and a 3 to 4 fold rise in high order births. This is due to increasing use of assisted reproduction techniques and in vitro fertilisation.[1,2]

Types of Twin Pregnancy

Monozygotic (Monovular) 30% of All Twins

- When there is one ovum fertilised and it divides early in development into two or more embryos
- (i) Cleavage before 5th day (33%)
  — Separate amnions and chorions

  (ii) Cleavage between 5–10 days (64%)
  — Separate amnions but a common chorion (placenta)

    (iii) Cleavage after 10th day (3%)
        — Common amnion and chorion

    (iv) Later division — many result in conjoined twins, where there is union between foetuses
- Always the same sex

Dizygotic Twins (Binovular) — 70% of Twins

- When two ova are fertilised, thus have two chorions and two amnions (dichorionic, diamniotic)
- Same or different sexes
- Factors affecting Dizygotic Twinning:
  - (i) More common in dark races
  - (ii) Maternal family history of twins/multiple pregnancy
  - (iii) Increased parity — more than 5
  - (iv) Increased maternal age (35 years)
  - (v) Higher fertility
  - (vi) Increasing use of ovulation induction drugs in assisted reproductive techniques
  - (vii) In vitro fertilisation (IVF)

Complications/Risk of Multiple Pregnancy

Maternal

Antenatal

- Excessive nausea/vomiting/hyperemesis gravidarum
- Pressure symptoms — oedema, haemorrhoids, varicose veins
- Miscarriage
- Anaemia
- Polyhydramnios
- Acute — in second trimester — associated with monozygotic twins
- Chronic — third trimester — associated with dizygotic twins
- Pregnancy-induced hypertension
- Antepartum haemorrhage — placenta praevia
                          — abruptio placenta
- Preterm labour
- Premature rupture of membrane

Intrapartum

- Malpresentation
- Cord prolapse
- Higher incidence of operative/assisted delivery leading to increased haemorrhage and infection

Postpartum

- Postpartum haemorrhage
- Anaemia
- Increased infection from assisted delivery
- Lactation issues
- Psychological effects

Foetal

- Prematurity as a result of preterm labour
- Intrauterine growth restriction
- Congenital anomalies
- Increased perinatal mortality — 2× greater in second twin due to growth restriction, malpresentation, assisted deliveries
- Others related to monochorionic, diamniotic twins e.g. twin to twin transfusion[3,4]

Clinical Features

History

- Uterus larger than date
- Exaggerated nausea/vomiting/hyperemesis gravidarum
- Pressure symptoms e.g. oedema, varicosities
- Complications of multiple pregnancy
    - (i) Miscarriage — threatened/actual
    - (ii) Pregnancy-induced hypertension
    - (iii) Anaemia
    - (iv) Polyhydramnios
    - (v) Antepartum haemorrhage
    - (vi) Preterm labour
    - (vii) Premature rupture of membranes

(viii) Malpresentation
(ix) Intrauterine growth restriction

Physical Examination

- Uterus larger than dates
- Abdominal girth >105 cm
- Three or more foetal poles
- Multiple foetal poles
- Two simultaneous foci of foetal heart rates that vary by 10 beats
- Other associated complications of multiple pregnancy

Investigations

Ultrasound is the most reliable method.

Antenatal screening/diagnosis

Early Ultrasound Assessment is crucial in the management of multiple pregnancy:

- Diagnosis: Only safe and reliable method for definitive diagnosis of twin gestation
- Dating: Accurate estimation of gestational age (measurement of largest baby is used to estimate gestational age)
- Chorionicity: Assessment of chorionicity: using the lambda or T-sign (V shaped extension of placental tissue into the base of the inter-twin membrane is referred to as the "lambda" and this determines dichorionicity. T shaped extension of the inter-twin membrane or the absence of the "lambda" determines monochorionicity. The number of placental masses, discordant foetal sex and membrane thickness (less than 14 weeks) are also used to determine chorionicity. Accuracy of determining chorionicity via ultrasound (if done before 14 weeks) has a sensitivity of 100% and a specificity of 99%.[5]
- Nomenclature: Assign nomenclature to foetus (e.g. upper/lower, left/right) to ensure consistency of management throughout pregnancy
- Screening for aneuploidy using nuchal translucency (NT): When crown-rump length measures from 45 mm to 84 mm (approximately 11w 0d to 13w 6d). NT when used as a screening tool for trisomy is similar between DC twins and singletons. The false-positive rate of screening becomes higher when performed on MC twins. See below for combining NT and serum testing.

- Prediction for Twin to Twin Transfusion Syndrome. See serial growth scans.

Serum screening in multiple pregnancies for aneuploidy is not as reliable as in singletons. Screening of choice is nuchal translucency and accuracy can be improved if combined with serum screening. This allows for calculation of an individual risk for each foetus. The false positive rate, likelihood of offering invasive testing and complications of invasive testing are higher. The NICE guidelines recommend referral to a foetal medicine specialist in women with a Down syndrome risk threshold of 1:150. The application of non-invasive prenatal testing is still at an early stage of development, but generally effective in monochorionic twins (due to doubling of amount of cell-free foetal DNA) and complicated in dichorionic twins (discordant DNA makes analysis difficult).

Amniocentesis in twins carries a similar loss rate compared to singletons. No data exists for higher order twins. Chorionic villus sampling (CVS) carries a higher loss rate and the problem of up to 4% incidence of co-twin contamination. In dichorionic twins, both foetuses need to be sampled. However, if the placentas are close together, CVS becomes difficult.

Antenatal monitoring

Foetal anomaly scan should be undertaken between 18–20 weeks. More time should be awarded for each consultation or scan appointment.

Serial growth scans looking for intrauterine growth restriction and growth discrepancy: Estimate foetal weight discordance using two or more biometric parameters at each ultrasound scan, every 28 days from 20 weeks. Consider a growth discrepancy of more than 25% between foetuses as an indicator for intrauterine growth restriction. For monochorionic twins, start diagnostic monitoring for TTTS from 16 weeks. Repeat monitoring every two weeks until 24 weeks. Features of TTTS on ultrasound include:

- Absent/small bladder in donor, large bladder in recipient
- Oligohydramnios in donor (maximal vertical pocket (MVP) of 2 cm) and Polyhydramnios in recipient (MVP of 8 cm)
- Blood flow in umbilical cord and foetal ductus venous reveals abnormal patterns
- Foetal hydrops
- Foetal death

Doppler assessment and cardiotocogram
In monochorionic twins, if one twin is smaller, assessment of foetal circulation and well-being should be performed weekly to biweekly

Management of Multiple Pregnancy

Management

- Early diagnosis is important
- Prevention of antenatal complications or early detection and treatment of complications

    (i)   Look for anaemia — early supplementation with iron and folic acid

    (ii) Hypertensive disorder in pregnancy
        — Detect early
        — Advice to take 100 mg of aspirin daily from second trimester if any of the following risk factors
        (a) First pregnancy
        (b) Previous pregnancy more than 10 years of age
        (c) Age 40 years or older
        (d) Family history of pre-eclampsia
        (e) Past history of eclampsia
        (f) BMI of 35 kg/m^2 at first visit

    (iii) Preterm Labour
        Preterm birth (birth <37 weeks) occurs in more than 50% of multiple pregnancies.[6] 10% deliver before 32 weeks. Preterm pre-labour rupture of the membranes also occurs more frequently. Maternal risks include hospitalisation, use of tocolytic drugs including its side effects and psychological sequelae. A foetal fibronectin test may be performed to assess the risk of preterm birth. A course of prenatal corticosteroids should be administered to women at risk of preterm birth less than 34 weeks. The risk is higher for monochorionic compared to dichorionic twins.

    (iv) Intrauterine growth restriction
        Incidence of small for gestational age (SGA) babies (birthweight <10 percentile) is 27% in twins[1] and 46% in triplets.[7] A foetus is considered SGA if the abdominal circumference or effective foetal weight are below the 10 percentile. Foetal risks are similar to singletons with growth restriction: intrauterine foetal demise and neurological morbidity.

    (v)   Growth discordance
        The definition of growth discordance is when the weight difference between foetuses is 25% or more. Growth discordancy increases the risk for adverse perinatal outcomes, and the possibility of TTTS needs to be ruled out.

Classification of growth restriction or growth discordance can be based on Doppler characteristics of the umbilical artery, in addition to the gestational age at first presentation.[6] The goal of management is to prevent intrauterine demise and long-term neurological damage.

(vi) Congenital abnormalities
There is an increased incidence of structural and chromosomal abnormalities, more evidently in monochorionic twins. Common abnormalities include: neural tube defects, facial clefts, gastrointestinal defects, anterior abdominal wall defect and cardiac anomalies. Screening and diagnostic tests are more complex as mentioned above. Management is complicated with medical and ethical dilemmas and include conservative, selective feticide or termination of whole pregnancy.

(vii) Single foetal death
Incidence of dying in utero is increased in multiple pregnancies and the risk increases with number of foetuses.[5] Early demise is termed "the vanishing twin" and occurs in 25% of cases. Demise beyond 12 weeks puts the remaining twin at risk of a poorer outcome. Management is conservative with serial ultrasound scans. Risks in all multiple pregnancies include miscarriage and severe preterm birth. Risks specific to monochorionic twins includes co-twin demise (12%) and neurological abnormality (18%).[8] Management is conservative and comprises of MCA doppler studies to exclude foetal anaemia associated with TTTS. A thorough neurodevelopmental assessment and follow-up is necessary after birth. Prognosis is determined by chorionicity and gestational age.

(viii) Twin anaemic-polycythaemic sequence
This condition is unique to monochorionic twins and refers to the discordance in haemoglobin between a monochorionic pair (Hb < 11 g/dL in donor and Hb > 20 g/dL in the recipient) in the absence of amniotic fluid discordance. The pathophysiology is again due to an imbalance in intertwin transfusion resulting in haemoglobin discordance. TAPS can occur spontaneously or after incomplete laser ablation for TTTS. Diagnosis is made via MCA Doppler suggestion anaemia and polycythaemia respectively. Anaemia results in hydrops and intrauterine death of donor, while polycythaemia causes cardiac failure and death in the recipient. Management includes elective delivery, cord occlusion or fetoscopic laser.

(ix) Twin-twin transfusion syndrome
TTTS is unique to monochorionic pregnancies and is caused by imbalance in net flow of blood transfused across arteriovenous anastomosis. This results in hypovolaemia, oliguria and oligohydramnios in the

donor twin; and hypervolemia, polyuria and polyhydramnios, fluid overload and hydrous in the recipient twin. Diagnosis is via ultrasound monitoring (see below). Untreated TTTS bears a mortality of almost 100%. Morbidity of survivals includes cerebral and cardiac sequelae owing to chronic haemodynamic imbalance in utero. Conservative management offers low survival rates. Management is via amnioreduction or laser ablation. The Eurofetus trial favours laser ablation, with fewer neonatal deaths, perinatal deaths and neurological abnormality after six months.[3]

(x) Cord entanglement
Cord entanglement is unique to monochorionic twins and incidence varies from 42% to 100%.[8,9] This may contribute towards intrauterine death. Therapy to reduce incidence of cord entanglement includes elective preterm delivery, oral sulindac therapy to reduce foetal urine production, liquor volume and foetal movement. Literature thus far had been biased in reporting, with a lack of safety evaluation of sulindac. Delivery at 32 weeks need to be balanced with the likelihood of respiratory distress syndrome and neonatal mortality.[9,10]

Timing of Delivery

Twin pregnancy: 60% will deliver spontaneously before 37 weeks' gestation.
Triplet pregnancy: 75% will deliver spontaneously before 35 weeks' gestation.
Uncomplicated monochorionic twin pregnancy: Aim to deliver by 36 weeks after a course of corticosteroids.
Uncomplicated dichorionic twin pregnancy: Aim to deliver by 37 weeks.
Uncomplicated triplet pregnancy: Aim to deliver by 36 weeks after a course of corticosteroids.
Monochorionic monoamniotic twin pregnancy: Aim to deliver at 32 weeks.

Mode of Delivery

Based on the presentation of first twin.

- Vertex-vertex — Vaginal Delivery recommended
- Vertex-Breech/Transverse Lie

> — Optimal mode is unknown. Literature supports both Vaginal Delivery and Caesarean Section
> — Management of second twin includes external cephalic version/internal podalic version and breech delivery

- Leading twin is non cephalic:
  Caesarean section recommended
- Very Low Birth Weight Infants (<1500 gm)
  Optimal mode unknown. Generally caesarean section recommended to reduce foetal trauma. However, there is little evidence on any differences in perinatal outcome
- Monochorionic/monoamniotic twin pregnancy
  Caesarean section recommended to prevent intrapartum cord complications
- Triplet or higher order pregnancies
  Optimal mode unknown. Generally Caesarean section, based on difficulties in monitoring

Intrapartum Management of Twin Pregnancy — Leading Twin is Cephalic

Stage I of Labour

- Blood for Group and Cross Matched, as there is increased incidence of operative delivery and subsequent primary postpartum haemorrhage.
- Set up intravenous line — will permit oxytocin infusion when required.
- A twin CTG machine should be used for continuous CTG monitoring throughout the intrapartum period. This includes continuous CTG monitoring of the second twin after delivery of the first twin.
- Epidural anaesthesia should be encouraged, which is especially useful for internal podalic version of second twin
- Multi-disciplinary approach should be ensured: a senior obstetrician, anaesthetist, neonatologist, midwife and paediatric nurses.

Stage II of Labour

- Send to assisted delivery or operating theatre when os is fully dilated
- Anaesthetist/neonatologist on standby

Delivery of First Twin

• Upon crowning perform a episiotomy under local anaesthesia (if epidural anaesthesia has not already been given)
• Deliver foetus
• Clamp and cut off cord of first twin
• Transfer care of neonate to paediatrician

Delivery of Second Twin

• Palpate the abdomen to determine lie of second twin
• If transverse lie, perform external version to bring one pole over the cervix. Preferably convert to breech presentation if extraction of second twin is likely. It is easier to bring down the legs of a breech then to apply forceps or ventouse to a very high floating head.
• Continuous foetal heart monitoring
  (i) To detect foetal distress that warrants immediate delivery
  (ii) Causes of foetal distress:
    — Decreased uterine volume after first twin delivery
    — Separation of placenta on which second twin depends
    — Cord prolapse

• Commence intravenous oxytocin drip to establish uterine contraction
• Confirm presentation per vaginally
• With uterine contractions and descent of presenting part, deliver second twin according to presentation of foetus (vertex or breech)
  * If second twin is cephalic and no descent of head, resort to Caesarean section as there is no place for High forceps or vacuum
  * If second twin is Breech, may consider Breech Extraction if the obstetrician is experienced. If not, resort to Caesarean section
  * If second twin remains in transverse lie — may consider Internal Podalic version with Breech extraction if membranes are intact and the obstetrician is experienced. If not, resort to Caesarean section

Stage III of Labour

• Ensure complete emptying of uterus
• Check placenta and membranes are delivered completely
• Ensure uterus is well contracted
  (i) Reduce the risk of primary postpartum haemorrhage
  (ii) Give intravenous Ergometrine/Syntocinon after delivery of second twin
  (iii) Set up prophylactic Syntocinon in drip

Puerperium

- Observe for postpartum haemorrhage
- Treatment of anaemia
- Management of lactation and breastfeeding
- Psychological support
- Treatment of neonatal problems
- Family planning advice

References

1. Louik C, Hernandez-Diaz S, Werler MM, Mitchell AA. (2006) Nausea and vomiting in pregnancy: maternal characteristics and risk factors. *Paediatr Perinat Epidemiol* **20**(4):270–278.
2. Platt MJ, Marshall A, Pharoah PO. (2001) The effects of assisted reproduction on the trends and zygosity of multiple births in England and Wales 1974–99. *Twin Res* **4**(6):417–421.
3. Cohen M, Kohl S, Rosenthal A. (1965) Foetal interlocking complicating twin gestation. *Am J Obstet Gynecol* **91**:407–412.
4. Hanson J (1975). Incidence of conjoining twinning. *Lancet* **2**(7947):1257.
5. Stenhouse E, Hardwick C, Maharaj S, *et al.* (2002). Chorionicity determination in twin pregnancies: how accurate are we? *Ultrasound Obstet Gynecol* **19**:350–352.
6. Krafft A, Breymann C, Streich J, *et al.* (2001). Hemoglobin concentration in multiple versus singleton pregnancies — Retrospective evidence for physiology not pathology. *Eur J Obstet Reprod Biol* **99**(2):184–187.
7. Campbell DM, Templeton A. (2004) Maternal complications of twin pregnancy. *Int J Gynaecol Obstet* **84**(1):71–73.
8. RCOG greentop guidelines no. 37A. (2009) Reducing the risk of thrombosis and embolism during pregnancy and the puerperium.
9. Elliott JP. (2005) High-order multiple gestations. *Semin Perinatol.* **29**(5):305–311.
10. Laws PJ, Hilder L. (2008) Australia's mothers and babies 2006. *In Unit NPS* (*ed*), Australian Institute of Health and Welfare, Sydney.

33

PRETERM LABOUR AND PRE-LABOUR RUPTURE OF MEMBRANES

Citra Mattar

Introduction

Preterm delivery is a major obstetric complication that affects 5–10% of live-births, although the incidence in developing countries may be significantly higher. It is a primary contributor to perinatal morbidity and mortality, as well as iatrogenic maternal complications, and creates significant medical and socio-economic burdens. Preterm labour is a common encounter in the delivery suite. While true labour is diagnosed in 50% of pregnancies <37 weeks' gestation, approximately 30% of preterm contractions resolve spontaneously. Fewer than 10% of women with preterm contractions will deliver within a week of onset, and 50% of women hospitalised for preterm labour will deliver at term. Key issues in management of patients with suspected or diagnosed preterm labour are the objective diagnosis of preterm labour, maternal and foetal assessment, decisions on tocolysis and conservation of pregnancy where appropriate, and technical aspects of delivering a preterm baby.

Preterm Labour

Definition and Incidence

Active labour diagnosed in a gestation <37 completed weeks.

Preterm labour precedes 50% of pregnancies which are eventually delivered <37 weeks. Preterm labour is diagnosed in the same way as labour in term pregnancies. Effacement and dilatation of the cervix should be documented together with regular uterine contractions. "Threatened" preterm labour is a term used colloquially to denote a patient suspected but not confirmed to be in labour, who has uterine contractions but no cervical changes indicating impending or active labour.[1-3]

Causes and Risk Factors

Risk factors can be identified in approximately 50% of patients experiencing preterm labour. In the remainder, there are rarely identifiable risk factors.

Factors which are strongly associated with preterm labour are:

- Extremes of maternal age (<18 or >35 years)
- Preterm delivery in a previous pregnancy
- Multiple gestations
- Over-distention of the uterus by liquor (polyhydramnios) or masses (uterine fibroids)
- Maternal habits of cigarette-smoking and/or
- Recreational drug use

Other factors positively associated with preterm labour include:

- Use of assisted reproductive techniques
- Congenital structural uterine anomalies (bicornuate or septate uterus)
- Subclinical lower genital tract infections including bacterial vaginosis
- Shortened cervix (due to deficiencies in extracellular matrix or preceding surgical trauma)
- Infections in adjacent organs (urinary or gastrointestinal tracts)
- Placental haemorrhage/antepartum haemorrhage
- Genetic and environmental influences
- Maternal medical conditions that necessitate iatrogenic preterm delivery and
- Low socio-economic group/poor healthcare may contribute

Often a single factor cannot be isolated, as the aetiology of preterm labour is multifactorial in most cases.

Maternal Complications

The main complications are related to prolonged hospitalisation and medical intervention aimed at avoiding labour and conserving the pregnancy. Examples of these include:

- Prolonged bed rest, leading to elevated risk of venous thromboembolism
- Constipation
- Chest infection
- Muscle atrophy
- Adverse effects of tocolytics
- Deranged blood sugar in diabetic women given corticosteroids.

The psychological and economic burdens should not be underestimated. If operative delivery is required, maternal surgical complications can be encountered.

Foetal Complications

Burden of preterm delivery

The common neonatal complications are

- Respiratory distress syndrome due to pulmonary surfactant deficiency
- Intracranial haemorrhage with the antecedent risks of cerebral palsy and other long-term neurological damage
- Necrotising enterocolitis
- Retinopathy of prematurity
- Low birth-weight, hypoglycaemia
- Poor temperature regulation
- Increased risk of mortality
- Birth trauma/perinatal asphyxiation due to technical complications at delivery, such as cord prolapse secondary to membrane rupture with the foetus in an abnormal lie or presentation, or the difficulty often encountered at caesarean section delivering a small foetus from a uterus with an ill-defined lower segment.

Perinatal survival depends on gestational age and birth-weight, the availability of antenatal corticosteroids, access to tertiary-level perinatal care and multidisciplinary management.

History and Physical Examination

The diagnosis of preterm labour is made in the same ways as term labour when the gestation is <37 weeks. Symptoms and risk factors should be documented, with particular attention to frequency and intensity of contractions, foetal movements and amniotic leak. Uterine contractions should be observed (palpated), and cervical changes affirmed. The symphysial-fundal height, foetal lie and presentation, and absence or presence of membranes should be documented.

Few investigations are needed to make the diagnosis of preterm labour. It is a clinical diagnosis and a composite of the subjective (symptoms) and objective (signs) evidence. If a patient is in active labour at a preterm gestation, ancillary investigations can determine the presence of a concomitant risk factor that, if treated, may reduce the risk of the labour progressing to delivery; e.g. urinary tract infection (urine microscopy and culture/sensitivity), bacterial vaginosis (vaginal swab for relevant organisms e.g. *Gardnerella, Mobiluncus*). If the membranes are ruptured, additional biochemical evidence of systemic infection may be sought (see section on pre-labour rupture of membranes). However, the collection of samples should not in any way delay the initiation of treatment once the clinical diagnosis has been made.

Prediction of delivery in a patient with suspected or "threatened" labour

Sometimes it may be a challenge to distinguish between actual labour and suspected "threatened" labour, where there are no cervical changes in the presence of symptomatic and/or palpable contractions. Because the subjective symptoms may be quite distressing for the patient, even if labour changes are not evident at the present time, management decisions rest on the likelihood of active labour commencing in the next few days.[4]

Investigations

While the diagnosis is a clinical one, certain bedside investigations may make a difference in management.

A number of biochemical and ultrasonographical markers have been evaluated for prediction of preterm labour in women in whom the diagnosis is not clear.[5]

Foetal fibronectin (fFN)

This large molecular weight glycoprotein occurs in the extracellular matrix (ECM), and is responsible for cellular adhesion at the utero-placental interface. It is always present in amniotic fluid and in cervicovaginal secretions prior to 22 weeks. When the ECM is disrupted by uterine activity or cervical change, there is a release of fFN, which forms the basis of the fFN test. In a symptomatic woman with "threatened" preterm labour in whom the amniotic membranes are intact, a sample of secretion is collected from the posterior fornix following a speculum examination. Vaginal/cervical digital examination should be avoided prior to this, due to the possibility of a false positive. The swab is placed in a proprietary solution according to the manufacturer's instructions and the result read. False positive results can also be caused by semen within the prior 24 hours or blood. This test is useful for its negative predictive value — the ability to forecast the risk of delivery based on the fFN result. A negative test result predicts that the probability of delivery within 7 days of testing is only 2.5% (negative predictive value, NPV, i.e. 97.5% of symptomatic women will not deliver within this period). A positive result predicts that the probability of delivery is approximately 25% (positive predictive value, PPV, i.e. 75% of symptomatic women are not expected to deliver). Although the fFN test carries a generally poor positive predictive value and has limited application, it does show a high PPV in populations with a high prevalence of preterm delivery, and high NPV in low prevalence populations. Cost, availability and false positive results are the downsides of this test.

Cervical length

This measurement may improve the prediction of delivery in symptomatic women, especially in combination with fFN. Normal cervical length of >30mm predicts a low likelihood of delivery (<5%) within the next 7 days. Short cervical length of <20 mm predicts a high likelihood of delivery (>25%). The prediction of delivery in women with intermediate cervical length of 20–30 mm can be improved with concomitant fFN testing, which helps to reduce uncertainty and the possibility of unnecessary intervention.

Biomarkers

Due to the heterogeneity of clinical presentations the development of a single prognostic or predictive biomarker is difficult. Risk assessment in future may require combined analyses of several markers and the development of multivariate classification models for diagnosis.

Pre-Labour Rupture of Membranes at Preterm Gestation

Definition and Incidence

Preterm pre-labour rupture of membranes (PPROM) refers to amniotic membrane rupture which occurs between 24 and <37 weeks of gestation, starting from the limit of viability.

PPROM affects 3–5% of pregnancies and complicates approximately 33% of preterm deliveries.

Causes and Risk Factors

Like preterm labour and delivery, the aetiology is multifactorial and the same risk factors described earlier apply. A history of PPROM in a previous pregnancy, lower genital tract infection (particularly bacterial vaginosis), antepartum haemorrhage and cigarette smoking provide especially strong associations.

Maternal Complications

These are related to

- Ascending infection
- Intra-amniotic infection (chorioamnionitis)
- Endometritis
- Septicaemia, with higher incidence at earlier gestation.

Foetal Complications

Foetal complications usually outweigh maternal complications. Foetal complications are greater at an earlier gestational age of PPROM. Intra-amniotic infection may lead to foetal tachycardia and distress in utero (including meconium-stained amniotic fluid) and even perinatal demise. Placental abruption (affects 2–5% of PPROM pregnancies) and umbilical cord prolapse (especially with non-cephalic presentations) result in acute hypoxia. Foetal malpresentation is common, especially with extremely preterm foetuses, which increases the risk of birth trauma. Prolonged severe oligohydramnios which occurs prior to 28 weeks is a factor for pulmonary hypoplasia, which may be fatal after birth. Foetal exposure to intrauterine inflammation is associated with elevated risk of neurodevelopmental impairment.

History and Physical Examination

- The typical symptom reported is a "gush" of fluid, usually unprovoked, but women can also describe intermittent leaking.
- There may also be infrequent mild uterine contractions, or light vaginal bleeding.
- Direct observation, via sterile speculum examination, of amniotic fluid pooling in the posterior fornix is sufficient for diagnosis. If it is not immediately visible, the woman is asked to cough, whereupon the fluid may be noticed leaking from the cervix.
- The cervical dilatation should also be noted, where possible, as digital examination is contraindicated due to the risk of intra-amniotic infection. The presence of cord or small foetal part prolapse, or uterine bleeding, is notable.
- The diagnosis is clinical, based on visualising amniotic fluid in the vagina.

Investigations

Again, the diagnosis is clinical, and investigations serve to monitor the mother and baby for adverse outcomes. Investigations may be required to confirm the diagnosis if the signs are equivocal.

Fern test

The simplest test is the "fern test," or arborisation, witnessed when the fluid from the posterior fornix is spread on a glass slide and allowed to dry completely, leaving a fine ferning pattern visible under a light microscope. False negative/positive results occur in 5 hours; cervical discharge, semen or soap may lead to false positive results.

Amnicator® test

This is a sensitive pH test which uses a simple colour change of Nitrazine yellow to detect the presence of amniotic fluid. Normal vaginal fluid is usually at pH 7.0–7.5, while amniotic fluid has a pH of 6.4–6.8. This test is said to reliably distinguish the slightly alkaline amniotic fluid from acidic cervical/vaginal fluid or urine.

Insulin-like Growth Factor Binding Protein 1 (IGFBP-1) test (ActimPROM)

This is a commercially available bedside test kit that detects the IGF-1 binding protein secreted by decidual and placental cells, the concentration of which is high in amniotic fluid. The test is most accurate when applied as early as possible after membrane rupture and is not affected by blood, semen or cervicovaginal secretions. This test has 95–100% sensitivity at detecting amniotic fluid.

Ultrasound assessment of amniotic fluid

This is performed to look for reduced liquor volume, but may not be a very useful diagnostic test. This is because the liquor volume often remains in the normal range in normally-grown pregnancies despite a loss through PROM, unless the loss of amniotic fluid is severe and has resulted in oligohydramnios. This test is useful in severely preterm PPROM, as part of longitudinal foetal surveillance.

Screening for treatable infections

Group B streptococcus and bacterial vaginosis screening may guide antibiotic choices.

Management

Clinical Course

The majority of pregnancies with PPROM deliver within one week of occurrence; the duration of latency period (between membrane rupture and delivery) correlates inversely with gestational age at which PPROM occurred. As management is often complex with consideration of multiple factors, the details and nuances are outside the scope of this chapter. Only the principles and key points will be discussed.

Expectant Versus Active Management

In most women the leaking will usually be continuous, although the volume lost may fluctuate daily. In some women, the leaking stops spontaneously if the membranes seal (e.g. after amniocentesis). The ruptured membranes expose the sterile intrauterine environment (including the foetus and membranes) to ascending infection from the flora of the lower genital tract, thus intra-amniotic infection is the bane of expectant management.

Expectant management is aimed at allowing the pregnancy to carry on until term, with the goals of achieving foetal maturity and normal foetal weight. This is possible for all pregnancies affected by PROM remote from term, in the absence of the following risk factors: intra-amniotic infection (chorioamnionitis), cord prolapse, foetal distress, foetal demise, active labour with contraindications to tocolysis, antepartum haemorrhage from placental abruption, or maternal complications where preservation of pregnancy is contraindicated. If the mother and foetus are stable, pregnancy may be prolonged until at least 34 weeks of gestation have been completed.

The principles of management are:

- Administration of corticosteroids to accelerate foetal physiological maturity
- Antibiotic coverage to prevent intra-amniotic infection. Additional medications to relieve contractions or abort active labour (in the absence of contraindications) may be considered.
- Active management of PPROM is necessary when a complication has occurred compelling delivery e.g. intra-amniotic infection or foetal distress. In the presence of such complications, the patient may already be in labour, or labour may begin spontaneously and should not be inhibited for the sake of pregnancy preservation, if the risks of immediate serious foetal/maternal morbidity or mortality outweigh the likelihood of foetal maturity.

What is the Role of Corticosteroids?

Corticosteroids are the key intervention in a preterm pregnancy complicated by labour or PPROM. Because of the high likelihood of delivery at <37 weeks, the priority is to optimise the probability of foetal maturity. Corticosteroid use, particularly below 34 weeks, significantly reduces neonatal acute respiratory distress syndrome, intraventricular haemorrhage, necrotising enterocolitis and overall mortality. Drug regimens include betamethasone 6 mg 12 hourly for 4 doses, or two doses of dexamethasone 12 mg either 12 hourly or 24 hourly. The effect of the corticosteroids on pulmonary maturity is anticipated to be complete within 48 hours.

What is the Role of Tocolysis?

The primary aim of tocolytic use is to postpone delivery for at least 48 hours to allow the corticosteroids to take effect. The secondary aim of tocolysis is to gain maximum time for the foetus to develop and grow in utero, as the perinatal risks associated with prematurity decrease with increasing gestation.

What is the role of antibiotics in preterm labour with intact membranes?

Antibiotics are not indicated in preterm labour with intact membranes, in the absence of clinical evidence of infection.

Preterm ruptured membranes without concomitant labour

Antibiotic therapy is only indicated for PPROM, with or without labour.

- In PPROM without labour, if the patient is assessed to be suitable for expectant management, prophylactic antibiotics are indicated to prolong the latency period and reduce the risk of ascending infection and the resultant maternal and foetal complications. These are started in the *absence* of an active infection. Additionally, judicial antibiotic use significantly reduces the risks of preterm delivery within 48 hours of membrane rupture, neonatal infection, neonatal oxygen therapy or neonatal neurological impairment. The preferred antibiotic regimen is erythromycin 250 mg 4 times a day for 10 days. The use of co-amoxiclav is associated with an increased risk of neonatal necrotising enterocolitis, and is thus avoided for prophylaxis.
- For established or suspected ascending infections, appropriate antibiotics to cover the major pelvic pathogens should be chosen. There are several appropriate regimens. Examples include intravenous ampicillin 2 g as a loading dose followed by 1 g 4 hourly (chemoprophylaxis for GBS), co-amoxiclav 1.2 g 8 hourly, ceftriaxone 1 g 12 hourly. Anaerobic cover can be provided with metronidazole 500 mg 6 hourly. Antibiotic duration is typically 7–10 days, depending on severity. In cases of suspected infection, delivery should be considered and the pregnancy managed actively.

Preterm ruptured membranes with suspected or established labour

In the absence of clinical evidence of intra-amniotic infection, if labour is suspected, the patient is preferentially given GBS prophylaxis of intravenous ampicillin 2 g loading dose and 1 g 4 hourly after the appropriate lower vaginal swab has been taken for GBS screening. If the screen is negative, the ampicillin can be stopped in favour of erythromycin orally if the labour is aborted. If labour progresses, or if evolving infection is suspected, the GBS regimen may be continued or can be changed to a broader spectrum regimen as described above.

For How Long Should the Pregnancy be Prolonged?

What are the clinical aims?

In pregnancies complicated by preterm labour or PPROM, the aim is to maximise foetal maturity prior to delivery, as the majority of pregnancies end prior to 37 weeks. Even with corticosteroids administered, in utero development and growth, including weight gain, are critical factors in perinatal survival and good outcomes. A more mature gestation and heavier birth weight are associated with a lower risk of acute and long-term complications. Thus, with extreme preterm pregnancies (<32 weeks), the aim is to achieve 34 completed weeks if possible, or at least 32 weeks, at which perinatal survival approaches 100% (at a tertiary level neonatal care facility). Beyond 34 weeks, if the pregnancy is still stable with a reassuring foetus status, it is beneficial to prolong gestation to approach term (≥37 weeks). Every week gained in utero will reduce the chance of the baby requiring special or intensive neonatal care, which will reduce hospitalisation stay and cost.

What are the possible adverse effects of preserving the pregnancy?

Although causes of preterm labour and PPROM cannot always be identified, underlying subclinical infection or placental vasculopathy may initiate these processes. Thus, labour and/or membrane rupture may be symptomatic of pathologies which could adversely affect the foetus. Tocolysis and pregnancy conservation may mask these symptoms. Exposure to lower genital tract flora (via ruptured membranes) leaves the PPROM pregnancy at constant risk of intra-amniotic infection, which can escalate quickly to a life-threatening septicaemia. Prolonged hospital stay for the mother can also bring about depression and anxiety.

How is maternal and foetal surveillance conducted in preserved pregnancies?

Mothers should be evaluated for adverse effects related to multidrug use, prolonged bed rest (e.g. venous thromboembolism), emotional complications, and ascending infection in PPROM by clinical and biochemical assessment. Foetuses should be reviewed daily for changes in heart rate and movements, and periodically for growth and well-being e.g. weekly ultrasound assessment for AFI and umbilical artery Doppler studies, three weekly assessment of growth.

When Does Delivery Become Necessary?

Once term or near-term gestation is completed (36 weeks onwards) when there is no longer a benefit to preserving the pregnancy, or in the event of complications threatening the well-being of either the mother or foetus, the pregnancy should be ended and the foetus delivered in the most appropriate way. Vaginal deliveries are the aim, although some complications e.g. acute foetal distress may require emergency caesarean section.

Preterm Delivery and Associated Problems

Mode of Delivery

This depends on the presence of abnormal lie and/or malpresentation. The aim is to deliver the foetus vaginally unless a contraindication exists.

Malpresentation

There is a higher risk of this complication in extreme preterm gestations. This is an important factor in determining mode of delivery.

Immediate Prenatal Care and Long-Term Outcomes

The neonate must be attended to by the neonatal team and may require immediate resuscitation or support.

Communication

Multi-Disciplinary Team Approach

Patients should be managed by a team consisting of neonatologists, anaesthetists, nurse specialists and psychologists/emotional support team, headed by specialists in maternal-foetal medicine. The patient and her partner should be in constant and regular contact with the neonatologist who will counsel them on neonatal outcomes, which will vary with gestational age. The couple should also be briefed on the expected cost of neonatal care. Emotional support is essential particularly if prolonged hospitalisation or extreme preterm delivery is anticipated.

References

1. Robinson JN, Regan JA, Norwitz GR. (2001) The epidemiology of preterm labor. *Semin Perinatol* **25**(4):204–214.
2. Georgiou HM, Di Quinzo MKW, Permezel M, Brennecke SP. (2015) Predicting preterm labour: current status and future prospects. *Disease Markers* **2015**:435014.
3. Norwitz ER, Robinson JN. (2001) A systematic approach to the management of preterm labor. *Semin Perinatol* **25**(4):223–235.
4. Simhan HN, Caritis SN. (2007) Prevention of preterm delivery. *N Engl J Med* **357**(5): 477–487.
5. Goldenberg RL, Gopefart AR, Ramsey PS. (2005) Biochemical markers for the prediction of preterm birth. *Am J Obstet Gynaecol* **192**(5):536–546.

34

MALPRESENTATION AND ABNORMAL LIE

Su Lin Lin

Introduction

Foetal presentation refers to the leading anatomical part of the foetus, the part that is closest to the pelvic inlet. Malpresentation is therefore defined as any presentation other than a vertex presentation.

Types of Malpresentation

- Breech presentation
- Transverse lie
- Face presentation
- Compound presentation

Causes of Malpresentation

The most common cause of malpresentation is preterm gestation. Before 24 weeks of gestation, the proportion of breech and cephalic presentations are similar. The incidence of cephalic presentation increases during the second period, lasting from 25th to 35th gestational week, with a concomitant decrease in breech presentation. At term, the incidence of breech presentation is approximately 4%.

Other causes of malpresentation include: foetal abnormalities, amniotic fluid abnormalities including both polyhydramnios and oligohydramnios and placenta location.

Uterine abnormalities such as bicornuate uterus and leiomyomata also increase the risks of malpresentation.

Breech Presentation

Breech presentation is the most common type of malpresentation. It is divided into three groups:

- Frank breech — buttocks presenting with legs flexed at the hip and extended at the knees. This is the most common type of breech presentation.
- Complete breech — buttocks presenting with legs flexed at hips and knees.
- Footling breech — one or both feet presenting with the buttocks at higher position.

Variations of the breech presentation

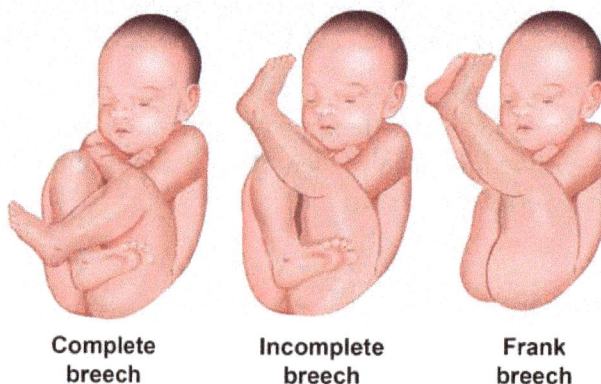

| Complete breech | Incomplete breech | Frank breech |

FIGURE 34.1 ■ Variations of the breech presentation.

Management

Preterm gestation

No active intervention is necessary for foetus diagnosed to be in breech presentation before 36 weeks' gestation. This is to allow time for spontaneous version to cephalic presentation.

At term

Counselling is important if the foetus remains in the breech presentation near or at term.

The options of management include:

- External cephalic version
- Elective caesarean section
- Vaginal breech delivery (if the obstetrician is experienced)

External Cephalic Version (ECV)

External cephalic version is the procedure in which the foetus is rotated from the breech to the cephalic presentation by manipulation through the mother's abdomen. The aim of ECV is to maximise the chance of normal vaginal delivery of a foetus in a cephalic presentation. Informed consent should be obtained for women undergoing the procedure and they should be informed regarding the nature of the procedure, the efficacy and the risks entailed.

Systematic review of seven randomised trials of ECV at term was published in 2012.[1] The pooled data from the studies show a statistically significant and clinically meaningful reduction in non-cephalic birth (risk ratio 0.46, 95% confidence interval 0.31–0.66) and caesarean section (risk ratio 0.63, 95% CI 0.44–0.90) when ECV was attempted. The pooled success rate of ECV was 58% in a 2008 systematic review of 84 studies including almost 13,000 version attempts at term.[2]

Contraindications for external cephalic version should be investigated, which include indications for caesarean section, severe oligohydramnios and non-reassuring foetal monitoring. Factors associated with lower ECV success rates are nulliparity, oligohydramnios and maternal obesity.

ECV, if indicated, should be performed near term to maximise the chance of spontaneous version. The foetus is likely to remain cephalic after successful ECV at this gestation. Should complications arise and emergency caesarean section is needed, foetal maturity is not a significant concern.

A 2015 systematic review of six randomised trials of ECV with or without tocolysis using beta-agonist concluded that tocolysis was associated with an increased prevalence of cephalic presentation in labour and a reduction of caesarean delivery rates. This reduction is seen in both nulliparous and multiparous women.[3]

Elective Caesarean Section

An international randomised controlled trial (Term Breech Trial) showed that elective caesarean section is associated with lower neonatal morbidity and mortality compared to vaginal breech delivery. Secondary analysis of the data showed that pre-labour caesarean section was associated with the best neonatal outcome and the rate of adverse neonatal outcomes increased with caesarean section in labour and vaginal breech delivery. For women undergoing vaginal breech delivery, labour augmentation, birthweight of less than 2.8 kg, longer second stage of labour and the lack of an experienced clinician are all associated with adverse perinatal outcome.[4]

Vaginal breech delivery

Some women with breech presentation choose to deliver vaginally (Doyle). Table 34.1 shows the factors which are regarded as unfavourable for vaginal breech birth.

TABLE 34.1 Factors Unfavourable for Vaginal Breech Birth

Clinically inadequate pelvis

Footling breech presentation

Macrosomia (>3.8 kg)

Intrauterine growth restriction (<2.5 kg)

If a woman requests vaginal breech delivery following counselling, it should be conducted by an experienced obstetrician in a hospital with facilities for emergency caesarean section. Continuous electronic foetal heart rate monitoring should be offered to the woman in labour. Vigilant monitoring of the progress of labour is essential, and caesarean section should be considered should there be a delay in the descent of the breech during the second stage of labour.

At the time of delivery, episiotomy should be performed if indicated to facilitate delivery. Spontaneous delivery of the trunk and limbs is preferred to avoid excessive traction of the baby which can lead to unnecessary bruising. Lovset manoeuvre refers to the rotation of the baby when the scapulae are visualized to facilitate delivery of the arms. For delivery of the head, one of three manoeuvres can be attempted: (1) Forceps (2) Mauriceau — Smellie-Veit manoeuvre (3) Burns-Marshall method.

Transverse Lie

The foetus is in a transverse lie when its longitudinal axis is perpendicular to the long axis of the uterus. When the curvature of the foetal spine is oriented upward, it is known as "back-up" or dorsosuperior position. When the curvature of the foetal spine is oriented downward, it is known as "back-down" or dorsoinferior position.

The incidence of transverse lie is around 1 in 300.[5] Predisposing factors include multiparity, prematurity, placenta praevia, polyhydramnios and uterine anomalies. Predisposing factors were found in 66% of primiparas but only 33% of multiparas (Gemer *et al.*).

Diagnosis

Clinical diagnosis can be made through abdominal palpation. However, ultrasound imaging is invariably used for confirmation of diagnosis where it is available. As placenta praevia is a predisposing factor for transverse lie, vaginal examination is contraindicated until placenta praevia is excluded on ultrasound.

Management

Preterm gestation

Conservative management should be employed before term gestation due to the likelihood of spontaneous version to cephalic presentation.

Term gestation

Should the presentation of the foetus remains in transverse lie near or at term, counselling is needed with two options:

- External cephalic version: This procedure is performed in the same way as that for breech presentation. The success rate is likely to be higher for foetuses in transverse lie compared to those in breech presentation.
- Caesarean section: Associated risks of caesarean section should be made known to the patient.

Face Presentation

The incidence of face presentation is 1 in 600 to 1 in 800. In face presentation, the foetal neck is deflexed, allowing the occiput to touch the back and the face to present in the birth canal.

Risk Factors

One risk factor for face presentation is foetal abnormality such as anencephaly, hydrocephalus or anterior neck mass. Abdominal laxity in multiparous women may also predispose to face presentation.

Diagnosis

Diagnosis is usually made late in the first stage or in the second stage of labour. The typical landmarks on vaginal examination are the ability to palpate the orbital ridge and orbits, saddle of the nose, mouth and chin. These landmarks may occasionally be mistaken for breech presentation.

Labour Management

Close surveillance of the progress of labour is essential. Cephalopelvic disproportion is more likely as the trachelo-bregmatic diameter is 0.7 cm greater than the suboccipito-bregmatic diameter of a normally flexed vertex presentation. For mentum-anterior position, vaginal delivery is possible. However, for mentum-posterior position, the foetus will not deliver vaginally unless spontaneous rotation occurs or the foetus is very small.

References

1. Hofmeyr GJ, Kulier R. (2012) External cephalic version for breech presentation at term. *Cochrane Database Syst Rev* **10**:CD000083.
2. Grootscholten K, Kok M, Oei SG, *et al.* (2008) External cephalic version-related risks: a meta-analysis. *Obstet Gynecol* **112**(5):1143.
3. Cluver C, Gyte GM, Sinclair M, *et al.* (2015) Interventions for helping to turn term breech babies to head first presentation when using external cephalic version. *Cochran Database Syst Rev* **2**:CD000184.
4. Su M, McLeod L, Ross S, *et al.* (2003) Factors associated with adverse perinatal outcome in the Term Breech Trial. **189**:740–745.
5. Gemer O, Segal B. (1994) Incidence and contribution of predisposing factors to transverse lie presentation. *Int J Gynaecol Obstet* **44**:219.

35

PREVIOUS CAESAREAN SECTION

Tan Eng Kien

Introduction

Caesarean section (CS) is a common operation in obstetrics, comprising approximately 25% of deliveries. There are concerns regarding a rising caesarean section rate in hospitals around the world, because of decreasing experience in instrumental deliveries, and also increasing medical litigation.

Caesarean section can be planned (elective), or occur as an emergency during labour.

It is important in the management of a previous caesarean section to:

- Understand the common indications for Caesarean section (CS)
- Appreciate the intrapartum complications due to a previous CS
- Know how to monitor a woman with a previous CS during labour.

TABLE 35.1   Indications of Caesarean Section

Elective CS	Emergency CS
Maternal reasons	Maternal reasons
— Severe medical problems	— Poor progress in labour
— Social — maternal request	
— Previous CS	
Foetal reasons	Foetal reasons
— abnormal presentation (e.g. breech, transverse lie)	— Suspected foetal distress
— congenital abnormalities where vaginal delivery is contraindicated	— Malpresentation/malposition

Indications for Caesarean Section

These may be maternal or foetal.

Maternal

- Previous caesarean section is the most common indication
- Maternal medical conditions eg. severe medical cardiac disease may preclude labour as the significant haemodynamic changes during labour may put the woman's life at a greater risk
- Social reasons like maternal request for a convenient date and time are increasing and should be discouraged as caesarean section carries a higher morbidity (eg. infection or bleeding) than a vaginal birth

Foetal

- Abnormal presentation eg. face, breech, transverse lie
- Foetal distress during labour
- Severe prematurity
- Severe intrauterine growth restriction
- Foetal congenital abnormality eg. large foetal neck masses

Management of Patients with Previous CS

- Taking a detailed history in the circumstances leading to the previous caesarean section is important in deciding on the mode of delivery in the current pregnancy. Details of the previous labour including the onset and progress of labour, as well as the stage of labour are important.

  A woman, who has a previous caesarean section at full dilatation due to cephalopelvic disproportion, has a lower success rate of achieving a vaginal birth in her subsequent pregnancy (success rate 60%). In contrast, a woman who has a previous caesarean section for foetal distress, has a higher success rate of achieving a vaginal birth in her subsequent pregnancy (success rate 80%).

- A woman who has 1 to 2 previous caesarean sections may be offered a trial of a vaginal birth in her subsequent pregnancy. VBAC (vaginal birth after caesarean) is contraindicated in a woman who has 3 or more previous caesarean sections.

- Counselling for VBAC is important. In addition to determining the success rate based on previous history of the first labour, the woman should be made aware that there is a (1 in 200 risk) of scar rupture during a trial of VBAC.
- All women undergoing VBAC must be continuously monitored during labour with CTG. In addition, a scar rupture during labour may present with sudden pain or bleeding. Any abnormalities on the CTG or symptoms of pain/bleeding during labour may be signs of scar dehiscence/rupture, and should prompt an emergency delivery by caesarean section.
- Induction of labour in a woman undergoing VBAC increases the scar rupture risk. Induction with prostin gel may increase the scar rupture risk to 2%. Induction/augmentation of labour with syntocinon increases the scar rupture risk to 0.8%. Induction of labour in a woman undergoing VBAC should only be allowed after informed counselling of the woman by a senior obstetrician.
- Women who are not suitable for a VBAC are offered delivery by elective caesarean section. This is generally performed after 39 weeks, when the risk of transient tachypnea of the newborn is the lowest.[1-5]

References

1. Royal College of Obstetricians and Gynaecologists, Green-top Guideline No. 45. (2015) *Birth after Previous Caesarean Birth*. (https://www.rcog.org.uk/globalassets/documents/guidelines/gtg_45.pdf)
2. Royal College of Obstetricians and Gynaecologists. (2008) *Birth after Previous Caesarean, Information for you*. (https://www.rcog.org.uk/globalassets/documents/patients/patient-information-leaflets/pregnancy/birth-after-previous-caesarean.pdf)
3. American Congress of Obstetricians and Gynecologists Practice Bulletin. (2010) *Vaginal Birth after Previous Caesarean Delivery*. (https://www.acog.org/Resources-And-Publications/Practice-Bulletins/Committee-on-Practice-Bulletins-Obstetrics/Vaginal-Birth-After-Previous-Cesarean-Delivery)
4. Society of Obstetricians and Gynaecologists Canada Guidelines. (2004) *Vaginal Birth after Previous Caesarean Birth*. (http://sogc.org/guidelines/guidelines-for-vaginal-birth-after-previous-caesarean-birth-replaces-147-july-2004/)
5. Obstetrical & Gynaecological Society of Singapore. (2015) Addendum to consent form vaginal birth after caesarean section (VBAC). (http://www.ogss.net/Portals/0/Documents/ADDENDUM-FOR-VAGINAL-BIRTH-AFTER-CAESAREAN-SECTION-VBAC_Hi-Res.pdf)

36

FOETAL DEMISE

Anita Kale

Introduction

Intrauterine foetal death (IUFD) or stillbirth is a very tragic event. Almost half of the late foetal deaths happen in uncomplicated low risk pregnancies. It triggers a change in the management and also in the patient's psychological needs. Investigations to determine the cause are essential for the successful management of future pregnancies.

The WHO defines stillbirth as a "foetal death late in pregnancy" and allows each country to define the gestational age at which a foetal death is considered a stillbirth for reporting purposes. As a result, some countries define stillbirth as early as 16 weeks of gestation, whereas others use a threshold as late as 28 weeks. In Singapore, the cut-off is at 24 weeks of gestation.

Pregnancy Management

The plan for delivery depends on the gestational age, placental localisation and parental wishes. Vaginal delivery is desirable as it carries less risk for the mother, even in the event of previous caesarean delivery.[1,2] Spontaneous labour usually begins in a week or two but conservative management carries with it a risk of developing disseminated intravascular coagulopathy (DIVC). Medical termination of pregnancy using prostaglandin analogues is the standard method below 24 weeks of gestation. Beyond 24 weeks, labour may be induced with usual regimens for induction of labour, as long as there is no contraindication for vaginal birth.

Investigations

The investigations of foetal death involve both the foetus and the mother. Whenever possible, effort should be made to decide the cause of death. Only then it is possible to assess the likelihood of recurrence. Common causes of foetal death are listed in Table 36.1 below.[3,4]

TABLE 36.1   Maternal and Foetal Causes of Foetal Death

Causes of Foetal Death
Maternal:
Diabetes mellitus
Hypertensive disorders: Pre-existing hypertension, pre-eclampsia
Connective tissue disorder
Thrombophilia
Foetal:
Infection — bacterial, viral
Foetal immune haemolytic disease
Cord accidents
Foetal malformations — structural and chromosomal
Placental dysfunction including intrauterine growth restriction, post maturity, abruption
Fetomaternal haemorrhage
Twin to twin transfusion syndrome

Often the cause of death can be decided by the gross and histopathological examination of the foetus and the placenta. Findings at the perinatal autopsy can change the clinical diagnosis or yield new information. Bacterial cultures performed on the placenta and/or amniotic fluid is an especially useful tool if autopsy permission is declined. Amniocentesis or chorionic villus sampling performed upon diagnosis of foetal demise appears to yield a higher rate of viable cells for successful culture and karyotyping than studies performed on the stillborn after delivery.

The optimal laboratory evaluation of the mother who has had a stillbirth is controversial. Many lists have been proposed, but the most cost-effective approach has not been determined. Below is the list of most relevant investigations:

- Kleihauer-Betke test to evaluate for fetomaternal haemorrhage
- Blood group antibody screen
- Fasting and post prandial blood glucose
- Anticardiolipin antibody, lupus anticoagulant
- Thrombophilia workup

Evaluation Prior to Future Conception

If the cause of death was ascertained, its implications for the future pregnancy should be discussed during follow up meetings postnatally and again prior to conception. Management will depend on the cause found. If no cause has been found, it should be impressed upon the patient and her husband that these events are usually quite unexpected and beyond anybody's control.

Psychosocial Care

Diagnosis of foetal death is a painful event for the patient, her family, as well as the doctor who has to break the news to them. Giving bad news puts one's professional skills to the test. If done poorly, the patient will never forgive and if done well, the patient will never forget. Many hospitals have a counsellor or psychologist to facilitate the grieving process. The couple may be put in touch with local support groups. The patient should be cared for in an isolated quiet room. Her husband should be encouraged to stay with his wife during the birthing process. They should be encouraged to view and hold the baby once born. Mementos should be offered in form of photos, footprints, and handprints.[5]

References

1. James DK, Steer PJ, Weiner CP, Gonik B. (2010) *High Risk Pregnancy Management Options*, 4th edn.
2. Edmonds K. (2012) *Dewhurst's Textbook of Obstetrics and Gynaecology*, 8th edn.
3. Fretts RC. (2015) *Fetal Demise and Stillbirth: Incidence, Etiology and Prevention*.
4. Robert DJ. (2015) *Evaluation of Stillbirth*.
5. Grunedaum A, Chervenak FA. (2015) *Fetal Demise and Stillbirth: Maternal Care*.

37

INDUCTION OF LABOUR

Ng Kai Lyn and Chong Yap Seng

Introduction

Induction of labour refers to the process of artificially starting the labour process. This chapter will cover the common reasons for offering induction of labour, methods of induction of labour, its processes, risks, alternatives, contraindications and induction of labour in special circumstances.

The indication for induction should always be documented, and discussion with the woman and her partner should include the reason for induction, method, and risks involved.

Reasons for Induction of Labour

Maternal Indications

○ ***Postdates pregnancies*** (i.e. pregnancies that have progressed beyond 42 weeks gestation). This is the most common indication for induction of labour. The incidence of postdates pregnancies range from 6–12% of all pregnancies. Perinatal mortality rates are known to be two to three times higher in post-date pregnancies and is postulated to be related to the declining function of the ageing placenta. There is also a link between postdates pregnancies and foetal macrosomia, which in turn leads to increased risk of shoulder dystocia and birth trauma.[1] Thus induction of labour should be offered between 41 weeks to 42 weeks of gestation. This is to reduce perinatal morbidity with minimal impact on the rates of caesarean section.

○ ***Other medical conditions.*** Certain maternal medical conditions may necessitate the delivery of the foetus at recommended gestations; this may include diabetes,[2] hypertension/pre-eclampsia/eclampsia,[3] obstetric cholestasis,[4] suspicion of infection or chorioamnionitis.

Foetal Indications

○ *Preterm pre-labour rupture of membranes (PPROM)*

Where there is evidence of preterm rupture of membranes with no signs of labour, induction of labour may be considered and offered, particularly if the pregnancy is beyond 34 completed weeks of gestation and a course of intramuscular steroids for foetal lung maturation has been completed. This is particularly the case if the mother is known to have carriage of group B Streptococcus.[5]

○ *Pre-labour rupture of membranes at term (PROM)*

Women with PROM at term (37 weeks and beyond) may be offered expectant management versus immediate induction of labour (e.g. with vaginal prostaglandins). Induction of labour is also appropriate 24 hours after PROM.[6]

○ *Intrauterine growth restriction (IUGR)*

IUGR is diagnosed when the foetal measurements lie below the 10th centile for a given gestational age, or when they cross centile lines.[7] IUGR may be associated with other signs like oligohydramnios and abnormal foetal Dopplers.

Foetal doppler ultrasound serves to detect changes in the pattern of blood flow through the foetal circulation; in particular, the umbilical artery of the foetus. As reduced or intermittently absent flow is associated with higher rates of foetal distress and compromise, induction of labour may be considered when foetal lung maturity has been achieved. However in certain situations (see following section: induction of labour in special circumstances), induction of labour may not be appropriate.

○ *Foetal conditions*

Certain foetal conditions (e.g. twins past 38 weeks gestation) and anomalies (e.g. congenital complex cardiac disease, anencephaly etc.) and conditions (e.g. rhesus isoimmunisation with foetal anaemia,[8] hydrops etc.) may necessitate induction of labour to ensure delivery with availability of trained personnel.

Methods to Induce Labour

Using Medications

○ *Vaginal prostaglandins*

These can come in the form of gel, tablets, and controlled release pessaries, which are inserted into the vagina to promote cervical ripening and encourage the onset of labour. Examples of prostaglandins include prostin, misoprostol and cervidil.

○ *Intravenous oxytocics*

This is a synthetic hormone that can be administered intravenously to augment uterine contractions, and is typically used in patients with ruptured membranes and favourable cervix (see section: modified Bishop's score below).

Using Mechanical Methods

○ *Surgical amniotomy of membranes*

This refers to the artificial rupture of membranes (ARM) in which the amniotic sac is deliberately ruptured, usually with a specialized tool like an amnihook. This is usually done when the cervix is favourable (see section: modified Bishop's score below). The release of the amniotic fluid encourages the release of endogenous prostaglandins and uterine contractions.

○ *Others*

Mechanical tools can sometimes be utilized to help dilate the cervical os. Examples include laminaria tents, which is a thin rod of dried laminaria that is inserted into the cervical os and subsequently expands by absorbing water with resultant cervical dilatation, and balloon catheters, which works by mechanical dilatation with inflation of the balloon.

Process of Inducing Labour

• Place

Induction of labour should be performed in the inpatient setting with availability of obstetrics, neonatal and anaesthetic support.

• Timing

Induction of labour should generally be performed in the morning for better patient satisfaction. However, in cases of foetal indications, considerations should be made to ensure availability of trained multidisciplinary personnel.

• Monitoring

The original Bishop score[9] was developed in 1964 as a predictor for successful induction, and has since underwent modifications (see Table 37.1: Modified Bishop score"). Assessment using this scoring system should be performed and recorded before induction of labour. As a general principle, a Bishop score of more than 6 is considered favourable and predictive of a successful vaginal delivery post-induction. The rates of failed induction and caesarean section is highest in women being induced with a poor Bishop score (0 to 3).[10]

Continuous electronic cardiotocography before, during and after induction of labour is required to confirm a reassuring foetal trace and contraction frequency.

Induced labour is likely to be associated with more pain as compared to spontaneous labour; pain relief options should be made available to patients who are being induced at all times.

TABLE 37.1   Modified Bishop Score

Score	2	1	0
Position of cervix	Anterior	Axial	Posterior
Length of cervix	Effaced <1 cm long	Partially effaced 1 cm long	Tubular 2 cm or more
Consistency of cervix	Soft, stretchable	Soft, not stretchable	Firm
Dilatation	≥2 cm	1 cm	0 cm
Station of presenting part	≤0	−1	−2

Risks Associated with Induction of Labour

○ *Hyperstimulation*

Hyperstimulation refers to a contraction frequency of five or more in 10 minutes. It can result in foetal distress, uterine rupture, placenta abruption or amniotic fluid embolism. This can be brought on by contractions arising from prostaglandin administration. In such cases, tocolytics (e.g. terbutaline) may be considered for reversal.

○ *Cord prolapse*

This refers to the condition where the umbilical cord prolapses out before the presenting part of the foetus.[11] Cord prolapse may occur at the time of amniotomy of membranes.

Amniotomy should hence be avoided if there is poor engagement of baby's head with a high station, or if there is umbilical cord presentation during preliminary vaginal examination.

○ *Failed induction*

This is defined as the failure of labour to start after induction of labour. It is generally agreed upon when there is a lack of cervical dilatation/ effacement associated with the absence of effective uterine contractions after administration of 3 consecutive prostaglandin doses.

Failure of induction is higher in women with a poor Bishop score, nulliparous patients and high body mass index (BMI). A thorough re-evaluation should be performed by an obstetrics consultant and a Bishop score recorded at this point, taking into account the patient's condition, her preferences, and foetal wellbeing.

Options for failed induction of labour include a further attempt to induce labour (e.g. insertion of prostaglandin) or a caesarean section.[6]

Alternatives to Induction of Labour

○ *Membrane Sweep*

A membrane sweep involves passing the examining finger through the cervix and rotating against the wall of the uterus in an attempt to separate the chorionic membrane from the decidua.

Women should be aware that this may be associated with discomfort and bleeding post sweep. A membrane sweep encourages the local release of natural prostaglandins that help initiate the onset of uterine contractions.

It is considered as an adjunct or alternative to induction of labour rather than a method of induction, and should be offered to all women prior to a formal induction of labour, as it has the potential to reduce formal induction of labour.[12]

○ Caesarean Delivery

Patients considering this should be counselled on the relevant risks of caesarean delivery as well as its impact on subsequent pregnancies.[13]

○ Await Onset of Spontaneous Labour (Expectant Management)

Patients considering this option should be counselled on the relevant risks, the need for increased foetal surveillance in the interim, and the symptoms that require immediate medical attention whilst awaiting spontaneous onset of labour.

Twice weekly cardiotocography and ultrasound estimation of maximum amniotic pool depth and Doppler studies should be undertaken in this group of patients who decline induction of labour beyond 41 weeks of gestation.[6]

Contraindications to Induction of Labour

• Patients with High Risk of Uterine Rupture

Such patients are prone to a higher risk of uterine rupture and induction of labour contraindicated[14]:

○ Prior classical caesarean section
○ High risk uterine incisions (e.g. inverted T or J incisions)
○ More than 2 previous lower segment caesarean sections
○ Previous uterine rupture
○ Previous myomectomy with significant breach of endometrial cavity

• Patients with Contraindications to Vaginal Birth

These patients are not suitable for a vaginal birth and caesarean delivery is the preferred mode of delivery:

• Placenta praevia
• Vasa previa

- Umbilical cord prolapse with non-imminent delivery
- Transverse foetal lie/ footling breech
- Non reassuring foetal trace
- Active primary maternal herpes infection
- Maternal HIV infection with high viral loads

Induction of Labour in Special Circumstances

• Patients with Previous Caesarean Scar

Patients wanting a trial of scar after caesarean (TOLAC) should be informed of a 1.5-fold increased risk of caesarean section with induction of labour as well as a two- to three-fold increased risk of uterine scar rupture (compared with spontaneous labours).[13]

In such cases, prostin remains the preferred agent for induction for labour as misoprostol is contraindicated.

• Intrauterine Death (IUD)

Women with confirmed cases of intrauterine foetal death should be offered induction of labour with the aim of achieving a vaginal delivery,[14] usually with misoprostol.

• Maternal Request

Induction of labour should not be routinely offered on social request alone.

• Breech Presentation

Induction of labour for breech presentation may be considered if individual circumstances are favorable[15,16] and must be decided upon by an obstetrics consultant and done in a centre experienced in handling breech deliveries.

• Severe IUGR and/or Abnormal Foetal Dopplers

Induction of labour is not recommended in cases where foetal compromise is already evident. This holds true particularly in cases with abnormal foetal Dopplers whereby there is absent or reversed umbilical arterial end diastolic flow, indicating that the foetus has little or no reserves; in such cases, an elective caesarean section is more appropriate.

• History of Precipitate Labour

Induction of labour for the purposes of avoiding an unattended birth should not be routinely offered to women with a history of precipitate labour.

• Suspected Foetal Macrosomia

Induction of labour for foetal macrosomia, diagnosed either clinically or on ultrasound estimation, should be individualized and decided upon on a case-by-case basis by an obstetric consultant.[11]

Conclusion

The rates of induction of labour continue to rise in most obstetrics units and in turn, remain a significant contributor to resultant caesarean deliveries. It is recommended that proper documentation and audit systems be put in place in all units offering induction of labour so as to ensure clinical governance of local practice.

References

1. Cunningham, Leveno, Bloom, *et al.* (2010). *Williams Obstetrics, 23rd edn*, United States: McGraw-Hill, pp. 832–835.
2. National Institute for Health and Clinical Excellence (NICE) Clinical Guidance [NG3]. (Feb 2015) *Diabetes in Pregnancy: Management of Diabetes and its Complications from Preconception to the Postnatal Period*. Available online at: https://www.nice.org.uk/guidance/ng3.
3. National Institute for Health and Clinical Excellence (NICE) Clinical Guidance [CG107]. (Aug 2010) *Hypertension in Pregnancy: The Management of Hypertensive Disorders during Pregnancy*. Available online at: https://www.nice.org.uk/guidance/cg107.
4. Royal College of Obstetrics and Gynaecology (RCOG). (May 2011) *Green-top Guideline No. 43. Obstetric Cholestasis*. Available online: https://www.rcog.org.uk/en/guidelines-research-services/guidelines/gtg43/.
5. Royal College of Obstetrics and Gynaecology (RCOG). (Jul 2012) *Green-top Guideline No. 36. Group B Streptococcal Disease, Early-onset*. Available online: https://www.rcog.org.uk/en/guidelines-research-services/guidelines/gtg36/.

6. National Institute for Health and Clinical Excellence (NICE) Clinical Guidance [QS60]. (Apr 2014) *Induction of Labour*. Available online: https://www.nice.org.uk/guidance/qs60.

7. Royal College of Obstetrics and Gynaecology (RCOG). (Mar 2013) *Green-top Guideline No. 31. Small-for-Gestational-Age Foetus, Investigation and Management.* Available online: https://www.rcog.org.uk/en/guidelines-research-services/guidelines/gtg31/.

8. Royal College of Obstetrics and Gynaecology (RCOG). *Green-top Guideline No. 65. The Management of Women with Red Cell Antibodies during Pregnancy.* Available online: https://www.rcog.org.uk/en/guidelines-research-services/guidelines/gtg65/.

9. Bishop EH. (1964) Pelvic scoring for elective induction. *Obstet Gynecol* **24**:266–268.

10. Society of Obstetricians and Gynaecologist of Canada (SOGC). (Sept 2013) *Guideline No. 296. Induction of Labour.* Available online: http://sogc.org/wp-content/uploads/2013/08/September2013-CPG296-ENG-Online_REV-D.pdf.

11. Royal College of Obstetrics and Gynaecology (RCOG). *Green-top Guideline No. 50. Umbilical Cord Prolapse.* Available online: https://www.rcog.org.uk/en/guidelines-research-services/guidelines/gtg50/.

12. World Health Organisation (WHO) *WHO Recommendations for Induction of Labour.* Available online: http://www.who.int/reproductivehealth/publications/maternal_perinatal_health/9789241501156/en/.

13. National Institute for Health and Clinical Excellence (NICE). (Nov 2011) *Clinical Guidance [CG132]. Caesarean section.* Available online: https://www.nice.org.uk/guidance/cg132.

14. Royal College of Obstetrics and Gynaecology (RCOG). (Feb 2007) *Green-top Guideline No. 45. Birth after Previous Caesarean Birth.* Available online: https://www.rcog.org.uk/en/guidelines-research-services/guidelines/gtg45/.

15. Royal College of Obstetrics and Gynaecology (RCOG). (Nov 2010) *Green-top Guideline No. 55. Late Intrauterine Foetal Death and Stillbirth.* Available online: https://www.rcog.org.uk/en/guidelines-research-services/guidelines/gtg55/.

16. Royal College of Obstetrics and Gynaecology (RCOG). *Green-top Guideline No. 20b. Management of Breech Presentation.* Available online: https://www.rcog.org.uk/en/guidelines-research-services/guidelines/gtg20b/.

38

NORMAL AND ABNORMAL LABOUR

Mahesh Choolani

Introduction

Labour is a normal physiological process women experience, usually at term, which culminates with the birth of the baby and expulsion of the placenta. Labour is characterised by the onset of regular, painful uterine contractions progressively increasing in frequency and intensity, and is associated with concomitant efface-ment and dilatation of the cervix. Two phenomena commonly associated with labour, but not necessary for the diagnosis of labour, are bloody show and leakage of amniotic fluid. Bloody show is the passage of the mucus plug mixed with a small amount of blood; this may precede the onset of labour by hours or days. Amniotic fluid leaks when the foetal membranes rupture; this may happen during labour or precede the onset of labour by up to a week.[1-3]

Stages of Labour

Labour is a continuous process, but it has been divided into three stages to facili-tate its study and understanding, and to aid in its management.

First Stage of Labour

The first stage of labour is the interval between the onset of labour and full cervical dilatation. The onset of labour is difficult to determine with precision. Two com-monly used methods to define the onset of labour are (1) the clock time when painful contractions become regular, or (2) time of admission to the labour ward in established labour. The first stage of labour ends with full dilatation of the cervix.

The first stage of labour is divided into two phases based upon the rate of cervical dilatation.

- The **Latent Phase** is of variable duration, and is that phase between onset of labour and established labour i.e. from when the cervix is closed at the beginning of labour until 3 cm dilatation, where the rate of cervical dilatation accelerates.
- In the **Active Phase**, the cervix dilates at approximately 1 cm/hour.

In general, the first stage of labour in multipara is faster than that in nulliparous women.

Second Stage of Labour

The second stage of labour is the interval between full dilatation (10 cm) and the birth of the infant. During this time, the foetus descends through the maternal pelvis, and the expulsion is aided by maternal straining ("pushing") efforts. The shape of the maternal pelvis e.g. Gynaecoid/Android could influence the duration of the second stage of labour.

Third Stage of Labour

The third stage of labour is the time from the delivery of the baby to the expulsion of the placenta. This is usually complete within 60 minutes from birth of the baby, but intervention to facilitate the delivery of the placenta may begin at 30 minutes.

In understanding labour, we need to appreciate both the mechanics that underpin the labour process, and the mechanism of the labour itself.

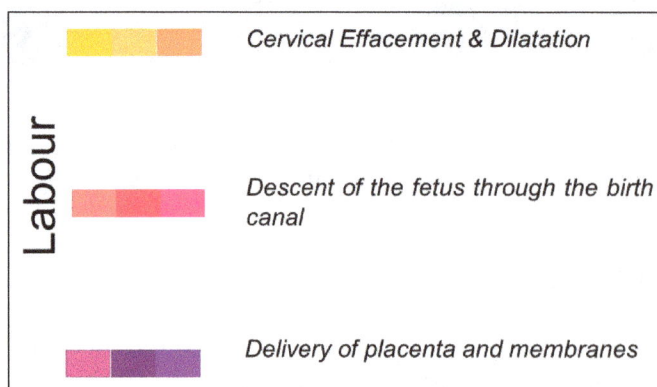

Cervical Effacement & Dilatation

Descent of the fetus through the birth canal

Delivery of placenta and membranes

FIGURE 38.1 ■ The 3 stages of labour.

Mechanics of Labour — The 3Ps

The two main functions of uterine contractions during the first and second stages of labour are to dilate the cervix and to push the foetus through the birth canal, respectively. The successful culmination of the birthing process is governed by a complex integration between three mechanical factors: the passage, the powers, and the passenger — the "3Ps."[4,5]

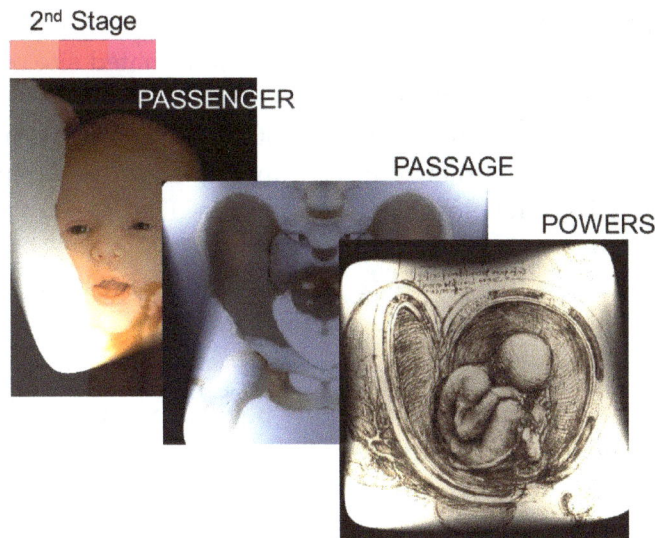

FIGURE 38.2 ■ The 3Ps in labour.

- **Powers** — uterine contractions — refers to the force generated by the uterine contractions to force the cervix open and the foetus through the birth canal. These forces can be measured by using an intrauterine pressure transducer and calculated quantitatively as Montevideo units, but this method is invasive and generally reserved for research use only. In everyday clinical practice we assess uterine activity qualitatively by palpation of the uterine fundus through the maternal abdomen, or by cardiotocography (CTG). The "toco" in cardiotocography refers to external tocodynamometry.

We are interested in the frequency, intensity and duration of the contractions. The frequency is measured as the number of contractions in an average 10 minute window, usually 2–4/10 min. In active labour the contractions increase in intensity over time, and last for approximately 20 seconds in early labour and 40–90 seconds in the active phase of labour.

- ***Passenger*** — refers to the foetus, and there are several foetal variables that can affect the course of labour:

  - Number — singletons, twins or multiples are associated with different problems that could affect the course of labour and delivery.
  - Size — small foetuses negotiate the birth canal readily; large babies could lead to cephalopelvic disproportion.
  - Lie — the long axis of the foetus relative to the long axis of the uterus, which is often dextro-rotated. Foetal lie can be longitudinal, oblique or transverse.
  - Presentation — the part of the foetus that directly overlies the pelvic inlet. It is usually cephalic (vertex), breech, or shoulder.
  - Position — this is the relationship of a nominated site of the presenting part of the foetus with respect to the denominating location on the maternal pelvis.
  - Station — is the degree of descent of the leading edge of the presenting part of the foetus, approximated in centimetres from the ischial spines e.g. 1–3 cm above, or 1–2 cm below the ischial spines. These are annotated as –3 to –1, and +1 to +2, respectively.
  - Anomalies — the presence of foetal anomalies could obstruct labour e.g. Hydrocephalus, Sacrococcygeal teratoma.

- ***Passage*** — this comprises the bony pelvis, and the soft tissues of the uterus e.g. cervix and pelvic floor muscles. The bony pelvis can be gynaecoid, anthropoid, platypelloid, or android. The gynaecoid pelvis is the most common pelvic shape, and is best for vaginal delivery. The platypelloid and android pelves may lead to obstructed labour.

Mechanism of Labour — The Foetal Cardinal Movements in Labour

The cardinal movements of the foetal head in labour are necessary for the most common leading part of the foetus to negotiate the birth canal. The two key features of the foetal head that explain many of the movements are (1) pivoting of the foetal head at the atlanto-axial joint of the cervical spine, and (2) the natural tendency of the foetal head to return to its neutral position where the spine, shoulders and sagittal suture are all three in an orthogonal relationship.

Engagement — happens when the widest diameter of the presenting part passes below the plane of the pelvic inlet. In a cephalic presentation, this would refer to the biparietal diameter. It is generally measured as fifths palpable above the pelvic brim, and the head is said to be engaged if three or more fifths are past the pelvic inlet.

7 Cardinal Movements of Labour

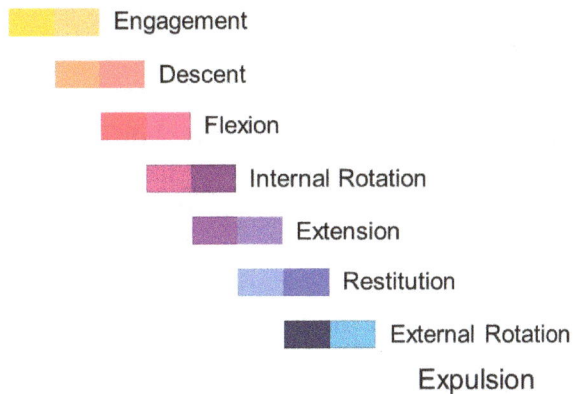

Engagement

Descent

Flexion

Internal Rotation

Extension

Restitution

External Rotation

Expulsion

FIGURE 38.3 ■ The 7 Cardinal movements of labour.

Descent — refers to the downward passage of the presenting part within the maternal pelvis.

Flexion — of the foetal head happens as the head meets resistance against the pelvic floor muscles, and the head pivots about the atlanto-axial joint. This allows the presentation of the smallest sagittal diameter of the foetal head — the suboccipitobregmatic diameter, and coronally, the biparietal diameter.

Internal rotation — of the foetal head occurs passively from a sagittal-transverse alignment of the foetal head in the maternal pelvis at the pelvic inlet to a sagittal-anteroposterior orientation at the pelvic outlet. This happens passively as guided by the slanted bowl shape of the pelvis which points downwards, inwards and forwards, and the similar orientation of the sling of pelvic floor muscles.

Extension — of the foetal head occurs once the foetus has passed the resistive forces of the pelvic floor musculature. Continued uterine contractions and maternal expulsive efforts continue to provide downward pressure onto the foetus, and the birth canal has an upward curve at the very end. Once pass the introitus (crowning), the foetal head extends to return to its neutral orientation with respect to its spine.

Restitution — is when the foetal head turns 45° to restore its normal orthogonal relationship with the shoulders. This is an active movement by the foetus carried out after all resistive forces by the maternal pelvis and pelvic floor musculature have been removed.

External rotation — Within the pelvis, the shoulders repeat the corkscrew action of the foetal head, but in a laterally-inverted fashion. So, if the foetal head had started from a Left-Occiput-Anterior position, the shoulders would start from a Right-biacromial-Anterior position. As the shoulders rotate internally within the pelvis, the foetal head continues to rotate externally, outside of the introitus. In other words, external rotation of the foetal head is merely an external representation of the internal rotation of the foetal shoulders within the maternal pelvis, all this while the foetal head maintains its orthogonal relationship with the shoulders and spine.

Expulsion — is the delivery of the rest of the foetal body, first with the anterior shoulder of the foetus just below the pubic symphysis, and then by a sweeping motion towards the maternal abdomen, posterior shoulder and the rest of the foetal torso.

Delivery of the Placenta and Perineal Repair

After the baby has been delivered, the umbilical cord is cut between clamps. The mother is usually administered oxytocin parenterally, to cause uterine contractions and facilitate the delivery of the placenta, and prevent the likelihood of postpartum haemorrhage. The placenta is then delivered by controlled cord traction by the Brandt-Andrews method to reduce the likelihood of uterine inversion.

At the time of crowning the perineum would commonly tear, or a mediolateral episiotomy might have been made just prior to crowning. These are repaired using a rapidly absorbable 2/0 suture.

In the immediate postpartum period, adequate analgesia and perineal toilet is encouraged.

Pain Management During Labour

Some women prefer a medication (analgesia)-free labour. These women would benefit from adequate psychological preparation, continuous support throughout the labour by the partner or a trained professional, and relaxation techniques such as meditation, massage, immersion in water during the first stage of labour and acupuncture.

Alternatively, there are different measures for pain control of varying degrees of success:

Transcutaneous electrical nerve stimulation (TENS)

ENTONOX® — a 50/50 mixture of nitrous oxide and oxygen, colloquially known by midwives as "gas and air."

Opioids such as pethidine, morphine and fentanyl could be used, but may cause respiratory depression in the neonate if given too close to birth.

Epidural analgesia is a popular medical pain control method in hospitals where regional anaesthetic services are readily available. It is an effective form of pain management that is not associated with an increased risk of caesarean section or depressed Apgar scores.

Pain Relief in Labour

- TENS, Acupuncture
- 'Entonox' (50/50 O$_2$/Nitrous oxide)
- Pethidine, Morphine
- Epidural analgesia

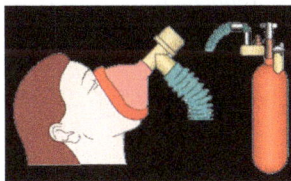

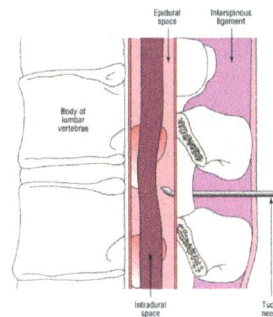

FIGURE 38.4 ■ Pain relief in labour.

Abnormal Labour and Delivery

Induction of Labour — In some circumstances e.g. insulin dependent diabetes mellitus, it is preferable that the baby be delivered by 38 weeks amenorrhoea. Often, labour would not have started spontaneously by then. Labour can then be induced to start by the use of vaginal prostaglandins, artificial rupture of membranes or intravenous oxytocin. Depending upon the Bishop Score (cervical score), any of these could be used alone or in combination to start active labour.

Prolonged Labour — Labour could be prolonged in either the first stage or the second stage. It is less common in multipara than in nullipara. It may occur due to poor (hypocontractile) uterine activity, persistent occiput posterior position (OP position), or cephalopelvic disproportion (CPD). The use of oxytocin to augment labour may be an appropriate action for the first two conditions, but could be dangerous in the presence of CPD and may cause a uterine rupture. Therefore, the use of oxytocin in a labouring parturient must be done only after careful evaluation of the full clinical picture, and a reasonable assessment of the underlying cause of delay.

References

1. Edmonds K. (2012) *Dewhurst's Textbook of Obstetrics and Gynaecology*, 8th edn.
2. Hanretty KP. (2009) *Obstetrics Illustrated*, 7th edn.
3. Oats JN, Abraham S. (2010) *Llewellyn Jones Fundamentals of Obstetrics and Gynaecology*, 9th edn.
4. Cohen WR, Friedman EA. (2011) *Labour and Delivery Care A Practical Guide*.
5. O'Driscoll K, Meagher D. (2003) *Active Management of Labour*, 4th edn.

39

COMPLICATIONS AT DELIVERY

Tan Eng Kien

Introduction

The second stage of labour begins when the cervix is fully dilated, and ends with the delivery of the foetus.

During the passive phase of the second stage, the foetal head descends to reach the pelvic floor.

During the active phase of the second stage, the foetal head descends low onto the pelvic floor, and the mother develops a strong urge to push.

During the second stage of labour, the foetal head descends into the pelvis with the head in the occipito-transverse direction. As the foetal head descends onto the pelvic floor, the head rotates normally into the occipito-anterior position, and ends with the delivery of the baby's head. Following delivery of the head, the baby's shoulders restitute, so that the head is facing sideways, before the anterior and posterior shoulders are delivered.

The third stage in labour commences after the baby is born, and ends with the delivery of the placenta.

Active management of the third stage of labour involves using an oxytocic agent and gentle, controlled cord traction to achieve delivery of the placenta.

It is thus important to:

- Recognize obstetric emergencies that can occur at delivery
- Anticipate potential complications in high risk situations
- Understand the principles of management of such emergencies

Complications of Second Stage of Labour

Prolonged Second Stage

The second stage of labour is considered prolonged if delivery of the baby has not taken place within three hours (or two hours) of starting the active second stage of labour, in nulliparous and parous women respectively.

Foetal Distress

Foetuses are at risk of being distressed in the second stage of labour, due to cord compression and prolonged pushing. This is manifested by an abnormal looking CTG in the second stage of labour.

Maternal Exhaustion/Poor Effort

Prolonged pushing may result in maternal exhaustion.

Shoulder Dystocia

The baby's head is delivered, but the shoulders become stuck behind the pubic symphysis, and fail to deliver. This is an obstetric medical emergency, as failure to deliver a stuck shoulder promptly and effectively may subject the foetus to hypoxic damage and birth injuries. Various manoeuvres may be utilised to effect delivery of the impacted shoulders. This may involve hyperflexing the maternal thighs so that the mother's knees are pointing towards her face; this McRobert manoeuvre helps to flatten the lumbar spine lordosis, and widens the pelvic inlet. In addition, suprapubic pressure may be employed to dislodge the impacted anterior foetal shoulder from the pubic symphysis. The McRobert manoeuvre and suprapubic pressure helps to deliver an impacted shoulder in 80% of cases of shoulder dystocia. Additional manoeuvres involve putting the operator's hands into the vagina to rotate the baby's shoulders sideways, and may be required if the McRobert and suprapubic pressure manoeuvre fails.[1]

Shoulder dystocia cannot be predicted. Although diabetic mothers with big babies are at higher risk of shoulder dystocia, more than 50% of shoulder dystocia occur in normal weight babies. Therefore, being prepared for this emergency in the form of emergency drills training is important for every birth attendant.

Complications of Third Stage of Labour

Primary Postpartum Haemorrhage (PPH)

Definition

A primary PPH is defined as a blood loss of 500 mL or more within 24 hours of delivery.

PPH occurs in 5% of all births, and is more common in multiparous women with prolonged labour and polyhydramnios.

Causes of PPH "4 Ts":

- Tone — Poor uterine tone accounts for the majority of PPH, and can be improved by using oxytocics in the active management of the third stage of labour
- Tissue — Retained placenta tissue and placental membranes can prevent adequate contraction of the uterus. Therefore, inspecting the placenta for missing cotyledons after birth is important to exclude retained tissue as the cause of bleeding after delivery
- Trauma — Bleeding from the vaginal wall and cervical tears, and from episiotomy wounds can be significant. Tears must be repaired promptly
- Thrombin — Abnormal coagulation (Disseminated Intravascular Coagulation) may happen as a result of maternal sepsis or placental abruption

Management

Uterine Atonia

Oxytocic agents in the active management of the third stage of labour are effective in reducing blood loss at delivery.[2] Rub uterus to ensure it is contracted. Give ergometrine/syntocinon intravenously or in a drip. To ensure sustained uterine contraction Misoprostol can be given per rectally or Carboprost intramusculary.

Birth Canal Trauma

Tears can occur to the vaginal wall and cervix during delivery. In addition, the anal sphincter can also be damaged during delivery, resulting in tears termed "third degree tears."

Trauma to the birth canal must be repaired promptly to reduce the amount of bleeding. Third degree tears must be repaired carefully to prevent later complications of faecal incontinence.

Lighting may not be sufficient in the labour room to allow tears higher up in the vagina to be visualised. Consideration should always be made to having the tears repaired in theatre, with better lighting and anaesthesia.[3,4]

Retained Placenta

The placenta may fail to deliver spontaneously, despite active management of the third stage. Retained placenta complicates 2% of all deliveries, and may result in heavy postpartum bleeding.

Arrangements should be made to manually remove any placenta fragments in surgical theatre under adequate anaesthesia and antibiotic cover.

Uterine Inversion

Uterine inversion occurs when the placenta fails to detach from the uterus during controlled cord traction in active management of the third stage. As a result, the inside surface of the uterus becomes exteriorised, with the whole uterus inside out. This is a rare complication, occurring in 1/2000 deliveries, and is associated with significant postpartum haemorrhage and shock. Prompt resuscitation is needed. The inverted uterus may be replaced with hydrostatic pressure in the vagina, achieved by pumping massive amounts (3 litres) of warm normal saline into the vagina. Adequate relaxation of the uterus may be required with tocolytics and general anaesthesia. In severe cases, a laparotomy may be needed to correct the inversion.[5]

A summary of the management of primary postpartum management is shown in Table 39.1.

TABLE 39.1   Summary of Primary Postpartum Haemorrhage Management

Scenerio	Action
1. Is Patient in shock?	a. Rub uterus
	b. Set intravenous line
	c. Group and cross match
	d. Give appropriate oxytocic agents
	e. Give blood if needed
	f. Monitor vital signs
2. Is Placenta delivered	a. If not delivered then deliver by control cord traction
	b. If retained arrange to remove it manually in theatre

(Continued)

TABLE 39.1 *(Continued)*

Scenerio	Action
3. Is there birth canal trauma	a. Look at perineum and vaginal examination for tears b. Repair any tears and if needed repair in theatre with better lighting and anaesthesia
4. Is there abnormal coagulation	a. Take blood for coagulation profile and DIVC screen b. Give fresh frozen plasma/fresh blood platelets *(Abnormal coagulation could be the cause of PPH or may result from prolonged bleeding)*
5. Primary Postpartum Haemorrhage of undetermined etiology	If bleeding persist despite of measurements taken above then take patient to operating theatre and consider a. uterine packing b. Bakri balloon c. Internal iliac ligation d. Hysterectomy as last resort

References

1. Royal College of Obstetricians and Gynaecologists. (2009) *Postpartum Haemorrhage, Prevention and Management (Green-top Guideline No. 52).* (https://www.rcog.org.uk/en/guidelines-research-services/guidelines/gtg52/).
2. Royal College of Obstetricians and Gynaecologists. (2012) *Shoulder Dystocia (Green-top Guideline No. 42).* (https://www.rcog.org.uk/en/guidelines-research-services/guidelines/gtg42/).
3. Royal College of Obstetricians and Gynaecologists. Green-top Guideline No. 29. (2015) *The Management of Third and Fourth Degree Perineal Tear.* (https://www.rcog.org.uk/globalassets/documents/guidelines/gtg-29.pdf)
4. *Managing Obstetric Emergencies and Trauma, The MOET Course Manual.* (2014) 3rd edn, Cambridge University Press.
5. *The Practical Obstetric Multi-Professional Training (PROMPT) Course. Manual,* (2014) 2nd edn, Cambridge University Press.

40

THE PUERPERIUM AND BREASTFEEDING RELATED PROBLEMS

Naushil Randhawa and Chong Yap Seng

Introduction

The puerperium stems from the Latin word *"puerpera,"* which means a woman in childbirth.[1] It typically refers to the first six weeks after childbirth.[2] Many physical and psychological events occur during this period and the new mother remains vulnerable to pathology.

Physical and Psychological Changes in Puerperium

Uterus

The uterus begins a process of involution. At the two week postnatal review, it is typically just palpable above the pubic symphysis. The cervical os closes after about a week.[2]

Pelvic Floor

Pelvic floor damage is a common phenomenon, often associated with urinary and faecal incontinence. Long term consequences include pelvic organ prolapse. Risk factors include: a prolonged second stage, instrumental delivery, macrosomia, shoulder dystocia, advanced maternal age, obesity and multiparity.[2] Current advice for all primigravida women is to be taught and commence pelvic floor exercises in the antenatal period so as to reduce the incidence of incontinence and prolapse.[3]

Vaginal Loss

The passage of lochia postpartum is physiological, but postpartum haemorrhage must always considered in the event of excessive lochia, as haemorrhage remains one of the leading causes of maternal death.

Gastrointestinal Tract

The relaxed lower gastroesophageal sphincter (secondary to progesterone effects during the pregnant state) returns to normal within a few days postpartum.[2]

Cardiovascular System

In the pregnant state, the plasma volume increases by 50%, causing dilutional anaemia and reduced oxygen carrying capacity.[2,4] The red cell mass also increases by approximately 25%, which returns to normal with 48 hours of childbirth.[2] After the third stage of labour, the plasma volume expands and then reduces due to diuresis, blood loss and excretion of extracellular fluid.

Fertility

In a non-breastfeeding mother, ovulation can return as early as day 28. Hence, fertility and contraception is an essential subject to discuss with the new mother upon childbirth and at their first postnatal visit. The choice of contraception and time of commencement will vary depending on several factors. The combined hormonal contraceptive method should be avoided in the first three weeks because of the increased risk of venous thromboembolism. The intrauterine systems should only be inserted after four weeks because of the risk of expulsion. For more details, the Faculty of Sexual and Reproductive Health provides is a good source of information for all contraceptive providers.

Psychological

The puerperium is a period of many changes and can be overwhelming for the new mother. The demands of a newborn, pain from perineal tears or a surgical scar and lack of sleep often makes the new mother vulnerable. Up to 80% of mothers will experience "baby blues" after day three of birth. These feelings typically resolve within two weeks as the mother settles into her new role.

However, a small percentage will progress onto a more severe grade of depression and anxiety. Also of importance is postpartum psychosis, which is strongly associated with suicide. In the latest confidential enquiry into maternal deaths[6] in the United Kingdom (2009–2012), mental health was highlighted as a key feature responsible for a significant number of maternal deaths. At the first postnatal visit, it is paramount to enquire about mental health and follow up accordingly where indicated.[5]

Haematological

Haemostatic changes during pregnancy result in a hypercoagulable state which persists on into the puerperium. In fact, the incidence of venous thromboembolism is highest during the puerperium. Pulmonary embolism remains a leading cause of maternal death. This can be significantly reduced through proper implementation of protocols to identify those at high risk during booking and thoughout the pregnancy. Risk stratification should also be employed upon admission of any pregnant women. Those at higher risk may require TED stockings or prophylactic low molecular weight heparin, and simple measures such as early mobilisation and adequate hydration are important.[6]

Sepsis

Puerperal sepsis remains the leading cause of maternal death in the latest confidential enquiry into maternal deaths.[7] Risk factors that predispose the new mother to puerperal sepsis include anaemia, prolonged rupture of membranes, trauma due to the birth, instrumentation and bacterial colonisation of the vagina which ascends to the genital tract. Group A *Streptococcus* is amongst the most common offending organisms.[7]

The Surviving Sepsis Campaign comprises of six basic steps in the management of the septic mother, which have been shown to reduce mortality and morbidity. These include prompt collection of cultures, administration of antibiotics within 1 hour, measurement of lactate and appropriate fluid resuscitation and monitoring of fluid balance.[7]

A multidisciplinary approach is key, with the involvement of the microbiologist and infectious disease team, as well as the paediatrician as neonatal prophylaxis may be required.[7]

The above highlights some of the main issues in the puerperium but is not exhaustive. Every new mother needs to be assessed, counselled and managed as an individual holistically. This cannot be emphasised enough.

Breastfeeding Problems

In strong support for breastfeeding, the World Health Organisation and UNICEF launched the Baby-friendly Hospital Initiative in 1991. Its basis is to protect, promote and support breastfeeding. This followed an abundance of research proving the enormous benefits of breast milk to a baby. The WHO recommends exclusive breastfeeding for the first six months, after which appropriate complementary foods can be introduced.[8]

As a result, the percentage of women who initiate breastfeeding has increased significantly globally. However, many new mothers have faced problems with breastfeeding, which result in them stopping short of their goals. Many of these problems can be tackled with patient education and appropriate management.

Cracked and Sore Nipple

This is typically due to incorrect attachment of the baby. Correct positioning and latching is fundamental to successful breastfeeding. Simple advice to rest the cracked nipple, and express milk from that breast for a few days until the crack heals, is usually all that is needed. Ointments are typically not necessary and a little expressed breast milk massaged over the cracked nipple aids in healing.

Breast Engorgement

Incorrect positioning or attachment, which leads to reduced frequency and duration of feeding at the breast, can lead to breast engorgement. Management involves unlimited access to the breast. If this is not possible, the milk should be expressed to relieve the discomfort. Antipyretics may be required as breast engorgement may be associated with pyrexia.

Mastitis

This usually occurs secondary to obstructed milk drainage, which in turn may be due to blocked ducts, restricted feeding, incorrect positioning or attachment.[5] The mother typically presents with a tender, red, oedematous breast associated with pyrexia. Management involves treating the pyrexia with hydration, cold compress and antipyretics. The obstructed milk flow needs to be relieved by correct positioning, attachment, unrestricted feeding and expression of the milk. In the infected breast, the most common offending organism is *Staphylococcus aureus*.[5] Hence, appropriate antibiotics would include penicillinase-resistant penicillins, such as flucloxacillin. Cephalosporins are an alternative.[5]

Breast Abscess

If not managed promptly and correctly, mastitis can progress on to a breast abscess, which requires involvement of breast surgeons and surgical drainage under antibiotic cover. While continued breastfeeding is encouraged in mastitis, in severe cases of a breast abscess, breastfeeding on the affected side may need to stop.[5]

Insufficient Milk

This is seen in less than 1% of women. Management includes hydration, adequate nutrition and reducing stress factors. Pharmacological interventions include dopamine antagonists, thyrotropin-releasing hormone, and oxytocin.

Drugs that reduce breast milk production should be stopped, or replaced as appropriate. This includes progestins, oestrogens, ethanol, bromocriptine, ergotamine, carbegoline and pseudoephedrine.

Conclusion

Early detection and prompt management of breastfeeding problems will increase the rates of continued successful breastfeeding. Hence, breastfeeding is a key topic to approach with the new mother. Specially trained lactation specialists and midwives are available to guide in the immediate puerperium. Correct positioning and attachment should be ensured prior to discharge. At every follow up, the mother should be asked how the baby is fed and if there are any issues. Mothers should be provided with written and verbal information on how to seek advice if needed.

While the pregnancy has ended, the puerperium remains a critical period, and if the mother's health is compromised, this would directly affect the well-being of the newborn and its survival.

References

1. O'Connor V, Kovacs G. (2003) *Obstetrics, Gynaecology and Women's Health*, 1st edn.
2. Royal College of Obstetricians and Gynaecologists. (2011) Greentop Guideline No. 56. *Maternal Collapse in Pregnancy and the Puerperium*.
3. Collins S, Arulkumaran S, Hayes K, Jackson S, Impey L. (2011) Normal changes in the puerperium. *Oxford Handbook of Obstetrics and Gynaecology*, 2nd edn.
4. MBRACE-UK (2014) Confidential Enquiry in Maternal Mortality and Morbidity: Saving Lives, Improving Mothers' Care.

5. NICE Clinical Guidance CG 192. (2014) *Antenatal and Postnatal Mental Health.*

6. Royal College of Obstetricians and Gynaecologists. (2015) Greentop Guideline No. 37a: *Thrombosis and Embolism during Pregnancy and the Puerperium, Reducing the Risk.*

7. Royal College of Obstetricians and Gynaecologists. (2012) Greentop Guideline No. 64b, *Bacterial Sepsis following Pregnancy.*

8. World Health Organistation (WHO). (1991) *Evidence for the ten steps to successful breast-feeding.* www.who.int/child-adolescent-health/

Part VI

MATURE WOMEN AND FUNCTIONAL AGING

Introduction

The lifespan of women has been increasing steadily over the years. In the 18th century, women can expect to live to 45 years. In Singapore, the life expectancy for women has increased from 63 years in 1957 to 85 years in 2014. The average age of menopause in Singapore is 49 years. Therefore, women can expect to spend more than 40 years and are more than a third of their lives in the post reproductive period.

Despite recording one of the longest life expectancies in the world and facing over half a lifetime in the menopausal transition and menopause, the health problems and challenges faced by Singaporean women in this ageing cohort are largely unmet. There is an urgent need to prioritise older women's health in an integrated and multidisciplinary manner.

Besides health issues arising from the menopause and rapid estrogen drop, other domains such as osteoporosis, sexual health, urogenital atrophy, osteoporosis causing hip fractures and consequent immobility become increasingly problematical. Gestational diabetes and pregnancy-induced hypertension are risk factors for the development of type II diabetes and hypertensive disorders in later life. As we age, cancer risk increases and part of the role of the gynaecologist is to encourage cancer health prevention through adequate evidence proven health screens such as PAP cervical smear and mammography.

Psychiatric issues such as anxiety, depression, and poor sleep become important. Obesity and related health issues crop up for many. Solutions for these probelms have common roots such as healthy diet and adequate exercise.

Clinicians need to deliver these health-care solutions in a one-stop multidisciplinary manner. By addressing woman-specific concerns in a holistic manner, clinicians, whether gynaecologists or in other medical disciplines, will play an important role in disease identification and prevention, health promotion and lifestyle modification for the rapidly ageing women of Singapore and beyond. The chapters in this section outline an approach to how every clinician can deliver a holistic, comprehensive, lifecourse approach to care of women after the reproductive period.

41

MENOPAUSE

Susan Logan

Introduction

This chapter on Menopause will encompass the following:

- Know the consequences of menopause — short and long term
- Know about health screening of menopausal women
- Know risks and benefits of hormone replacement therapy (HRT)

Normal Physiology of Menopause

Menopause is defined as the permanent cessation of menses. It is diagnosed retrospectively after a woman has experienced 12 months of amenorrhoea without any other reversible cause.

Globally, the age of natural menopause occurs consistently at 49–51 years. In contrast with males, women are born with all their oocytes and menopause reflects the near or complete depletion of these. With no follicles for the pituitary hormones to stimulate, oestrogen and progesterone levels fall. With no feedback to the pituitary, the gonadotrophins (FSH and LH) increase to try and stimulate the non-functioning ovary. The resulting hypoestrogenemia and high FSH concentrations can be detected by blood tests. Another blood test that reflects ovarian reserve is anti-mullerian hormone (AMH), secreted by the granulosal cells in the ovary. Low levels reflect declining ovarian reserve and impending menopause.

The **menopausal transition**, or perimenopause, occurs after the reproductive years, but before menopause, and is characterised by irregular menstrual cycles, endocrine changes, and symptoms such as hot flushes.

Menopause is increasingly recognised as an important life stage. Globally, and particularly in Singapore, the population is aging and Singaporean women currently live, on average, to 85 years. This equates to 35 years or 52% of a woman's life in the transition and menopause stages. Care can be broken down into short term management of menopausal symptoms and long term strategies to promote functional aging — health promotion and prevention of diseases manifesting primarily in the menopause, such as osteoporosis, cardiovascular disease, diabetes, hypertension and cancer.[1]

Note: Menopause before age 40 years is abnormal and is referred to as **primary ovarian insufficiency** (POI; formerly premature ovarian failure) and is secondary to primary ovarian failure, surgery, chemotherapy or radiotherapy. All women with POI have increased risk of cardiovascular disease, osteoporosis, dementia and early death if oestrogen is not replaced.

History

The diagnosis of menopause should be borne in mind with any woman who presents with irregular or infrequent menses or secondary amenorrhoea. It can occur at any age. The menopause transition usually predates the final menses by 4–5 years. While the menopause is natural, hormonal fluctuations produce the following symptoms thought to be due to the body's sensitivity to low oestrogen levels:

- *Bleeding*: Irregular menses or secondary amenorrhoea
- *Vasomotor symptoms* in the form of hot flushes and night sweats
  - Hot flushes are among the most recognised symptom of the menopause, yet only a minority of women seek medical attention. Symptoms tend to be worse in the late menopause transition. Compared to sweating in hot weather, hot flushes start at the chest/face and spread, lasting 2–5 minutes on average. The heated feeling is associated with perspiration, palpitations and then followed by feelings of cold and anxiety. Frequency and intensity varies between individuals. Most will stop within eight years but a minority will continue to have symptoms long term.
- *Psychological changes*
  - Anxiety and depression symptoms increase in the menopause transition and may be of new onset. These may affect memory and concentration
  - Anxiety: Heart beating quickly and strongly, feeling tense or nervous, difficulty in sleeping, excitable, attacks of panic, difficulty in concentrating

- Sleep may be disturbed by vasomotor symptoms, psychological symptoms, medical problems and relationship issues. In general, sleep difficulties increase in the perimenopause and menopause
- Depression: Feeling tired or lacking in energy, loss of interest in most things, feeling unhappy or depressed, crying spells, irritability
- *Physical symptoms*: Feeling dizzy or faint, pressure or tightness in head or body, parts of body feeling numb or tingling, headaches, muscle or joint pains, loss of feeling in hands or feet and breathing difficulties
  - Joint pain is the most common symptom experienced by Singaporean women and is often worse in obese and depressed women
  - Headaches often increase during the menopause transition
- *Sexual dysfunction*
  - Oestrogen depletion leads to thinning and friability of the tissues. Symptoms of itch, dryness, discomfort and dyspareunia are common and worsen through the menopause. Many women complain of loss of desire, vaginal dryness and dyspareunia and orgasmic difficulties. Continued sexual activity can prevent deterioration in symptoms
- *Urogynaecological symptoms* are often a later presentation. Symptoms of an overactive bladder (frequency, urgency, urge incontinence and nocturia) are common. An increase in urinary tract infections, stress incontinence and dysuria reported
- Brittle nails, thinning of skin, hair loss

While not life-threatening, these symptoms can have considerable impact on quality of life and should be sensitively explored in the history.

Menses

Ask about LMP, cycle length, skipped menses, length of bleeding, heaviness of bleeding and dysmenorrhoea. A menstrual calendar is a helpful pictorial overview of a woman's bleeding.

Note: The **STRAW (Stages of Reproductive Aging Workshop) staging system** provides a framework for assessing fertility and symptoms (Fig. 41.1).

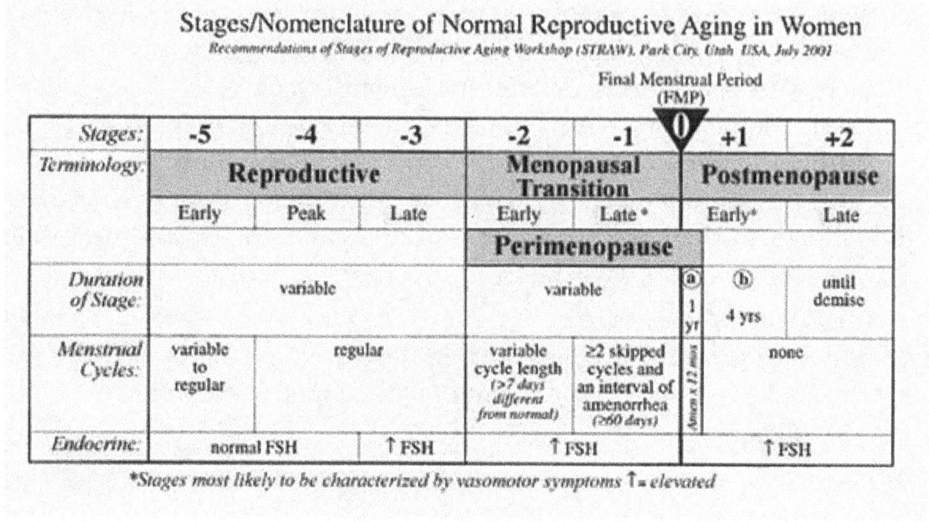

Stages/Nomenclature of Normal Reproductive Aging in Women

Recommendations of Stages of Reproductive Aging Workshop (STRAW), Park City, Utah, USA, July 2001

Stages:	-5	-4	-3	-2	-1	0	+1	+2
Terminology:	Reproductive			Menopausal Transition			Postmenopause	
	Early	Peak	Late	Early	Late *		Early*	Late
				Perimenopause				
Duration of Stage:	variable			variable		(a) 1 yr	(b) 4 yrs	until demise
Menstrual Cycles:	variable to regular	regular		variable cycle length (>7 days different from normal)	≥2 skipped cycles and an interval of amenorrhea (≥60 days)	Amen x 12 mos	none	
Endocrine:	normal FSH		↑ FSH	↑ FSH			↑ FSH	

*Stages most likely to be characterized by vasomotor symptoms ↑ = elevated

FIGURE 41.1 ■ The stage/nomenclature of normal reproductive aging in women — the STRAW staging system.[2]

Late Reproductive Years — Usually age 40+, FSH increases, oestradiol remains steady and luteal progesterone decreases. Ovulation occurs but the follicular phase (1st half) shortens, so overall cycle length decreases e.g. 28 to 23 days.

Menopause transition — typically occurs around 47 years of age.

Early transition — As ovarian follicular depletion continues, FSH levels fluctuate and cycle length increases from 3–4 weeks to 5–7 weeks.

Late transition — Usually lasts 1–3 years and reflects increasing anovulation and fluctuations in FSH and oestradiol. Cycle length increases further with skipped months and episodes of amenorrhoea. Bleeding can be light or heavy, short or prolonged. Anovulation will contribute but fibroids, adenomyosis and precancerous/cancerous endometrial changes may play a role.

Menopause: The final menses is determined in retrospect. FSH levels are high and sustained.

Past medical history — chronic medical conditions may relate to current physical and psychological symptoms. Ask about conditions that may affect your approach to treating menopausal symptoms — cancer, cardiovascular disease, venothromboembolism (VTE), osteoporosis/fracture, migraines, liver disease, gall stones, etc. Document gynaecological and non-gynaecological operations.

Family medical history — ask about cancer, especially breast, ovarian and bowel; heart disease, stroke/VTE, high blood pressure, diabetes and hip fracture.

Social history — ask about smoking and alcohol. Is she married and sexually active? Any issues? Is she working? Does she look after children/elderly relatives?

Note: Most patients will not bring up sexual problems unless asked directly. This is a private but important area to explore. Approach sensitively and after building rapport.

Other symptoms: Ask about bleeding (especially postmenopausal), urinary, bowel and prolapse symptoms and abdominal/pelvic pain.

Note: Have a low threshold to examine women with pelvic/abdominal pain, abdominal swelling, bloating, urinary urgency or increased frequency, a feeling of fullness and a loss of appetite and unexplained weight loss or gain. These symptoms are associated with ovarian cancer.

Examination

General Examination. Record height, weight, body mass index (BMI) and blood pressure. Waist circumference is increasingly being recorded. Grip strength, measured by dynamometer, can predict poorer health outcomes in the long term. General survey may point to physical signs that signal the need for further questioning and investigation.

Breast. Women who are symptomatic with breast concerns (skin distortion, nipple discharge, pain, lumps) need to be examined in a systematic way covering inspection and palpation of the breast, areola, nipple, axilla and supraclavicular fossa. In asymptomatic women, examination should at least be offered.

Abdominal Examination. Women who are symptomatic should be examined and scars, areas of tenderness and masses or fluid recorded. Examination can be difficult in obese patients.

Pelvic Examination. Women who are symptomatic should be examined and findings reported in a systematic way. Record positive findings in the vulva, perineal body, vaginal walls and cervix on speculum examination, and uterus and adnexae on vaginal examination (VE). In asymptomatic women, examination can be offered.

Investigations

Bloods to Confirm Menopausal Status. Routine FSH estimation in older women with regular menses is unreliable as levels fluctuate in the menopause transition. Changes in menstrual pattern are a more reliable predictor of a woman's menopausal staging. It is appropriate to check an amenorrhoea panel (+/− thyroid panel) in younger women with irregular menses or secondary amenorrhoea as it may confirm a diagnosis of premature ovarian insufficiency. FSH estimation is clinically useful in women where the menstrual cycle cannot be assessed e.g. hysterectomy, endometrial ablation or amenorrhoea associated with progesterone only contraception (IUS and Depo-Provera). Regarding contraception, women who are amenorrhoeic can have their FSH levels checked. If the level is in the menopausal range, it should be repeated after six weeks. *Note: FSH measurement is unreliable if a woman is taking combined hormones as gonadotrophins are typically suppressed. Stop the pill/patch/ring for 2–4 weeks to test. Remind her to use condoms or abstain during this time.*

Note: *Always consider the possibility of pregnancy in sexually active women with secondary amenorrhoea.*

Screening

CervicalScreen Singapore is Singapore's national cervical cancer screening program. Women who have been sexually active in the past or who are currently sexually active are invited to attend for a **Pap smear** once every three years from 25 years of age up until the age of 69 years. Screening beyond this age is by patient choice. This is discussed in the chapter on Cervical Cancer and Prevention Screening.

BreastScreen Singapore is Singapore's national breast cancer screening program. Women aged 50 years and older are invited to have screening **mammograms** once every two years. Those aged between 40 to 49 years old can participate in this program after discussion on risks and benefits, but should undergo a screening mammogram once a year until the age of 50 years. Benefits are greater in those with a higher risk of breast cancer — high breast density, family history of breast cancer, and history of benign breast biopsy. Overall mortality is decreased. Risks include false positives and false negatives, the latter being more common with denser breasts. About 25% of cancers may be missed in younger women.

Breast Self-Aware — Encourage women to perform monthly breast self-examination so they are aware of any changes to their breasts.

Bone Mineral Density (BMD). There is no national screening program to measure BMD and predict fracture risk. Many guidelines recommend measuring BMD by DXA (Dual-energy X-ray absorptiometry) scan by the age of 65 years. Whether to undergo assessment earlier can be advised using OSTA (the **Osteoporosis**

—— What is the **OSTA?**——

The Osteoporosis Self-Assessment Tool for Asians (OSTA) is a guide to help assess an Asian woman's risk of osteoporosis. This is done simply by comparing her weight (in kilograms) to age. For example, if you are 60 years of age and weigh 50 kilograms, you come under the moderate-risk group (indicated in orange).

Age (Yr)	Weight (kg)							
	40-44	45-49	50-54	55-59	60-64	65-69	70-74	75-79
45-49								
50-54						Low Risk		
55-59								
60-64								
65-69			Moderate Risk					
70-74								
75-79	High Risk							
80-84								
85-89								

Understanding your OSTA score

Risk category	What does it mean?	What must you do?
High	Your risk of having osteoporosis is HIGH. About 61% of individuals in the high-risk group have osteoporosis. Consult your doctor to have your bone mass checked.	In addition to a diet with adequate calcium and regular weight-bearing exercises, you may require medicine/ supplements to strengthen your bones.
Moderate	Your risk of having osteoporosis is MODERATE. About 15% of individuals in the moderate-risk group have osteoporosis. See your doctor to determine whether you have any other risk factors.	In addition to a diet with adequate calcium and regular weight-bearing exercises, you may need to change your lifestyle (quit smoking, drink less alcohol) to reduce your risk.
Low	Your risk of having osteoporosis is LOW. Only about 3% of individuals in the low-risk group have osteoporosis. However, if you have any of the risk factors listed on page 3, please see a doctor.	You still need to maintain a diet with adequate calcium and do regular weight-bearing exercises to maintain bone mass.

FIGURE 41.2 ■ The osteoporosis self-assessment tool for asians.[1]

Self-assessment Tool for Asians[3]) (Fig. 41.2) which estimates risk based on age and weight into low, moderate and high risk categories. FRAX®, developed by the World Health Organisation, estimates risk based on age, sex, BMI, ethnicity, personal and family history of fracture, history of rheumatoid arthritis, use of corticosteroids, identification of secondary causes for osteoporosis and smoking and drinking. Once the BMD of the hip is measured, this figure can be re-entered into "FRAX® Singapore" to give an estimate of fracture risk over the next 10 years.[1]

---

[1] http://www.shef.ac.uk/FRAX/.

Encourage checks for glucose and lipids to test for diabetes or high cholesterol. Check BP and BMI at each visit and encourage Faecal Immunochemical Test (FIT) to screen for colon cancer.

Management of the Menopause

Menopause treatment should be discussed in a holistic way with non-directive counselling individualised to that woman.

Menopausal Symptoms

How much menopausal symptoms affects a woman is very individual. Symptoms tend to peak during the menopause transition and are worse if a surgical menopause (oophorectomy) has occurred. Symptoms may last 2–8 years.

Healthy lifestyle. Watch weight, limit alcohol and stop smoking. Take regular exercise and take adequate calcium and vitamin D.

General measures. Suggest wearing lighter layers that can be removed and replaced; sleep with air conditioning or a fan, avoid stress or reduce with yoga/ meditation; reduce spicy foods, caffeinated drinks and alcohol; stop smoking.

Non hormonal treatment

Tibolone (Livial) is a synthetic steroid with oestrogenic, progestogenic and androgenic effects. It reduces vasomotor symptoms (but not as well as oestrogen), increases BMD and may improve sex drive. There is a doubling of stroke risk with use beyond 60 years. It can be used in women who are postmenopausal, with or without a uterus. It is a no bleed preparation.

Selective serotonin reuptake inhibitors (SSRIs) and Serotonin and noradrenaline reuptake inhibitors (SNRIs). These antidepressant medicines reduce vasomotor symptoms (VMS) but not as well as oestrogen. Common side effects include nausea and reduced libido.

Gabapentin. This epilepsy and chronic pain drug can help with VMS. Drowsiness and dizziness are commonly reported.

Clonidine. This blood pressure drug may help with VMS. Dry mouth, dizziness and nausea are common side effects.

Herbal and complementary therapies. Remifemin, ginseng, evening primrose oil, kava, dong quai and red clover, among others, have been marketed for menopausal symptoms. While some women find them helpful for short term management, the evidence base and quality control in the manufacture of such herbal preparations is not robust. Full ingredients are unknown so they should be used with caution in women who cannot take oestrogen, and they may interfere with prescribed medication. Rarely, serious morbidity has been reported with use and long term safety has not been established.

Phytoestrogens are naturally occurring compounds found in plants that are structurally related to oestradiol. The main types are genistein, lignans and coumestans. Food rich in phytoestrogens include: soya beans, nuts and wholegrain cereals. They are widely available in concentrated tablet form over the counter in pharmacies and health shops.

Hormone replacement therapy (HRT)

Menopause transition with a uterus — monthly cyclical HRT where oestrogen is taken every day for 21–28 days and a progestogen is added in for 12–14 days. This causes a regular, light bleed.

Post-menopausal with a uterus — continuous combined HRT (CCHRT) is where both oestrogen and a progestogen are taken every day, so no bleeding occurs. CCHRT can be started after taking cyclical HRT for 12 months or if has been one year since last menses, or two years if under 50 years of age.

Perimenopausal/postmenopausal without a uterus — only oestrogen is required and taken daily.

Note: *A progestogen is only added to HRT so that the endometrium does not build up under the influence of unopposed oestrogen and undergo pre-cancerous and cancerous changes.*

Drug delivery

In Singapore, oestrogen can be taken as a pill, patch or gel. The progestogen can be delivered as a pill, capsule or the intrauterine system (Mirena®).

Benefits and risks of HRT

The risks and benefits of HRT will vary depending on her age and medical history. Counselling should be individualised and woman-centred. Most of the evidence comes from two large studies reported in the early 2000s: The Women's Health Initiative Study, a randomised controlled trial involving over 25,000 women aged 50–70 years of age, and the Million Women study, a population-based prospective cohort study of over a million UK women aged 50 and over.[4,5]

Benefits

- Hot flushes and night sweats — improved
- Vulval atrophy — reduces dryness, dyspareunia, UTIs and overactive bladder symptoms
- Mood — some evidence of improvement
- Sleep — some evidence of improvement
- Joint pain — some evidence of improvement
- Bone mineral density — improvement, with reduced fracture risk
- Coronary heart disease — observational studies suggest a "window of opportunity" if taken in the first 10 years of menopause/under 60 years of age. Oestrogen protects against atherosclerosis by increasing high density lipoprotein and decreasing low density lipoprotein-cholesterol transfer to the arterial wall

Risks

Breast cancer

HRT may be associated with a small increased risk of breast cancer, but this is influenced by the constituents of the HRT used:

- Combined (E2 and P) HRT has a higher risk
  - There is a higher risk of an abnormal mammogram because HRT increases breast density
  - The risk increases the longer the HRT is used
  - The risk reduces to that of non-use once HRT has been stopped for five years
  - If 10,000 women took combined HRT for a year, it would result in up to eight more cases of breast cancer. Most studies do not show an increased risk in the first five years of use
- E only HRT does not have an increased risk

   Note: *There is no increased risk of breast cancer when HRT is taken under the age of 50 years.*

Ovarian cancer

There may be a slightly increased risk (1 extra cancer/1,000 women over five years) with HRT use, that returns to baseline on stopping treatment.

Endometrial cancer

- The risk reduces considerably with the addition of progestogen in women with a uterus
- Risk is greater with long term (> five years) sequential HRT use compared to continuous combined

Stroke

- There may be a small risk of stroke associated with HRT use over the age of 60 years
- The risk of stroke appears to be related to dose, with lower doses conferring a lower risk
- There is no increased risk with TRANSDERMAL (patch, gel) preparations

Venothromboembolism

- There is an increased risk of VTE with the oral use of HRT (2–4×)
- The risk is higher with E + P HRT compare with E only HRT
- The risk is greatest in the 1st year of use
- The risk is greater if a woman has additional risk factors — obesity, age, immobility, smoking, associated medical conditions
- There is no increased risk with TRANSDERMAL (patch, gel) preparations

Bowel cancer

- Reduced incidence of colorectal cancer

Unclear effect

Dementia/Alzheimer's — evidence conflicting

Contraindications to HRT

Absolute:

- Hormonally sensitive cancer — breast, endometrial
- Pregnancy

Relative:

- Personal history of VTE
- Family history of VTE
- History of myocardial infarction, angina and stroke
- Uncontrolled blood pressure
- Severe liver disease
- Undiagnosed breast lump
- Uninvestigated vaginal bleeding

Common side effects

Most side effects are transient and settle by three months. They include break through bleeding, headaches, nausea, leg cramps, dry eyes and skin pigmentation.

Changing to a different preparation or delivery system may help.

Contraception

HRT is not contraceptive. The dose of oestrogen is not high enough to suppress gonadotrophins.

Contraception should be continued for two years after the last menses if the woman is under 50 years of age and one year if 50 years or above.

How long?

Women with POI should receive oestrogen replacement until the average age of the menopause, 50 years of age.

For women taking HRT beyond 50 years of age, the most consistent advice is to take the lowest dose possible for the shortest time. Most menopausal symptoms improve over 1–3 years, so HRT can be stopped to assess current symptoms. It is recommended to start at a low dose and increase if symptom control is not achieved. Stopping may produce a temporary rebound effect on symptoms. Some women choose to continue HRT for longer term health benefits. The individual benefits and risks of this approach should be discussed at each annual review with the woman.

Genital symptoms only

Vaginal dryness may benefit from:

- Personal lubricants: aqueous and silicone
- Vaginal moisturisers: last for 2–3 days

- Oils (e.g. olive, coconut)
- Vaginal oestrogen:
  - Available as a cream or tablet
  - Administered per vagina
  - Minimal absorption systemically
  - Can be continued long term with no increased risk of endometrial or breast cancer or cardiovascular disease

Longer Term Issues

There are a number of long term effects of oestrogen deficiency:

Cardiovascular. The risk of cardiovascular disease (CVD) increases after the menopause with changes in lipid profiles — an increase in cholesterol, low density lipoprotein (LDL) and triglycerides and a gradual decrease in high density lipoprotein (HDL)

Dementia, degenerative arthritis and weight gain — there is currently insufficient evidence to link oestrogen depletion to these health issues.

Osteoporosis (OP)

Definition. a progressive, systemic skeletal disease characterised by reduce bone density (mass). Reduced bone mineral density (BMD) is one of the main risk factors for fracture. This needs to be looked into and managed. It is discussed in greater detail in the chapter on Well Women Screening.

References

1. O'Reilly B, Bottomley C, Rymer J. (2012) *Essentials of Obstetrics & Gynaecology*, 5th edn. Saunders Elsevier, Philadelphia, pp. 173–182.
2. Harlow SD, *et al.* (2012) Executive summary of the stages of reproductive aging workshop + 10: Addressing the unfinished agenda of staging reproductive aging. *J Clin Endocrinol Metab* **97**(4):1159–1168.
3. Koh LKH, Ben Sedrine W, Torralba TP, Kung A, Fujiwara S, Chan SP, Huang QR, Rajatanavin R, Tsai KS, Park HM, Reginster JY. (2001) A simple tool to identify Asian women at increased risk of osteoporosis. *Osteoporosis Int* **12**(8):600–705.

4. Panay N, Hamoda H, Arya R, Savvas M. (2013) The 2013 British Menopause Society & Women's Health Concern recommendations on hormone replacement therapy. *Menopause Int* **19**(2):59–68.

5. Ministry of Health. (2009) *Singapore Clinical practice Guidelines on Osteoporosis.* https://www.moh.gov.sg/content/dam/moh_web/HPP/Doctors/cpg_medical/current/2009/CPG_Osteoporosis_Booklet_Jan2009.pdf.

42

WELL WOMEN SCREEN

Anupriya Agarwal

Introduction

Gynaecologists are quite likely to see the "well woman" as she attends the clinic for gynaecological problems and routine tests like the Pap smear, and this provides a unique opportunity for well woman screening of these women. In this chapter we will discuss the various screening tests and their indications.

Pap Smear for Cervical Cancer

This is the most common test performed for cervical cancer and pre-cancer. Information regarding the pap smear test is provided in the chapter on Cervical Cancer Prevention and Screening.

Breast Cancer

Breast cancer is a malignant tumour of the breast tissue and is the most common cancer in women in Singapore. More than 25% of all cancers diagnosed in women are breast cancers. Between 2009 and 2013, almost 1,800 women were diagnosed to have breast cancer in Singapore each year.

Breast cancer is usually a slow growing cancer and early detection can increase the chances of survival. Hence, the value of screening for breast cancer in every woman aged 40 and above.[1]

Risk Factors

The majority of breast cancers are dependent on oestrogen and progesterone. Hence, the longer the exposure to these hormones, the higher the chance for development of breast cancer. Between 5–10% of all breast cancers are caused by genetic factors. The BRCA1 and BRCA2 genes have found to be associated with breast cancer, occurring in approximately half of all families with a very strong history of breast and/or ovarian cancer.

The chances of getting breast cancer increase with age. Other risk factors for breast cancer include:

- Having a family history of breast cancer in a first-degree relative
- A history of malignant or benign (non-cancerous) breast disease
- A history of ovarian cancer
- Early onset of menstruation
- Late menopause
- Having first completed pregnancy after the age of 30
- Nulliparity
- Hormone replacement therapy — oestrogen and progesterone therapy
- Weight gain, especially after menopause

Breast cancer risk prediction tools — these risk prediction tools combine major risk factors and serve to stratify women into risk categories to enable optimisation of screening. The most widely used tool to calculate breast cancer risk is the Breast Cancer Risk Assessment Tool (BCRAT), also called the Gail Model, which takes into consideration race and ethnicity as well as age, history of breast disease, age at onset of menses, parity and family history, and is available online at www.cancer.gov/bcrisktool/.

Screening for Breast Cancer

- Regular mammography remains the mainstay of screening for breast cancer, as demonstrated by several randomised controlled trials.
- Breast Self-Examination (BSE) is recommended to be done from age 30 onwards and may help women detect changes in their breasts in between regular mammograms.

How often should screening be done?

The Singapore Health Promotion Board has the following screening guidelines for different groups of healthy women:

Women above 50 years

Screening every two years is recommended. A systematic review of screening mammograms concluded that, with at least 11 years of follow-up, the pooled relative risk for breast cancer mortality was 0.86 (0.75–0.99) for women 50 to 59 years of age, and 0.68 (0.54–0.87) for women 60 to 69 years of age.

Women between 40–49 years

Annual screening is recommended as younger women have faster growing cancers. A systematic review and meta-analysis of eight RCTs found a 15% reduction of breast cancer mortality in women of this age group who were randomly assigned to mammographic screening (RR 0.85, 95% CI 0.75–0.96). However, the sensitivity of mammography is lower in younger women. Benefits for screening women in their 40s are more favourable when considered from the perspective of years of life saved.

Women below 40 years

There is no need for women in this age group to go for screening unless in the high risk group.

Women with germline mutations

Germline mutations that increase the risk of cancers — only about 5% of all breast cancers are associated with germline (inherited) genetic mutations, the most common of these being mutations of BRCA1 and BRCA2 genes. Testing for mutations in these genes is available and should be offered to patients who have clustering of breast, ovarian or colonic cancers in their families.

Women with BRCA1 or BRCA2 mutations are at a high risk of both breast and ovarian cancer. Such women should be referred for appropriate counselling to consider options for reducing risk and intensified surveillance. For women with an inherited predisposition, guidelines from major groups like the American Cancer Society recommend a combination of annual mammography and breast MRI for breast cancer surveillance. These women should be referred to breast specialists for further management.[2]

Practical advice to women undergoing mammography for breast cancer screening

- For premenstrual women the best time for doing a mammogram is in the post-menstrual phase, as the breasts will be less tender and swollen and the quality of images will be better.
- Patients should be advised to disclose history of breast implants, if any.

- Patients should be advised not to wear any deodorant, perfume, lotion, or powder under your arms or on your breasts on the day of the mammogram, as these can cast shadows and reduce the quality of the mammogram image.
- Previous mammogram images should be brought along for comparison.

Benefits and harm of mammograms

TABLE 42.1   Benefits and Risks of Screening Mammography[3]

Benefits	Harms
*Among 1000 **40-year-old** women undergoing annual mammography for 10 years:*	
0.1–1.6 Woman will avoid dying from breast cancer	510–690 Women will have at least 1 "false alarm" (60–80 of whom will undergo a biopsy)
	?-ll Women will be overdiagnosed and treated needlessly with surgery, radiation, and/or chemotherapy
*Among 1000 **50-year-old** women undergoing annual mammography for 10 years:*	
0.3–3.2 Women will avoid dying from breast cancer	490–670 Women will have at least 1 "false alarm" (70–100 of whom will undergo a biopsy)
	3–14 Women will be overdiagnosed and treated needlessly with surgery, radiation, and/or chemotherapy
*Among 1000 **60-year-old** women undergoing annual mammography for 10 years:*	
0.5–4.9 Women will avoid dying from breast cancer	390–540 Women will have at least 1 "false alarm" (50–70 of whom will undergo a biopsy)
	6–20 Women will be overdiagnosed and treated needlessly with surgery, radiation, and/or chemotherapy

Osteoporosis

Definition. It is a progressive systemic skeletal disease characterised by reduced bone density (mass). Reduced bone mine density (BMD) is one of the main risk factors for fracture.

TABLE 42.2   Risk Factors for Osteoporosis, Falls and Fractures

---

A. Risk Factors for Osteoporosis and Fractures

Non-modifiable

- Personal history of previous fragility fracture as an adult
- Height loss of more than 2 cm over three years
- History of fracture in a first-degree relative (especially maternal)
- Low body weight — BMI less than 19 kg/m^2
- Increasing age

Potentially-modifiable

- Lack of regular physical exercise
- Prolonged immobilisation
- Current cigarette smoking
- Alcohol abuse
- Low calcium intake (< 500 mg/day)

Secondary Osteoporosis

- Drugs e.g. corticosteroids (equivalent to prednisolone > 7.5 mg/day for more than six months), anticonvulsants.

- Ongoing disease conditions e.g. hypogonadism, anorexia nervosa, hyperthyroidism, hyperparathyroidism, Cushing's syndrome, chronic obstructive airways disease, liver disease, malabsorption, chronic renal failure, rheumatoid arthritis, organ transplantation.
- Early natural or surgical menopause before age 45 years

B. Risk factors for falls and fracture

Patient factors

- One or more previous falls in the past year
- Impaired eyesight
- Certain medications e.g. sedatives, antihistamines, antihypertensives
- Gait abnormality associated with medical conditions e.g. stroke, parkinsonism, neuropathy or arthritis
- Reduced muscle strength and impaired balance due to ageing and lack of exercise
- Cognitive impairment

Environmental factors

- Slippery floors
- Obstacles on the floor e.g. uneven carpet, wires
- Inadequate lighting
- Inappropriate foot wear

Osteoporosis is the most common bone disease in humans, representing a major public health problem with significant medical, social and financial implications, as up to 30% patients who sustain a fracture do not return to their previous functional status and may require long term institutional or nursing care. The age-adjusted hip fracture rates among Singaporean women over the age of 50 years are about 450/100,000. Fracture of the lower limb ranks fourth in terms of the number of hospital inpatient discharges and direct hospital cost per year in Singapore.[1]

Screening for Osteoporosis

In the year 2006, a hip Bone Mineral Density (BMD) measurement study estimated that there were about 55,000 female Singaporeans above the age of 50 who are suffering from osteoporosis. This problem will, of course, increase over time as the population ages rapidly. The numbers of hip fractures per year in Singapore are projected to increase from 1,300 in 1998 to 9,000 in 2050 because of the aging of the population. In Singapore, the incidence of hip fracture has increased five times in women since the 1960s, similar to trends seen in the West.[4]

According to the WHO, osteoporosis is defined by a bone mineral density (BMD) at the hip or lumbar spine which is less than or equal to 2.5 standard deviations below the mean BMD of a young adult reference population. The risk of osteoporotic fractures is highest in those with the lowest BMD; however, most fractures occur in patients with low bone mass rather than osteoporosis, as this forms a much larger group of individuals. Osteoporotic fractures are a major health problem.

Osteoporosis is a silent disease, hence the need for timely screening. Early diagnosis of low bone mass can encourage modification of risk factors associated with osteoporosis such as smoking, heavy alcohol consumption and a sedentary lifestyle, and can help initiate timely and appropriate treatment which can then prevent the many sequelae associated with osteoporotic fractures.

Investigations

It is not recommended to screen the general population at normal risk for BMD. There are several tools that have been used for the risk assessment of osteoporosis:

Osteoporosis Self-Assessment Tool for Asians (OSTA)

The Osteoporosis Self-Assessment Tool for Asians (OSTA) is a simple tool based on age and weight which has been developed for the assessment of postmenopausal Asian women. This tool categorises women into high, moderate and low risk of being diagnosed with osteoporosis on subsequent bone mineral density (BMD) measurement (Table 42.3).

TABLE 42.3   The Osteoporosis Self-Assessment Tool for Asians[5]

Age (Yr)	Weight (kg)							
	40–44	45–49	50–54	55–59	60–64	65–69	70–74	75–79
45–49								
50–54								
55–59					Low Risk			
60–64								
65–69			Moderate Risk					
70–74								
75–79	High Risk							
80–84								
85–89								

Table 42.4 shows the suggested action based on osteoporosis risk from the OSTA.

TABLE 42.4   Suggested Action Based on Osteoporosis Risk

Osteoporosis Risk	Patient's Age (years) Minus Weight (kg)	Suggested Action
High	> 20	Measure BMD
Moderate	0–20	Check for risk factors or past history of fracture, measure BMD if either is present
Low	< 0	Can defer BMD unless assessed to have high risk of fracture. Start screening at 65 years

A long-term prospective study involving almost 5,000 women aged 67 years or older found that the interval between baseline testing and the development of osteoporosis in 10% of study participants was 16.8 years for women with normal bone density (T score above –1.00), 17.3 years for women with osteopenia (T score of –1.00 to –1.49), 4.7 years for women with moderate osteopenia (T score of –1.50 to –1.99), and 1.1 years for women with advanced osteopenia (T score of –2.00 to –2.49).

You should measure BMD once a year if the patient has osteoporosis. In osteopenic patients, the frequency of repeat BMD varies from 1–5 years, depending on the severity of osteopenia, and once in every five years if the bone mass is normal.[6]

There are other ways to assess fracture risk. The Facture Risk Assessment (FRAX®) Tool has been developed by the World Health Organisation (WHO) based on population-based cohorts from Europe, North America, Asia, and Australia. It is a simple, yet useful tool that incorporates the risks associated with clinical factors as well as bone mineral density at the femoral neck for each individual patient. FRAX models have been developed. FRAX algorithms give the 10-year probability of hip or major osteoporotic fracture (clinical spine, forearm, hip, or shoulder fracture). It is free software that is available at www.who-frax.org.[7]

Bone mineral density (BMD) measurement

BMD is a measurement which assesses the fracture risk. While there are many methods to measure BMD, the dual energy X-ray absorptiometry (DEXA) is the method of choice for measuring the BMD.

Hip measurements at the femoral neck and of the total hip joint are the best predictors of hip fracture, and are also good predictors of other osteoporotic fractures. Measurements are conventionally taken at the unfractured and non-dominant hip. Hip and spine measurements are obtained and reported as T and Z scores.

T-score

The values are measured using dual-energy X-ray absorptiometry (DEXA). T-scores are derived by comparing the bone density of an individual with the mean bone density of young healthy adults of the same gender. The result is expressed as the number of standard deviations (SD) from the mean. According to the WHO, the T-score is divided into 4 categories:

TABLE 42.5   T-Score Based on Bone Mineral Density

BMD T-Score (S.D.)		Definition
>−1	BMD greater than the lower level of normal, 1 S.D. below the adult reference mean.	Normal
<−1 to >−2.5	BMD between 1 and 2.5 S.D. below the adult reference mean.	Low bone mass (osteopenia)
<−2.5	BMD 2.5 S.D. or more below the adult reference mean.	Osteoporosis
<−2.5 + fragility fracture	BMD 2.5 S.D. or more below the adult reference mean.	Severe or established osteoporosis

Also consider testing erythrocyte sedimentation rate (ESR), full blood count (FBC), thyroid panel, renal panel, liver panel , calcium panel, parathyroid hormone (PTH) and vitamin D to identify underlying disease that is causing secondary osteoporosis.

Management

General measures to reduce fracture risk include the following:

- Weight bearing exercise — walking, jumping, aerobics, line dancing, Tai Chi
- Diet: Aiming for 1000–1200 mg calcium per day from milk, cheese, yogurt, sardines and Chinese greens
- Sunshine for 15–30 minutes 3–4× per week
- Stop smoking
- Reduce alcohol
- Fall reduction advise

Medication

Hormonal (HRT). Please refer to Chapter 41 for regimes.

Non-hormonal

- *Bisphosphonates.* Act by inhibiting osteoclasts and are usually used first-line, starting with the least expensive, alendronate. They are poorly absorbed with food and cause oesophageal irritation. As such, they are taken fasted, sitting up or standing with plenty of water. Ca and Vit D supplementation is co-prescribed. Risedronate is an alternative if gastrointestinal side effects are too great. Bisphosphonates are usually prescribed for 5–10 years with drug holidays in between. Longer term use has been associated with atypical hip fractures.

- *Raloxifene.* Is a selective oestrogen receptor modulator (SERM). It reduces postmenopausal bone loss, vertebral fractures and risk of breast cancer but has an increased risk of VTE and hot flushes as a side effect.

- **Tibolone** (Livial). Is a synthetic steroid with estrogenic, progestogenic and androgenic effects. It increases BMD. It is discussed in more detail in the Chapter on Menopause.

TABLE 42.6 Well Woman Screening Tests — Based on Health Promotion Board, Singapore Recommendations

Health Service	13–18 Years	19–39 Years	40–64 Years	65 Years and Older
Physical examination				
Height	✓	✓	✓	✓
Weight	✓	✓	✓	✓
BMI	✓	✓	✓	✓
Blood pressure	✓	✓	✓	✓
Tanner staging of secondary sexual characteristics	✓			
Breast exam		✓	✓	✓
Abdominal exam	✓	✓	✓	✓
Pelvic exam	If indicated	✓	✓	✓
		Age 21 and older		

Laboratory testing

Chlamydia

A woman 25 years or younger:
— Who has a new sexual partner
— Who has a partner with symptoms of an STD
— Who has had two or more sexual partners in the past 12 months
— Whose partner does not use condoms.
A woman who has gone through an abortion with the risk factors stated above.

For high risk women:

Gonorrhoea
— Those who exchange sex for money or drugs
— Those with repeated gonorrhoea infections
— Those who have had two or more sexual partners in the past year.

Test				
Syphilis	Screening is recommended for those who practice unsafe sex, including the following: • Those who exchange sex for money or drugs • Those who have other STDs (including HIV) and ulcers on the genitals • Those whose partners have syphilis. Screening should be done one month after possible contact, and again after three months.	√		
HIV	If sexually active √	All women who have ever had sex: √		
Pap smear	All women who have ever had sex: First Pap smear by 25 years of age. Low risk: Every three years	All women who have had sex: First Pap smear by 25 years of age. Low risk: Every three years High risk (immunosuppressed or HIV infection): yearly	Low risk: Every three years High risk (immunosuppressed or HIV infection): yearly	Can stop if the past Pap smears have been normal
HPV vaccination	√	Recommended up to the age of 26 years		
Fasting glucose	Consider screening at age 30 and older if high risk factors: Overweight or obese, Family history, PCOS, Coronary heart disease, abnormal lipids	Age 40 and older Every three years if normal results		

(Continued)

TABLE 42.6 *(Continued)*

Health Service	13–18 Years	19–39 Years	40–64 Years	65 Years and Older
Lipid profile		Consider screening at age 30 and older if high risk factors: Overweight or obese, Family history, PCOS, Coronary heart disease, abnormal lipids	Age 40 and older Every three years if normal results	
Mammography		Only if high risk	Age 40 to 49: annual. Age 50 and older: every two years	
BMD			Use OSTA/FRAX score to stratify risk — Yearly if osteoporosis or high risk — In 1–5 years if osteopenia — Once in five years if BMD is normal.	

Legend
STD — sexually transmitted diseases
HIV — human immunodeficiency virus
PCOS — polycystic ovarian syndrome
BMD — Bone mineral density
Modified from Health promotion broad, Singapore, heath screening guidelines

Morbidity and Mortality

Fragility fractures cause pain, deformity, disability and loss of quality of life. Hip and vertebral fractures are associated with reduced life expectancy. Hip fracture is the most severe, with hospitalisation guaranteed, loss of independence in half and a 20% mortality.

Other Screening Tests

There are other screening tests that may be appropriate for women of different age groups, for example screening for sexually transmitted diseases in sexually active women. For the purpose of simplicity, it is useful to divide the women according to their age group: ages 13–18, 19–39, 40–64, and older than 65 as it helps organise the approach to primary and preventive health care. Table 42.6 helps to highlight the common health problems that are most prevalent among women at each life-stage and also provides guidance for the clinical approach to physical examination, laboratory testing, and immunisation. While these guidelines are quite comprehensive, professional judgment must be used for each individual patient.

References

1. Nelson HD, Tyne K, Naik A, *et al*. (2009) Screening for breast cancer: an update for the U.S. Preventive Services Task Force. *Ann Intern Med* **151**:727.
2. American College of Obstetricians-Gynecologists (2011). Practice bulletin no. 122: Breast cancer screening. *Obstet Gynecol* **118**:372.
3. Welch HG, Passow HJ. (2014) Quantifying the benefits and harms of screening mammography. *JAMA Intern Med* **174**(3):448–454.
4. Ministry of Health Singapore Clinical Practice Guidelines on Osteoporosis. (2009) https://www.moh.gov.sg/content/dam/moh_web/HPP/Doctors/cpg_medical/current/2009/CPG_Osteoporosis_Booklet_jan2009.pdf.
5. Koh LKH, Sedrine WB, Torralba TP, *et al*. (2001) A simple tool to identify Asian women at increased risk of osteoporosis. *Osteoporosis Inter* **12**(8):600–705.
6. Gourlay ML, Fine JP, Preisser JS, *et al*. (2012) Study of Osteoporotic Fractures Research Group. Bone-density testing interval and transition to osteoporosis in older women. *N Engl J Med* **366**(3):225–233.
7. FRAX: WHO Fracture Risk Assessment Tool Web site. www.shef.ac.uk/FRAX/.

43

GENITAL PROLAPSE AND URINARY PROBLEMS

Ng Kwok Weng Roy

Introduction

In this chapter, the following aspects of genital prolapse and urinary problems will be discussed.

- To understand the health impact of pelvic organ prolapse (POP) and urinary incontinence (UI).
- To be able to elicit the symptoms of POP, recognise and appropriately counsel the options of treatment.
- To understand the different types of urinary incontinence and the approaches to management.

The Health Impact of Pelvic Organ Prolapse (POP) and Urinary Incontinence (UI)

Both pelvic organ prolapse and urinary incontinence are not directly life threatening but they can affect the quality of life of about 10–20% of women worldwide. POP impacts simple daily activities like sitting, standing, walking, working, exercising, micturating, defaecating and sexual intercourse. It alters the body image of affected women, reduces libido, causes dyspareunia or apareunia, which affects their psychological health, leading to depression and even suicidal tendencies.

When POP progresses it can cause cervical ectropion, abrasion, ulceration, bleeding and infection. A prolapsed bladder or cystocoele (anterior compartment

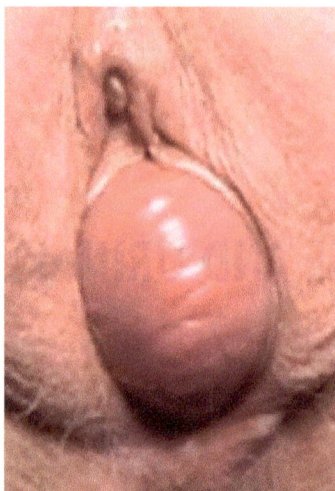

FIGURE 43.1 ■ Cystocoele.

prolapse) outside the vagina (Fig. 43.1) can kink the urethra causing voiding difficulty, residual urine, recurrent urinary tract infections and antibiotic resistance.

Similarly a large rectocoele (posterior compartment prolapse) can behave like a "road hump", causing obstructive constipation (Fig. 43.2). Such patients would need to use their finger/s to manually reduce or splint their cystocoele and rectocoele vaginally, to enable them to micturate and defaecate respectively.

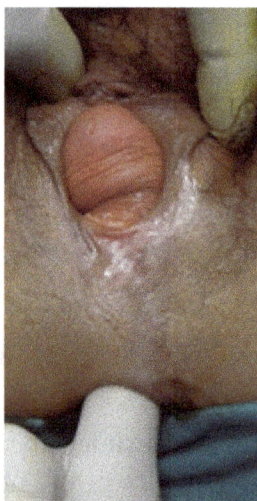

FIGURE 43.2 ■ Rectocoele.

Significant POP or procidentia (Fig. 43.3(a)) or complete eversion of the vagina can result in kinking of both ureters, causing bilateral hydroureters and hydronephroses (Fig. 43.3(b)), impairment of renal function, pyelonephritis and urological sepsis, which can be fatal if not managed aggressively with: pessary reduction of the POP, intravenous antibiotics, fluid and electrolyte correction; and surgical correction when they are fit for anaesthesia and surgery.

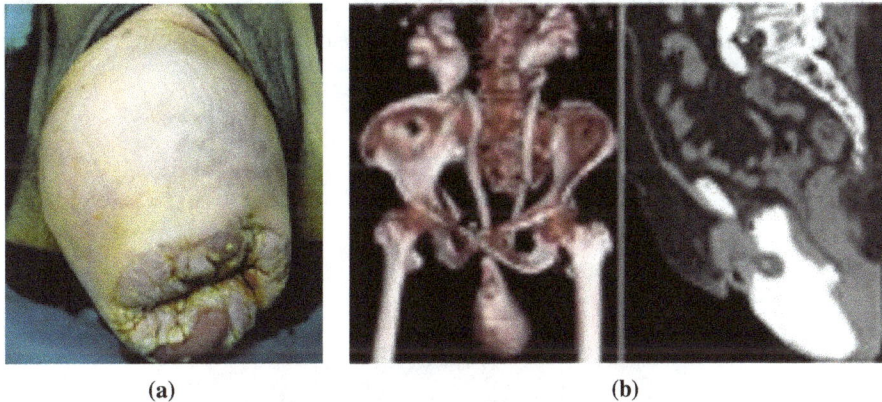

(a) **(b)**

FIGURE 43.3 ■ (a) Procidentia. (b) Model (left) and MRI (right) of hydroureters and hydronephroses caused by procidentia.

Urinary frequency, nocturia, urgency, urge and stress urinary incontinence can affect women's ability to work, fulfil their duties as partners, wives, mothers, play and interact. They become withdrawn and may eventually be prisoners in their own homes because of the fear, anxiety, shame and embarrassment from wetness and odour of urinary incontinence. Such significant impact on their physical, emotional, psychological and financial health can obviously affect their general wellbeing. Urinary incontinence can also cause nappy rash and infection; falls, fractures, hospital admissions, surgeries, morbidity and mortality, especially in the elderly, where urinary incontinence is more prevalent.

Normal Pelvic Anatomy and Support

In *Homo sapiens* the pelvic floor has evolved to accommodate our upright posture. It comprises of a sling of several muscle groups:[1]

(i) Pubococcygeus, from the symphysis pubis to the coccyx.
(ii) Iliococcygeus, from the ilium to the coccyx.
(iii) Coccygeus (previously known as ischiococcygeus) from the ischium to the coccyx.

(i) and (ii) collectively are also called Levator ani, and together with the Coccygeus the Pelvic diaphragm, which stretches from the symphysis pubis to the coccyx and from the side walls of the ilium and ischium. It is concave and funnelling downwards, it supports the abdominal and pelvic organs and contains three principal perforations through which the urethra, vagina and rectum pass (Fig. 43.4). The pelvic floor is innervated by the pudendal nerve (S2, 3, 4). Its damage during vaginal birth along the Alcock canal can cause pelvic organ prolapse and urinary incontinence.

Superior view

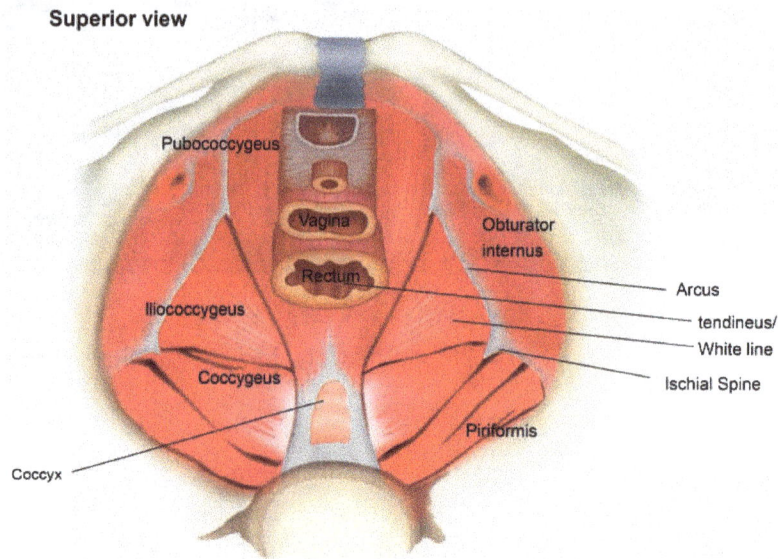

FIGURE 43.4 ■ Female pelvic floor — superior view.

The Pubocervical Fascia and Rectovaginal Septum

The pubocervical fascia is a thickening of the endopelvic fascia anteriorly. The endopelvic fascia is a layer of fibromuscular tissue (Fig. 43.5(b) — courtesy Gynecare, Ethicon, Johnson & Johnson, 2005) consisting of collagen, elastin and smooth muscle; it is a continuation of the abdominal transversalis fascia which includes the visceral and parietal component:

(i) The visceral layer lies immediately beneath the peritoneum and attaches to the bladder, vagina, uterus and rectum.
(ii) The parietal layer has areas of condensation, ligaments and septae which provide fixation to the pelvic floor.

The pubocervical fascia is attached:
(i) Distally to the symphysis pubis through the transverse perinei membrane
(ii) Proximally to the cervix (Fig. 43.6, under the rectovaginal septum).
(iii) Laterally to the white line, also known as the arcus tendineus fasciae pelvis, a linear thickening of the levator ani fascia from the ischial spine to the posterior aspect of the symphysis pubis (Fig. 43.5(a) — courtesy of Gynecare, Ethicon, Johnson & Johnson, 2005).

The pubocervical fascia supports the anterior compartment, in which lies the bladder and urethra. A defect of the pubocervical fascia can cause an anterior compartment prolapse or cystocoele.

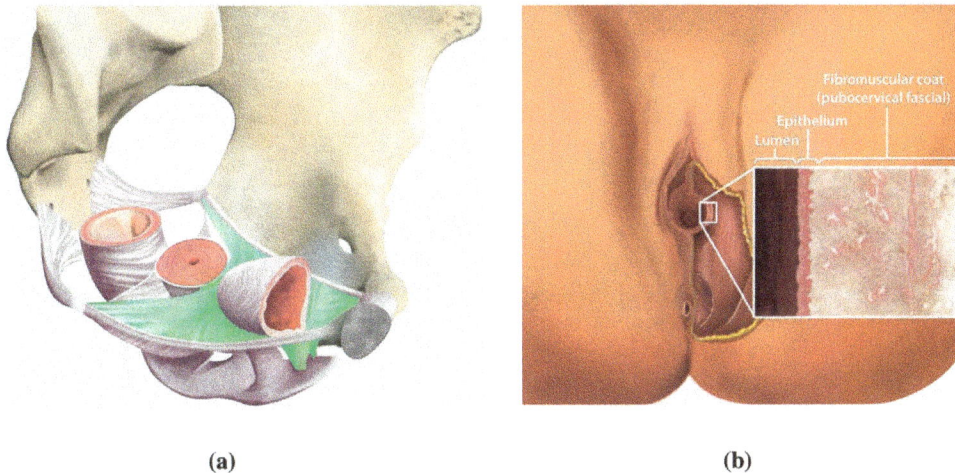

(a)   **(b)**

FIGURE 43.5 ■ (a) Arcus tendineus fasciae pelvis. (b) The endopelvic fascia.

The Rectovaginal Septum

The rectovaginal septum is a thickening of the endopelvic fascia posteriorly. It is attached:

(i) Proximally to the Pouch of Douglas and uterosacral ligaments
(ii) Distally to the perineal body.
(iii) Laterally to the white line, similar to the pubocervical fascia. The rectovaginal septum supports the posterior compartment, in which lies the rectum and Pouch of Douglas. A defect of the rectovaginal septum can cause a posterior compartment prolapse or rectocoele and/or enterocoele.

Physiology of Bladder Filling/Storage and Voiding

The urinary tract is controlled mainly by local innervation acting under central nervous system modulation. Local innervation is chiefly by parasympathetic and sympathetic autonomic and peripheral somatic motor and sensory system.

The sympathetic autonomic nerves to the bladder and urethra originate in cord levels T5 to L2. They innervate the beta (β) receptors in the detrusor muscle and alpha (α) receptors in the bladder neck and proximal urethra through the hypogastric nerve (Fig. 43.7).

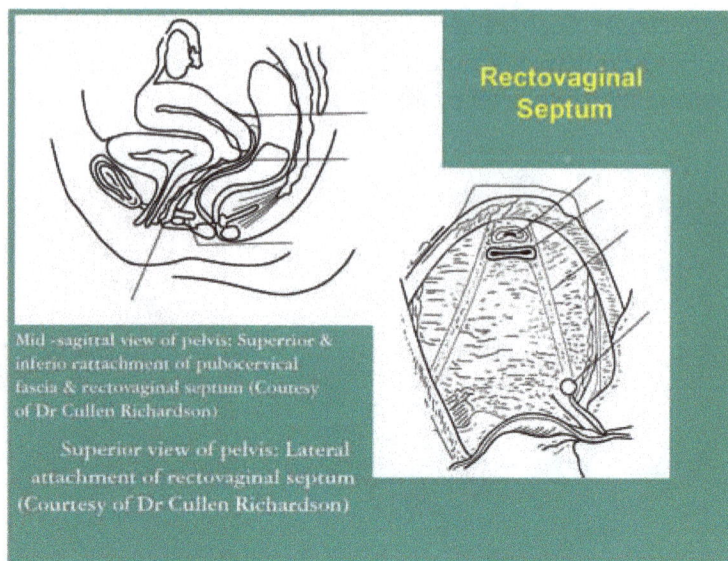

FIGURE 43.6[1] ■ The rectovaginal septum.

The parasympathetic autonomic nerves to the bladder originate in spinal segments S2 to 4 and innervate the beta (β) receptors in the detrusor muscle through the pelvic nerve and plexus (Fig. 43.7).

The pudendal nerve which originates from S2 to 4 is the somatic nerve supply to the striated urogenital diaphragm. It also innervates the perineal muscles and external anal sphincter.

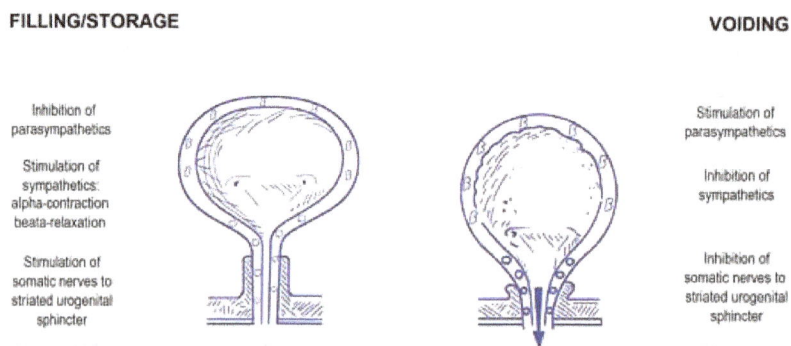

FIGURE 43.7[2] ■ Actions of the autonomic and somatic nervous system during bladder filling/storage and voiding.

Genital Prolapse or Pelvic Organ Prolapse (POP)

Types of POP

(i) Anterior compartment prolapse/prolapse of the bladder (cystocoele) (Fig. 43.1(a) and (b))

(ii) Posterior compartment prolapse/prolapse of the rectum (rectocoele) or Pouch of Douglas (enterocoele). Clinically, it is not possible to differentiate a rectocoele from an enterocoele or an enterocoele from a vault prolapse. The diagnosis of the latter can only be made either by perineal ultrasound scan. MRI, or during surgery when the enterocoele sac is identified.

(iii) Apical prolapse: (a) Uterine prolapse, usually with elongated cervix where the uterine fundus cannot be palpated outside the vagina (Fig. 43.8) or procidentia, where the fundus can be palpated outside the vagina (Fig. 43.3(a)).

(b) Vault prolapse after previous hysterectomy (Fig. 43.9).

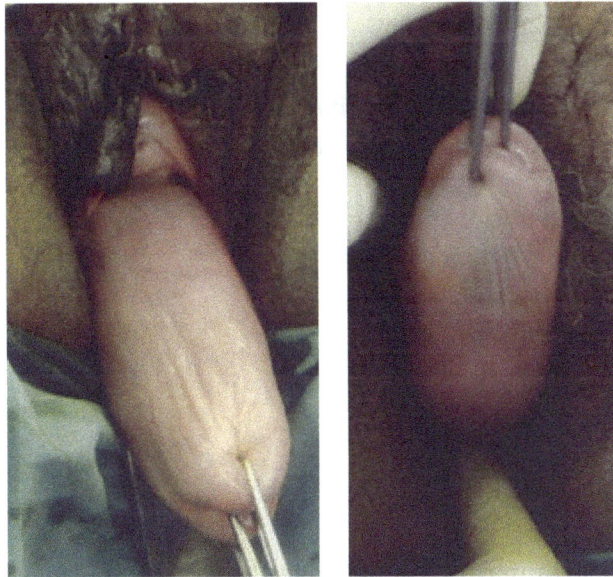

FIGURE 43.8 ■ Uterine prolapse anterior (left) and posterior (right) view.

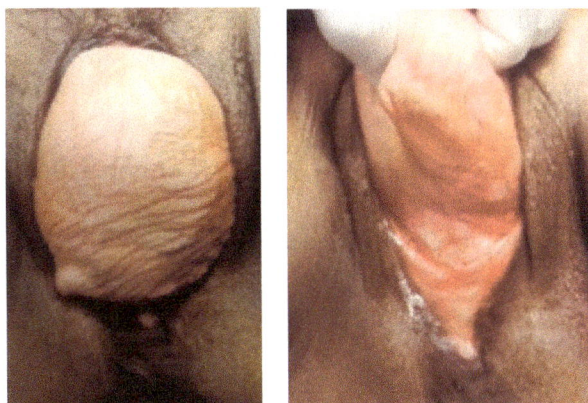

FIGURE 43.9 ■ Vault prolapse anterior (left) and posterior (right) view.

Aetiology of POP

- Congenital — related to collagen deficiency
- Joint hypermobility
- Pregnancy
- Vaginal births
- Ageing
- Menopause
- Chronic cough, constipation
- Occupations requiring heavy lifting

Symptoms of POP

- Something coming down/lump below
- Pain/pressure/discomfort/backache
- Difficulty in walking, sitting; having vaginal intercourse (or cannot have)
- Vaginal laxity
- Overactive bladder (urgency, frequency, nocturia)
- Urinary/faecal incontinence
- Voiding difficulty
- Vaginal discharge/bleeding
- Fear of growth/cancer
- Anxiety/shame/depression

Signs of POP

- Cystocoele (anterior compartment prolapse)
- Rectocoele/enterocoele (posterior compartment prolapse)
- Uterovaginal prolapse
- Procidentia
- Uterine/vaginal vault (apical) prolapse
- Abrasion/ulceration/cervical ectropion/oedema
- Vaginal discharge/bleeding
- Atrophic genitalia
- Stress urinary incontinence — revealed or concealed/occult
- Urinary retention
- Poor/absent pelvic floor/anal tone
- Vaginal laxity
- Torn anal sphincter (previously unrepaired/repaired inadequately)/short perineum
- Scarred vagina
- Drain-pipe urethra

Grading/Staging of POP

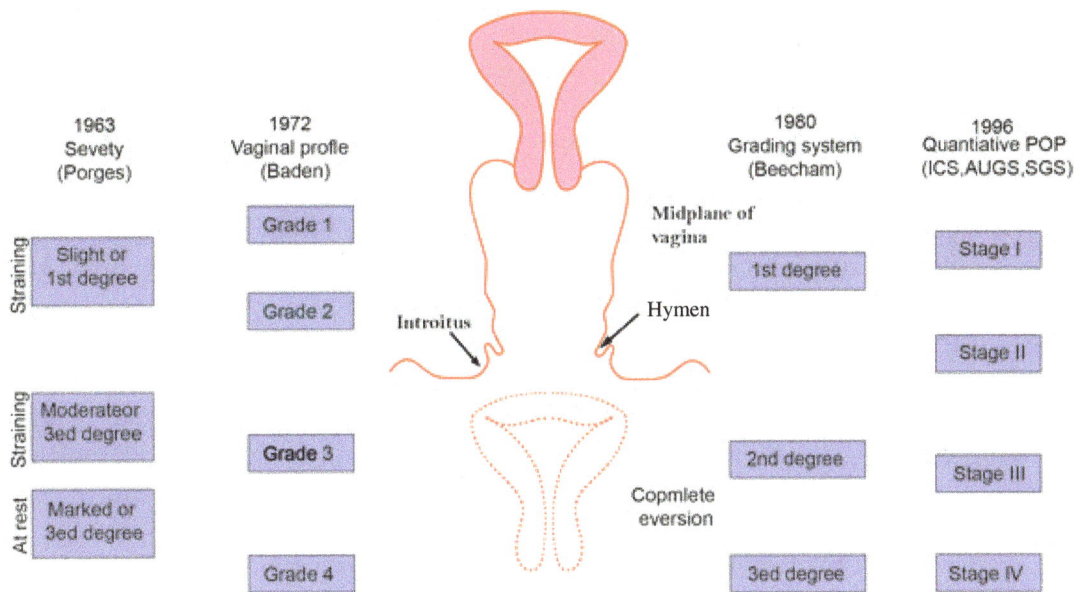

FIGURE 43.10[3] ■ Comparison of the four most commonly used pelvic organ prolapse (POP) grading.

Porges developed one of the earliest systems of evaluating prolapse in 1963. He used the *introitus* (defined as entrance into the vagina) as the reference point:

Slight or 1st degree = Prolapse to or above the introitus
Moderate or 2nd degree = Prolapse outside the introitus
Marked or 3rd degree = Complete eversion.
Porges recommended two separate sets of observations: *at rest* and with *straining*.
One of the most widely used grading systems currently in use was published by **Beecham** in 1980. The reference point for this grading system was also the *introitus*. The 3 grades used, 1st to 3rd degree, were similar to Porges' but only during *straining*.

In 1972, **Baden and Walker** proposed a method of classifying vaginal support by a site-specific examination during *straining*, in which six different anatomical reference sites were assigned a numerical value from 0 to 4, using the *hymen* as the reference point.

The *vaginal profile* evaluates four sites: urethrocele, cystocele, rectocele and uterine prolapse as:

0 = Normal
1 = Descent half way to the hymen
2 = Progression to the hymen
3 = Progression half way through the hymen
4 = Maximal progression through the hymen

The other two anatomical reference sites evaluated were enteroceles and perineal lacerations. I have excluded the former because it is very difficult to differentiate an enterocele from a rectocele clinically. The latter has also been excluded because the Sultan classification of perineal or obstetrical anal sphincter injuries (OASIS) is a more widely recognised system.

Quantitative pelvic organ prolapse (POP-Q) examination system, 1996[4]

The POP-Q system has been adopted by the International Continence Society (ICS), American Urogynecologic Society (AUGS) and American College of Obstetricians & Gynecologists (ACOG). It has been validated with high inter- and intra-observer reproducibility among examiners and can be learnt and performed rapidly. The remnant of the *hymenal ring* is used as the reference point and the examination is performed during *straining*.

Structures above the hymenal ring are measured in negative centimetres. Structures which prolapse beyond the hymenal ring are measured in positive centimetres. Any structure that descends to the level of the hymenal ring is measured as zero centimetres.[4]

The POP-Q system comprises: Six sites: two each on the anterior and posterior vaginal walls and apex. Three measurements: two externally and the total vaginal length, which is the only point or measurement measured at rest. These are depicted diagrammatically in Fig. 43.11(a) and recorded in a 3-by-3 grid box as shown in Fig. 43.11(b).

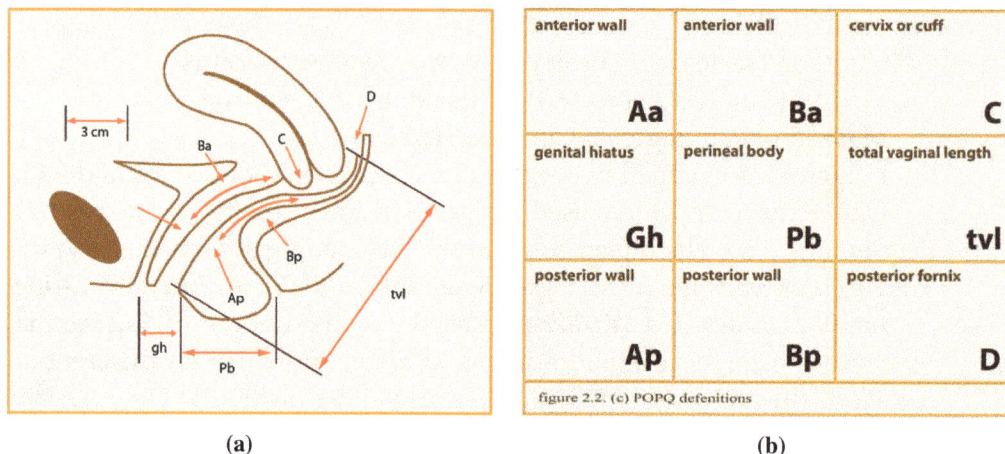

anterior wall	anterior wall	cervix or cuff
Aa	**Ba**	**C**
genital hiatus	perineal body	total vaginal length
Gh	**Pb**	**tvl**
posterior wall	posterior wall	posterior fornix
Ap	**Bp**	**D**

figure 2.2. (c) POPQ defenitions

(a)   (b)

FIGURE 43.11 ■ (a) 6 sites (points Aa, Ba, C, D, Bp and Ap), genital hiatus (gh), perineal body (pb), and total vaginal length (tvl) used for pelvic organ prolapse quantification (POP-Q) and 3 measurements used to quantify pelvic organ prolapse (POP-Q). (b) 3-by-3 grid for recording and quantitative description of pelvic organ support.

TABLE 43.1   Sites Measured in POP-Q

Point	Description
A anterior (Aa)	A point on the anterior vaginal wall 3 cm above the hymenal ring
B anterior (Ba)	Most dependent or distal point on the anterior vaginal wall between Aa and point C, or the cuff if subject is post hysterectomy
C	Anterior/posterior lip of the cervix, or the cuff if the subject is post hysterectomy
A posterior (Ap)	A point on the posterior vaginal wall 3 cm above the hymenal ring
B posterior (Bp)	Most dependent or distal point on the posterior vaginal wall between Ap and point D, or the cuff if the subject is post hysterectomy
D	Posterior fornix (this space is left blank if the subject is post hysterectomy)
Genital hiatus (gh)	Middle of external urethral meatus to posterior hymenal ring
Perineal (pb)	Posterior hymenal ring to middle of anal opening
Total vaginal length (tvl)	Hymenal ring to vaginal apex

TABLE 43.2   Staging of Pelvic Organ Prolapse

Stage	Description
0	No descensus of pelvic structures during straining
I	The leading surface of the prolapse does not descend below 1 cm above the hymenal ring
II	The leading edge of the prolapse extends from 1 cm above the hymen to 1 cm through the hymenal ring
III	The prolapse extends more than 1 cm beyond the hymenal ring, but there is not complete eversion
IV	The vagina is completely everted

In my opinion, and most educators', undergraduates are expected to know either the Porges or Beecham classification for POP. The POP-Q is an improved version of the Baden-Walker grading system and is widely accepted and used in publications on POP. Hence, if an undergraduate wishes to take up a Student Internship Program (SIP), intends to become a resident or widen his/her knowledge in Obstetrics and Gynaecology, he or she would find learning the POP-Q system beneficial.

Management of POP

The decision to treat POP very much depends on whether the patient with POP is symptomatic: troubled or bothered by her prolapse. Treatment for POP can either be conservative or surgical.

Conservative treatment for POP includes

- Pelvic floor muscle training or Kegel's exercises.
- Topical or vaginal oestrogen cream [conjugated oestrogen (Premarain)] 0.5 to 1 g and/or tablet [Oestradial 0.1 mg (Vagifem)] twice per week.
- Vaginal pessaries.

   There are a large variety of pessaries available for different types and combinations of POP which may or may not be associated with stress urinary incontinence. They are made of latex, silicone or PVC.

   (i) Ring pessary is used for 1st and 2nd degree POP (see Fig. 43.12).
   (ii) Gelhorn pessary is reserved for significant 2nd and 3rd degree POP.

Indications:

- Elderly and frail patient.
- Unfit for anaesthesia or surgery.
- Unwilling to have surgery.

Frequency of change of pessary: 3–4 monthly; can be washed and reused.
Complications: If too small, will fall out; if too big, will cause pain, ulceration, infection, discharge and bleeding.

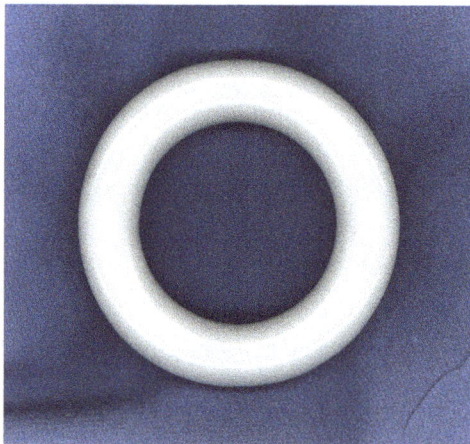

FIGURE 43.12 ■ Ring pessary.

Surgical treatment for POP

If conservative treatment for POP fails, surgical treatment can be offered. It includes the following operations for the different types of POP:

- Anterior vaginal wall repair or anterior colporrhaphy or vaginal cystocoele repair for anterior compartment prolapse or cystocoele.

- Posterior vaginal wall repair or posterior colporrhaphy/colpoperineorrhaphy or vaginal rectocoele repair/perineal repair for rectocoele.
- Vaginal enterocoele repair for enterocoele.
- Manchester repair for elongated cervix with minimal or no uterine prolapse.
- Vaginal hysterectomy, removal of the uterus performed vaginally for uterine prolapse. A McCall culdoplasty is usually done routinely to prevent vaginal vault prolapse. Anterior and/or posterior vaginal wall/enterocoele repair can be performed after vaginal hysterectomy if the patient has anterior and/or posterior compartment prolapse/enterocoele.
- Vaginal sacrospinous ligament fixation (Fig. 43.13) as a primary or secondary operation for procidentia or complete vaginal eversion or vaginal vault prolapse respectively.
- Abdominal/laparoscopic/robotic sacrocolpopexy (Fig. 43.14) (for similar indications as vaginal sacrospinous ligament fixation).

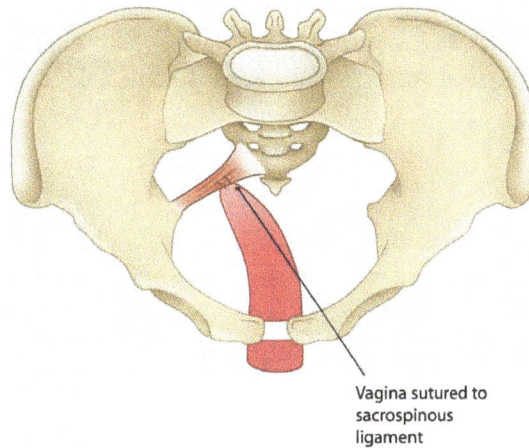

Vagina sutured to sacrospinous ligament

FIGURE 43.13 ■ Vaginal sacrospinous ligament fixation.

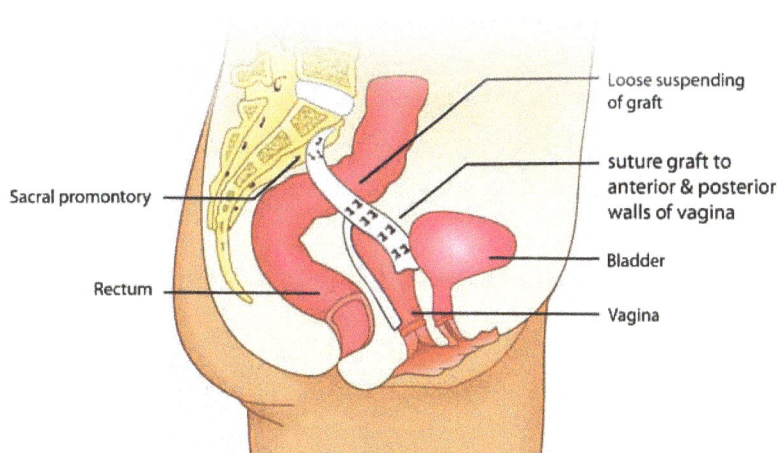

Loose suspending of graft

suture graft to anterior & posterior walls of vagina

Bladder

Vagina

Sacral promontory

Rectum

FIGURE 43.14 ■ Abdominal sacrocolpopexy.

- Colpocleisis or vaginal obliterative surgery as a primary or secondary operation in the elderly, frail and medically unfit patient who is no longer sexually active. Partial colpocleisis is performed for a patient with a uterus with significant 2nd or 3rd degree POP, and complete colpocleisis or colpectomy is for a patient with vaginal vault prolapse after a previous hysterectomy.
- Mesh augmented surgery for POP is usually reserved for failed/recurrent POP surgery or primary procidentia or complete vaginal eversion.
- Undergraduates do not need to know the steps of each of the above operations, only general principles will suffice. All operations have a known success rate and complications from the literature. The complications include anaesthetic, intraoperative (injury to the bladder, ureters, rectum, vessels, bleeding and nerves) and postoperative (bleeding, haematoma, infection, venous thrombopulmonary embolism, cardiovascular accidents and failure or recurrence of POP).

Stress Urinary Incontinence

Definition

(according to the International Continence Society, 2002):

Urinary incontinence: is the complaint of any involuntary leakage of urine.

Stress urinary incontinence: is the complaint of involuntary leakage on effort or exertion, or on sneezing or coughing.

Aetiology

- Congenital: weakness of muscles, ligaments and fascia; collagen deficiency
- Pregnancy, vaginal delivery
- Ageing
- Menopause
- Pelvic organ prolapse
- Conditions which predispose to raised intra-abdominal pressure: obesity, chronic cough, constipation, occupations requiring heavy lifting

How to Evaluate a Woman with Stress Urinary Incontinence?

- *Symptoms*:

History of involuntary leakage of urine while coughing, sneezing, running, exercising or lifting.

- *Sign*:

Stress urinary incontinence can be demonstrated with a reasonably full bladder (last voided about two hours previously) during coughing, when standing with both feet apart or in the dorsal supine positon, with both hips and knees flexed and apart.

- *Basic investigations*:
    (i) Urinalysis (dipstix, microscopy or culture and sensitivity) for urinary tract infection.
   (ii) Post-void residual urine measurement using ultrasound scan to exclude overdistension/overflow incontinence.
  (iii) Modified pad test: To qualify and quantify stress urinary incontinence by asking a patient to cough 10 times onto a pre-weighed incontinence sheet/ sanitary towel, while standing with both feet apart. Her bladder should be reasonably full (at least 250 mL), this can be ascertained using a portable bladder scan or transabdominal ultrasound scan. The difference in weight in grams is the amount or volume leaked as the specific gravity of urine is 1, i.e. $1 \text{ g} = 1 \text{ mL}$.

- *Urodynamic investigation* (filling and voiding cystometry): To diagnose urodynamic stress incontinence (Fig. 43.15) and exclude detrusor overactivity.

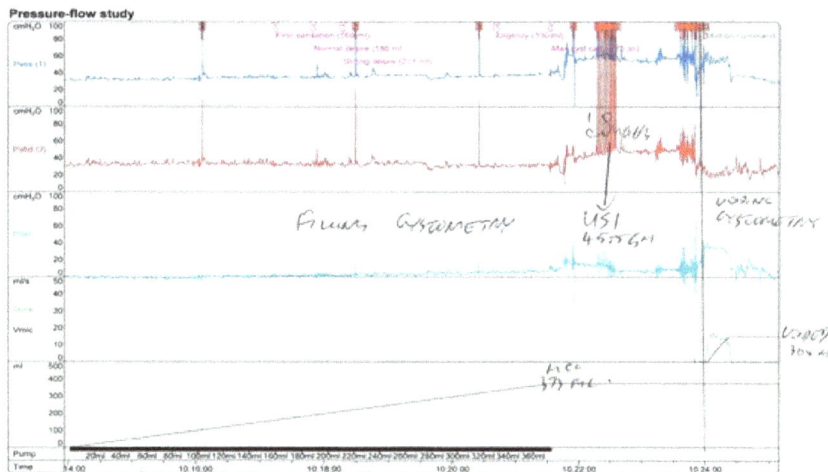

FIGURE 43.15 ■ Urodynamic trace (Filling and voiding cystometry) demonstrating urodynamic stress incontinence (USI): Defined as the involuntary leakage of urine during raised intravesical pressure secondary to increased abdominal pressure, in the absence of a detrusor contraction.

Pves: Vesical pressure, measured by catheter in the bladder
Pabd: Abdominal pressure, measured by catheter in the rectum, inserted through the anus

Pdet: Detrusor pressure: Pves – Pabd

MCC 375 mL: Maximum cystometric capacity of 375 mL, when the patient could not hold anymore. i.e. she needed to void.

USI 45.5 g: Urodynamic stress incontinence of 45.5 grams = 45.5 ml (SG of N.saline = 1) was elicited with the patient coughing 10 times, moderately hard, in the erect posture with her feet apart, at a MCC of 375 mL.

Treatment of Stress Urinary Incontinence

Conservative

The mainstay of conservative treatment is pelvic floor (Kegel's) exercises. Women with stress urinary incontinence should be taught to contract and strengthen their pelvic floor muscles. This is graded according to the Oxford subjective score: from 1 = flicker, 2 = poor, 3 = moderate, 4 = strong, 5 = strong and sustained. Pelvic floor exercises should be tried for at least 3–6 months, which results in at least a 50% cure or improvement rate in women with moderate to severe stress urinary incontinence.

Surgery

• *Burch colposuspension*

2–3 long-term absorbable or permanent sutures are inserted between the perivaginal fascia and the Cooper's ligament, medial part of the inguinal ligament, on each side to support the urethrovesical junction (bladder neck)[5] (Fig. 43.16).

Results: Cure or improvement rate — 80–90%.

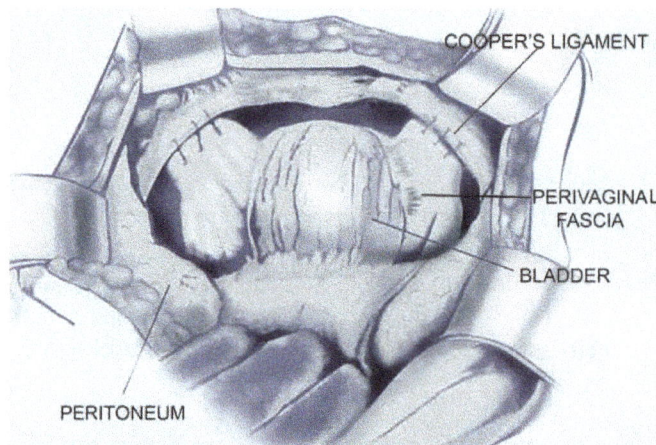

FIGURE 43.16[5] ■ Burch colposuspension.

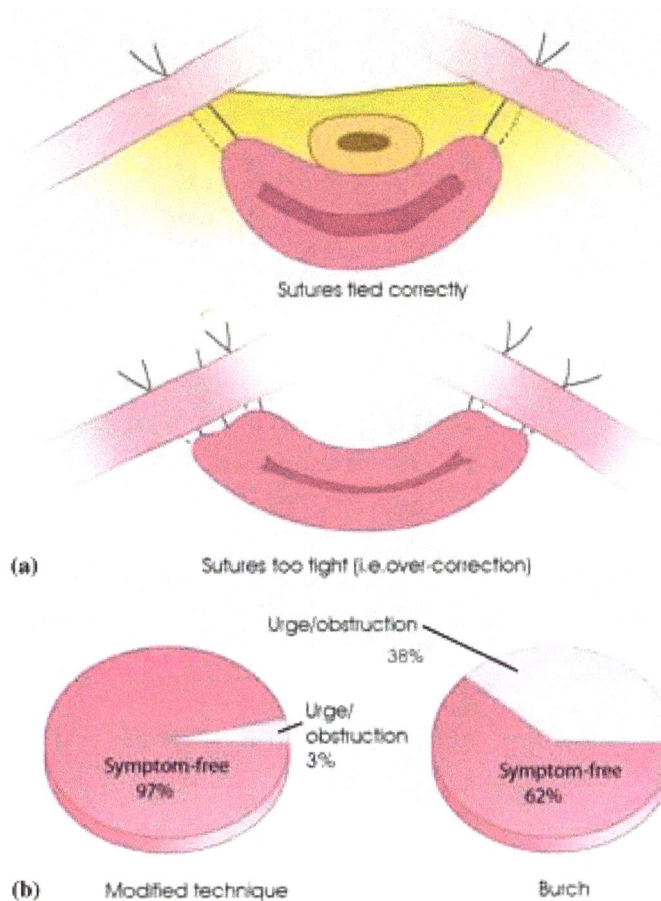

Sutures tied correctly

Sutures too tight (i.e. over-correction)

(a)

Urge/obstruction
38%

Urge/
obstruction
3%

Symptom-free
97%

Symptom-free
62%

(b)   Modified technique   Burch

FIGURE 43.17[6] ■ Possible urinary complication resulting from Burch colposuspension.

Complications: Voiding difficulty and overactive bladder secondary to tying the sutures too tightly without "bow-stringing," as clearly demonstrated in Fig. 43.17(a).

- *Mid-urethral tape* (*MUT*)
(i) Retropubic (Fig. 43.18) (ii) Trans-obturator (Fig. 43.19) A MUT procedure involves inserting a thin 11 mm width strip of Type I (monofilament, macroporous) synthetic polypropylene (prolene) tape beneath the mid-urethra from the vagina and exiting at the
(i) Superior border of the symphysis — Retropubic tape (TVT®) or
(ii) The infero-medial part of the obturator foramen through the upper inner thigh — Transobturator tape (TOT®, TVT-O®).

Results: Cure or improvement rate — 80–90%.

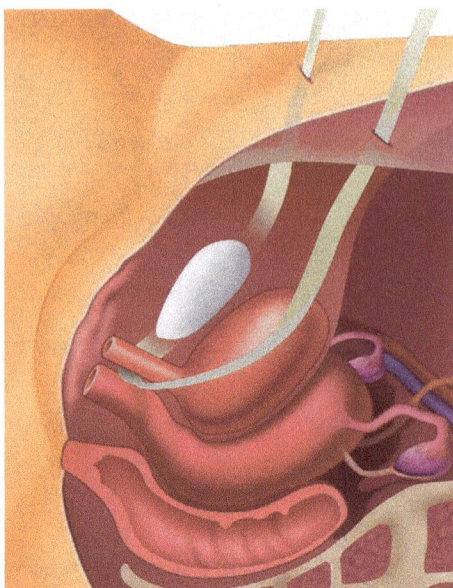

FIGURE 43.18 ■ Mid-urethral tape (Retropubic).

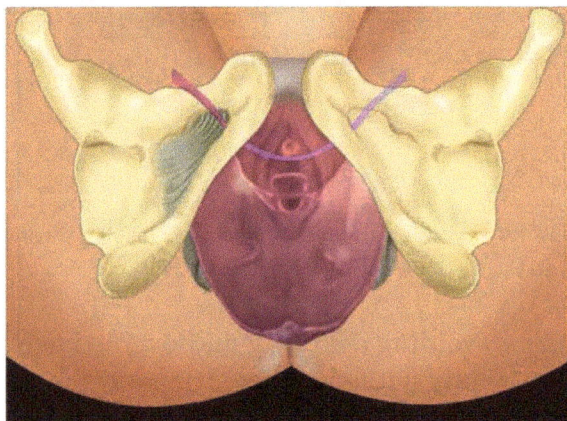

FIGURE 43.19 ■ Mid-urethral tape — Transobturator.

Complications:

(i) Mid-urethral tape: Bladder perforation, urethral, bowel and vascular injury.

(ii) Transobturator tape: Vaginal, bladder, urethral, vascular and nerve injury (Obturator). Both can cause voiding difficulty and OAB.

Overactive Bladder (OAB)

Overactive bladder is a clinical diagnosis characterised by urgency with or without urge incontinence (OAB wet or dry respectively), usually associated with frequency and nocturia, in the absence of pathologic or metabolic conditions that might explain these symptoms (International Continence Society Terminology, 2002).

Definitions

Urgency: the complaint of a sudden compelling desire to pass urine which is difficult to defer.

Urge urinary incontinence: the complaint of involuntary leakage accompanied by or immediately preceded by urgency.

Frequency: eight or more visits to the toilet in 24 hours. *Nocturia:* two or more visits to the toilet during sleeping hours.

Mixed urinary incontinence: is the complaint of involuntary leakage associated with urgency and also with exertion, effort, sneezing or coughing.

Investigations

INTAKE-FREQUENCY VOLUME CHART
(INTAKE-URINARY DIARY)

Instructions

Ideally this chart should be sent to the patient before the first consultation.

1. Please record whatever you drink and whenever you pass urine as shown in the chart below.

2. Measure your urine passed in ml using a measuring jug. If it is not possible to do so, just tick (√).

3. If you feel urgent (desperate) before you have to pass urine add (U) after the (√) or after the amount of urine passed, eg. 200 ml (U)

4. If you have any incontinent episodes write (W) under the appropriate headings: Urgency, Physical Activity (coughing, sneezing, laughing, running, walking, jumping, lifting), Neither (urgency nor physical activity), During sex (penetration or orgasm or both or Others (hand washing, in shower, in swimming pool).

5. Keep this chart for at least 2 to 3 days, to include one weekday and one weekend either before or immediately after your first consultation.

6. If you are given any treatment (eg. Physiotherapy or drugs) your doctor will advise you to repeat this chart just before your next follow-up appointment.

Date: _____   Name: _____

| Time | Fluid Intake | Urine Passed (in ml or √) if urgent (U) | Incontinent Episode (W) | | | | |
			Urgency	Physical Activity	Neither	Sex	Others
6.30 am		350 (U)	W				
7.00 am	1 cup coffee 1 cup water						
7.30 am	"	150					
8.30 am	"						
10.00 am	1 cup coffee						
11.00 am		√ (U)	W				
12.00 pm	1 can Coke						
2.00 pm		√					
3.00 pm	1 glass water						
4.30 pm		√					
6.00 pm				W			
6.30 pm		200 (U)					
7.00 pm	1 bowl soup 1glass water						
10.00 pm		300 (U)					
3.00 am							

FIGURE 43.20 ■ Intake-Frequency volume chart (Intake-urinary diary).

Apart from those performed for stress urinary incontinence:

- *Intake-frequency volume incontinence chart or intake urinary/bladder diary* is a very useful aid to diagnose OAB, stress urinary incontinence and mixed incontinence (See Fig. 43.20).

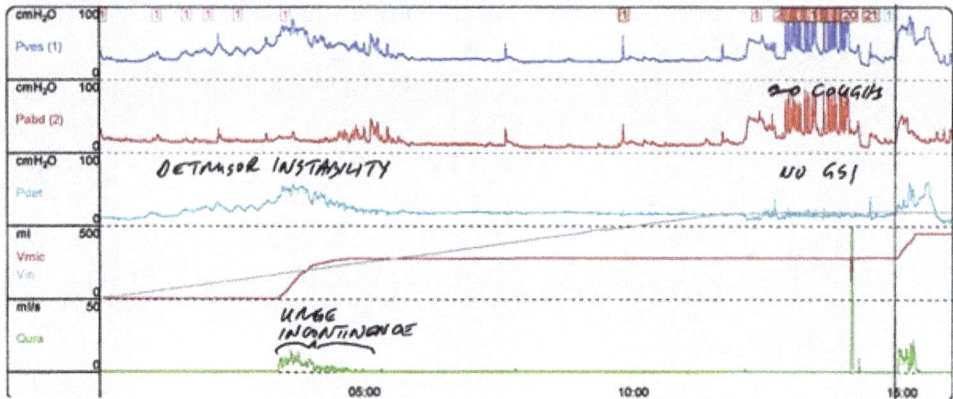

FIGURE 43.21 ■ Urodynamic trace [filling and voiding cystometry] demonstrating detrusor overactivity [previously known as detrusor instability] with urge urinary incontinence without urodynamic stress incontinence (previously known as genuine stress incontinence [GSI]). Detrusor overactivity is defined as: Involuntary contraction/s during the filling phase at any time prior to "permission to void" being given; the contractions may be of any size and may be associated with urinary incontinence.

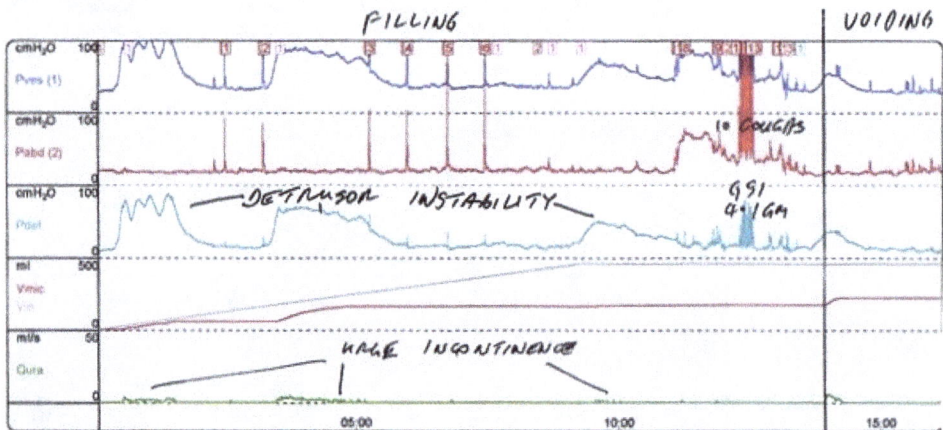

FIGURE 43.22 ■ Urodynamic trace [filling and voiding cystometry] demonstrating mixed detrusor overactivity [previously known as detrusor instability] associated with urge urinary incontinence and urodynamic stress incontinence [previously known as genuine stress incontinence (GSI)].

- **Urodynamics:** To diagnose detrusor overactivity (DO), previously known as detrusor instability (DI) (Fig. 43.21) and mixed DO with urodynamic stress incontinence (USI), previously known as genuine stress incontinence (GSI) (Fig. 43.22).

Management of OAB

Fluid management

- Advised to drink 1.5–2.0 litres or 7–8 cups or glasses of fluids per day; restricting coffee, tea to 1–2 cups or glasses and alcohol to 1–2 units.
- To stop drinking 2–3 hours before bedtime.

Pelvic floor exercises and bladder training

Patients should be taught pelvic floor exercises, so that they are able to perform bladder training until they can hold for about two hours before voiding.

Pharmacotherapy

The mainstay is antimuscarinic or anticholinergic drugs, which compete with acetylcholine at the muscarinic receptors at the neuromuscular junction. Hence their side-effects of visual disturbances, dry mouth, headaches, palpitations, gastrointestinal reflux, constipation and voiding difficulty.

References

1. Brubaker LT, Saclarides TJ. (eds.), (1996) *The Female Pelvic Floor: Disorders of Function and Support*. F.A. David Co., Philadephia, p. 20.
2. Benson JT, Wal``ters MD. (1999) Neurophysiology of the Lower Urinary Tract. In: Walters MD, Karram MM. (eds.), *Urogynecology and Reconstructive Pelvic Surgery*, 2nd edn. St Louis, pp. 15–24.
3. Swift S, Theofrastous J. (2001) Aetiology and classification of pelvic organ prolapse. In: Linda Cardozo L, Staskin D. (eds.), *Textbook of Female Urology and Urogynaecology*, 1st edn, London Isis Medical Media Ltd, pp. 580–585.
4. Bump RC, *et al.* (1996) The standardisation of terminology of female pelvic organ prolapse and pelvic floor dysfunction. *Am J Obstet Gynecol* **175**:10–17.
5. Burch JC. (1961) Urethrovesical fixation to Cooper's ligament for correction of stress urinary incontinence, cystocele and prolapse. *Am J Obstet Gynecol* **81**:281–290.

6. Petri E. (2001) Retropubic cystourethropexies. In: Cardozo L, Staskin D. (eds.), *Textbook of Female Urology and Urogynaecology*, 1st edn. London Isis Medical Media Ltd **41**:514–524.

44

CARCINOMA OF THE CERVIX

Pearl Tong and Joseph Ng

Introduction

The cervix lies at the opposite end of the vaginal canal from the vulva and vaginal opening or introitus. It is commonly referred to as the neck or mouth of the womb. It is the distal-most anatomical structure visible on a speculum examination of the vagina and the part of the anatomy that is brushed for cytological samples in Pap smear screening.

The cervix is covered by two distinct types of surface epithelium: squamous and columnar. The visible junction between these two epithelial types is therefore referred to as the **squamocolumnar junction** or **SCJ**. The SCJ is a dynamic margin, meaning that this border is constantly shifting over the course of a woman's lifetime depending on the relative proportions of squamous and columnar epithelium on the surface of the cervix at any one given time. Since there is a dynamic shift, there must be an original SCJ and a new SCJ. The area between the OSCJ and the NSCJ is referred to as the **transformation zone**.

The transformation zone is clinically important because most cervical dysplasias originate from and can therefore be found in this zone.

The transformation zone can therefore be thought of as the "soil" in which oncogenic "seeds" such as HPV (human papillomavirus) are planted and coaxed to grow into the terrible bloom of cancer by the "water and sunlight" of co-factors such as cigarette smoking, young age at first intercourse, multiple sexual partners and a history of sexually transmitted infections (STIs).[1]

Cervical cancer is the 10th most common cancer in Singaporean women. Its incidence has been steadily declining in Singapore over the past decades.[2]

History

The most common presenting complaint in cervical cancer is **persistent postcoital bleeding**. In postmenopausal women, cervical cancer can also present as postmenopausal bleeding. It is important to determine the onset of the postcoital bleeding, whether it occurs after every episode of penetrative intercourse and the amount of blood lost with each episode of postcoital bleeding.

A relevant history for a patient with cervical cancer will focus on the following risk factors:

- Early age at first intercourse
- Cigarette smoking
- Multiple sexual partners
- History of sexually transmitted infections
- Absence of regular Pap smear screening

Physical Examination

The physical examination of a patient presenting with postcoital bleeding should cover the following areas:

- Supraclavicular nodes. Palpation of the hollow in the neck just above the clavicles should be carried out to determine if any of these lymph nodes are suspiciously enlarged
- Abdominal examination. Although less likely to return with a positive finding, the abdomen should be examined for the presence of ascites and masses outside of the pelvis
- Pelvic examination. Special attention should be paid to the following areas:
  - Vulva and external genitalia. The examination should focus on possible sources of bleeding such as atrophy, trauma or malignant lesions
  - Vagina and cervix. The vagina and cervix should also be examined for possible sources of bleeding such as atrophy or trauma. Keep in mind that vaginal atrophy is the most common cause of postmenopausal bleeding. Contact bleeding and petechiae on the cervix and vagina on gentle insertion of the speculum are signs of significant atrophy
  - Vaginal vault. The vaginal vault and the cervical os should be examined for evidence of active bleeding or old blood. Blood noted at the external os suggests an endocervical or endometrial source
  - Cervix. The cervix should be examined for any irregular growths or suspicious lesions, especially those that bleed on gentle contact. The character of the cervix on palpation should also be noted to determine if it is harder than expected or the surface counter feels irregular or craggy

- Uterus and adnexae. The shape, size, and mobility of the uterus should be ascertained by bimanual examination. The presence of adnexal masses should also be determined at the same time
- Rectal examination. This facilitates examination of the Pouch of Douglas and rectovaginal septum for possible masses. It also allows a more complete assessment of the dimensions of a cervical mass and the involvement of the parametrium. The rectal mucosa should also be assessed for possible lesions or sources of rectal bleeding that could be mistaken for vaginal bleeding. It is also important to assess if a cervical mass has invaded into the rectum

Investigation

The next step in the evaluation of a patient with postcoital bleeding and cervical mass is a histological diagnosis. This is achieved by taking a biopsy of the cervical mass. This can be performed with punch biopsy forceps without anaesthesia in the outpatient setting. Sometimes, a cone biopsy of the cervix may be required to accurately evaluate the degree of invasion.

The next step after a histological diagnosis of cancer is made is to stage the cancer, as this would affect the management and prognosis. Cancer staging follows set rules laid out by FIGO, the International Federation of Obstetricians and Gynaecologists. FIGO staging of cervical cancer is arrived at by utilising the following:

- Examination under anaesthesia. This allows a more complete appreciation of the extent and size of the cervical mass and the involvement of the surrounding tissue
- Cystoscopy and Proctoscopy. These procedures are carried out as indicated based on clinical suspicion of bladder and rectal involvement respectively
- Chest X-ray. To determine the presence of gross lung metastases
- Intravenous pyelogram or urogram. To determine the presence of hydrone-phrosis or hydroureter. The presence of either of these findings suggests that the cervical cancer has reached the pelvic side wall and involved the ureter

You will notice that these modalities are relatively basic. This is because the burden of disease is heaviest in countries or clinical settings that do not have access to more sophisticated imaging and diagnostic equipment. Put simply, cervical cancer is most common in the third world.

However, in more developed settings, we utilise imaging modalities such as Computed Tomography (CT) scans of the thorax, abdomen, or even combined Positron Emission Tomography (PET)-CT and Magnetic Resonance Imaging (MRI) to aid in treatment planning. In general terms, CT scans are useful in detection of distant metastases whereas MRI offers superior imaging of soft tissue and is able to help delineate the extent of tumour spread, especially in areas where clinical examination is limited, for example the endocervical canal.

Basic blood investigations such as full blood count, renal and liver function tests should also be part of the workup. Not uncommonly, anaemia may be detected and this is due to the presence of prolonged bleeding per vaginum, or a deranged renal function test from advanced cases where bilateral ureteric blockages result in hydronephrosis, compromising kidney function. It will be vital to know these results, as anaemia should ideally be corrected prior to radiotherapy to ensure optimal response, and dosages of medications may need to be adjusted according to renal function.[3,4]

Staging

TABLE 44.1   The 2018 FIGO Staging of Carcinoma of Cervix

Stage 1 Tumour limited to the cervix

    IA   Diagnosis by microscopy

        IA1   Measured stromal invasion <3 mm

        IA2   Measured stromal invasion >3 mm and <5 mm

    IB   Macroscopic tumour or microscopic tumour with dimensions bigger than that of 1A

        IB1   Invasive carcinoma ≥5 mm depth of invasion, and <2 cm in greatest dimension

        IB2   Invasive carcinoma ≥2 cm and <4 cm in greatest dimension

        IB3   Invasive carcinoma ≥4 cm in greatest dimension

Stage 2 Tumour spread beyond body of uterus but not to pelvic wall or lower third of vagina

    IIA   Upper 2/3 of vagina, no parametrial involvement

        IIA1   Invasive carcinoma <4 cm in greatest dimension

        IIA2   Invasive carcinoma ≥4 cm in greatest dimension

    IIB   Tumour with parametrial involvement but not up to pelvic sidewall

Stage 3 Tumour extending to the pelvic wall and/or lower third of vagina and/or causing hydronephrosis/non-functioning kidney

    IIIA   Tumour involving lower third of vagina, no extension to side wall

    IIIB   Tumour extending to pelvic wall and/or causing hydronephrosis/non-functioning kidney

    IIIC   Nodal involvement (additional notations for *p* pathologically confirmed, *r* radiologically only, no pathology)

        IIIC1   Pelvic nodal metastasis only

        IIIC2   Para-aortic nodal metastasis

Stage 4 IVA   Tumour invades mucosa of bladder or rectum and/or beyond true pelvis

    IVB   Distant metastasis (including peritoneal spread, involvement of supraclavicular, mediastinal, para-aortic lymph nodes, liver, lung or bone)

Management of Cervical Cancer

Cervical cancer is largely managed according to stage.

Cervical cancer treatment is guided by the principle that patients should receive the ONE treatment with the best chance of cure. This principle translates into a treatment philosophy that all cervical cancer can be effectively treated with radiation and that, in select patients with early disease where clear surgical margins can be obtained, surgery can result in cure whilst sparing the patient the morbidity associated with radiation.[5]

TABLE 44.2 Management of Carcinoma of Cervix According to Stage

	Fertility Sparing	Non Fertility Sparing	Medically Inoperable Cases/ Non-Surgical Alternative
Stage IA1	Cone biopsy with clear margins	Simple hysterectomy	Observation after cone biopsy with clear margins
Stage IA2, IB2	Vaginal/Abdominal trachelectomy with pelvic lymph node dissection, with the following criteria fulfilled: 1. Tumours 2 cm or less 2. Squamous or adenocarcinoma cell types 3. No evidence of lymph node involvement/ distant metastases	Modified radical hysterectomy with pelvic lymph node dissection +/- para aortic lymph node dissection	Radiation therapy
Stage IB3, IIA	Not recommended	Modified radical hysterectomy with pelvic lymph node dissection +/- para aortic lymph node dissection	Concurrent chemoradiation
Stage IIB to IVA		Concurrent chemoradiation	
Stage IVB		Chemotherapy with individualised decision for radiation therapy	

Table 44.2 outlines the general principles of management according to stage. Each case should ideally be discussed at a multidisciplinary tumour board meeting for a consensus opinion.

Surgery

- A cone biopsy simply refers to excision of the cervix, which can be done by various means; with a cold knife, utilising a loop electrode (also known as LEEP, loop electrosurgical excision procedure), laser or needle with diathermy. **The most important principle is that clear margins should be achieved**
- Trachelectomy involves excision of the cervix and parametrium only, thus preserving the uterus, and is a fertility-sparing procedure. It is usually accompanied by a cervical cerclage which will necessitate future deliveries by Caesarean section. This is not without obstetric risks, such as increased risk of pregnancy losses in the first and second trimesters, and preterm deliveries
- A simple hysterectomy is also known as an extrafascial hysterectomy, where the uterosacral ligaments, uterine vessels and cardinal ligaments are divided just adjacent to the uterus
- A modified radical hysterectomy is one where much wider surgical margins are obtained. Part of the uterosacral ligaments, cardinal ligaments, and the part of the upper vagina are removed to provide a "margin" of normal tissue around the primary cervical tumour. Removal of normal ovaries is not essential; in fact ovarian transposition can be considered in younger patients who are undergoing pelvic radiation, in an attempt to prevent premature ovarian failure. Pelvic and para-aortic lymph node dissection involves the stripping of fatty nodal tissue surrounding the major blood vessels at the risk of vessel injury and haemorrhage. In addition, removal of lymph nodes can also impair lymphatic flow from the limbs and result in lymphoedema of extremities, with increased risk of cellulitis. Lymphatic fluid collection around the blood vessels can also cause symptoms like pain and get secondarily infected, requiring drainage. Hence lymph node dissection is a procedure not without its morbidities, and strategies such as sentinel lymph node biopsies are being employed nowadays to select only patients who require these procedures

Simple and radical hysterectomies can be carried out via open laparotomy, with laparoscopy or robotically.

Chemoradiation

In patients for whom surgery may be hazardous or whose tumours are unlikely to be resected with clear surgical margins, radiation therapy may be employed as definitive therapy. Radiation therapy employs two modalities: external beam radiation, where the radiation source is away from the area to be treated, and brachytherapy, where the radiation source is placed inside or next to the area requiring treatment. The addition of chemotherapy, which acts as a radio-sensitizer, improves the tumour's overall treatment response. The use of small amounts of chemotherapy and radiation together, or concurrently, is known as chemoradiation and is the current standard of care in the treatment of advanced cervical cancer.

Prognosis by Stage in Cervical Cancer

TABLE 44.3 Prognosis of Carcinoma of Cervix According to Stage of Disease

FIGO Stage	5 Year Survival (%)
I	90
II	60
III	40
IV	20

References

1. Rubin E, Farber JL. (1994) *Pathology*, 2nd edn.
2. National Registry of Diseases Office (2014). *Annual Registry Report. Trends in Cancer Incidence in Singapore 2009–2013*. Singapore Cancer Registry, Health Promotion Board, Singapore. https://www.nrdo.gov.sg/docs/librariesprovider3/default-document-library/cancer-trends-2010-2014_interim-annual-report_final-(public).pdf?sfvrsm=0
3. Philip J, Saia D, Creasman Wt. (2012) *Clinical Gynecologic Oncology*, 8th edn. Elsevier.
4. Berek JS, Hacker NF. (2014) *Berek & Hacker's Gynecologic Oncology*, 6th edn.
5. Morrow PC. (2013) *Morrow's Gynecologic Cancer Surgery*, 2nd edn.

45

CARCINOMA OF THE ENDOMETRIUM

Joseph Ng

Introduction

The endometrium is the lining of the uterine cavity. This is the same tissue layer that is shed during the menstrual period. It consists of two distinct tissue layers, the functional and the basal layers. A new functional layer grows from the basal layer over the course of each menstrual cycle. It is the functional layer that is shed.

Endometrial cancer therefore affects the lining of the uterine cavity. Common histological cell types in endometrial cancer are:

- Endometrioid
- Uterine papillary serous (UPSC)
- Clear Cell
- Mixed
- Mucinous
- Squamous
- Undifferentiated

Endometrial cancer is the most common gynaecological cancer in Singapore. It is also the fourth most common cancer among Singaporean women overall and follows Breast, Colon, and Lung respectively in incidence. Its incidence is increasing in Singaporean women.[1]

There are 2 types of endometrial cancer, and their characteristics are outlined in Table 45.1 below:

TABLE 45.1   Types of Endometrial Cancer and their Characteristics

	Type 1	Type 2
Age of Onset	50–60	70+
Prognosis	Good	Poor
Histology	Endometrioid, Grade 1	Endometrioid, Grade 3 Clear Cell Uterine Papillary Serous
Percentage of Endometrial Cancers	80%	20%
Endometrial Hyperplasia	Present	Absent
History of unopposed oestrogen exposure	Present	Absent

In most endometrial cancers the most common risk factor is a history of unopposed oestrogen exposure. This risk factor may be manifest in the following historical scenarios:

• Chronic anovulation. For example in conditions such as polycystic ovarian syndrome (PCOS).
• Oestrogen-only hormone replacement therapy.
• Oestrogen-secreting tumours.
• Metabolic syndromes resulting in obesity.
• Early menarche, late menopause.
• Nulligravidity.
• Not breastfeeding. Breastfeeding lowers a woman's lifetime risk of breast cancer.

Being on the combined oral contraceptive pill has been shown to lower a woman's lifetime risk of endometrial cancer.

History

The most common presenting symptom in endometrial cancer is abnormal vaginal bleeding. In premenopausal women in their 40's, the most common presenting complaint is persistent intermenstrual bleeding. In postmenopausal women, it is bleeding after menopause. Menopause is defined as 12 continuous months of amenorrhoea. All postmenopausal bleeding is cancer until proven otherwise.

TABLE 45.2   **Effective Screening Questions in Endometrial Cancer**

Effective Screening Questions in Endometrial Cancer	
Premenopausal	"Are you experiencing any bleeding in between normal periods?"
Postmenopausal	"Have you experienced any vaginal bleeding since you stopped having normal periods?"

The most common clinical presentation in endometrial cancer is postmenopausal bleeding. However, the most common cause of postmenopausal bleeding is not endometrial cancer, it is vaginal and lower genital tract atrophy.

The evaluation of a patient presenting with postmenopausal bleeding begins with a history that focuses on the above mentioned risk factors, that is risk factors that increase a woman's lifetime risk of unopposed oestrogen exposure.

Physical Examination

The physical examination of a patient presenting with postmenopausal bleeding should cover the following areas:

- Supraclavicular nodes. Palpation of the hollow in the neck just above the clavicles should be carried out to determine if any of these lymph nodes are suspiciously enlarged
- Breast examination. The breasts should always be examined for an incidental finding of concurrent breast cancers. It is interesting to note that both breast and endometrial cancers share quite a few common risk factors
- Abdominal examination. Although less likely to return with a positive finding, the abdomen should be examined for the presence of ascites and masses outside of the pelvis
- Pelvic examination. Special attention should be paid to the following areas:
  - Vulva and external genitalia. The examination should focus on possible sources of bleeding such as atrophy, trauma or malignant lesions
  - Vagina and cervix. The vagina and cervix should also be examined for possible sources of bleeding such as atrophy, trauma or malignant lesions. Keep in mind that vaginal atrophy is the most common cause of postmenopausal bleeding. Contact bleeding and petechiae on the cervix and vagina on gentle insertion of the speculum are signs of significant atrophy
  - Vaginal vault. The vaginal vault and the cervical os should be examined for evidence of active bleeding or old blood. Blood noted at the external os suggests an endocervical or endometrial source

- Uterus and adnexae. The shape, size, and mobility of the uterus should be ascertained by bimanual examination. The presence of adnexal masses should also be determined at the same time
- Rectal examination. This facilitates examination of the Pouch of Douglas and rectovaginal septum for possible masses. The rectal mucosa should also be assessed for possible lesions or sources of rectal bleeding that could be mistaken for vaginal bleeding

Investigations

Endometrial evaluation in Postmenopausal Bleeding

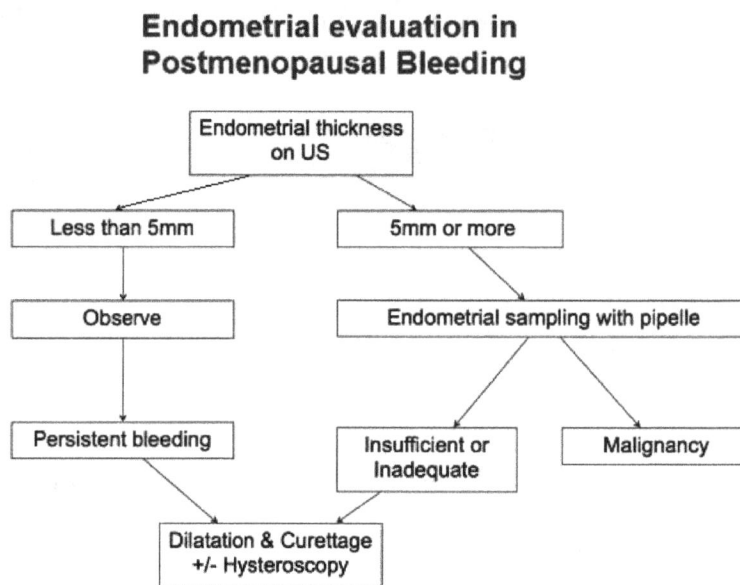

FIGURE 45.1 ■ The workflow for the investigation of postmenopausal bleeding.

Some other common investigations that you may see being performed are a CT scan of the thorax and abdomen along with an MRI of the uterus and cervix.

The CT scan of the thorax and abdomen is performed to evaluate these anatomical compartments for evidence of metastatic endometrial cancer in the soft tissue organs of the abdomen such as the liver, spleen and kidneys, and the lymph nodes of the abdomen and thorax.

The MRI of the uterus and cervix evaluates the size of the primary endometrial tumour, as well as the degree to which the tumour invades into the myometrium, and the presence of any obvious pelvic lymph node involvement.

Management of Endometrial Cancer

The foundation of the management of endometrial cancer is surgery: Surgery to remove the uterus, Fallopian tubes and ovaries, which is correctly termed a total hysterectomy and bilateral salpingo-oophorectomy (THBSO).

Endometrial cancer is staged surgico-pathologically. This means that the staging process involves surgery to remove the primary tumour and the tissues that it commonly spreads to, then histological evaluation of these tissues for the presence of tumour involvement to arrive at a disease stage. The FIGO staging system is most commonly used to stage endometrial cancer.

TABLE 45.3 2009 FIGO Staging for Endometrial Cancer

Note:
— Carcinosarcomas should be staged as carcinomas of the endometrium.
— Simultaneous tumours of the uterine corpus and ovary/pelvis in association with ovarian/pelvic endometriosis should be classified as independent primary tumours.

STAGE I Tumour confined to the corpus uteri
IA No, or less than half, myometrial invasion
IB* Invasion equal to or more than half of the myometrium

STAGE II* Tumour invades cervical stroma, but does not extend beyond the uterus**

STAGE III* Local and/or regional spread of the tumour
IIIA* Tumour invades the serosa of the corpus uteri and/or adnexae#
IIIB* Vaginal and/or parametrial involvement#
IIIC* Metastases to pelvic and/or para-aortic lymph nodes#
IIIC1* Positive pelvic nodes
IIIC2* Positive para-aortic lymph nodes with or without positive pelvic lymph nodes

STAGE IV* Tumour invades bladder and/or bowel mucosa, and/or distant metastases
IVA* Tumour invasion of bladder and/or bowel mucosa
IVB* Distant metastases, including intra-abdominal metastases and/or inguinal lymph nodes

*Either G1, G2, or G3.
**Endocervical glandular involvement only should be considered as Stage I and no longer as Stage II.
#Positive cytology has to be reported separately without changing the stage.

The risk of extrauterine spread is significantly increased in endometrial cancer with the following factors:

• Endometrial tumour larger than 2 cm
• Presence of High-risk histological factors:
  • Poorly-differentiated endometrioid adenocarcinoma (G3 endometrioid)
  • Clear Cell carcinoma

- Papillary Serous carcinoma
- More than 50% myometrial invasion by the endometrial tumour

In cases where there is a significant risk of extrauterine spread, the lymph nodes of the pelvis and along the para-aortic chain are removed by systematic lymphadenectomy. This allows accurate staging of the cancer by providing a more complete assessment of whether the cancer has spread outside of the primary organ (endometrium) and if so, to what extent. In the absence of risk factors, patients can forego the morbidity associated with lymphadenectomy due the low likelihood of extrauterine spread. Randomised trials have shown that the procedure of lymphadenectomy itself does not confer survival benefit.[2]

Eighty percent of endometrial cancer is detected in FIGO Stage I. This is because early cancerous changes, and even pre-cancerous changes such as endometrial hyperplasia, are usually associated with abnormal vaginal bleeding that prompts the patient to seek medical attention and evaluation.

Almost all women with endometrial cancer are physiologically unaffected by the disease. This means that other than abnormal vaginal bleeding, women with endometrial cancer are functionally well. This should be taken into consideration when considering the mode of surgery, as surgical options that result in a significant loss of function can reasonably be perceived by the patient to be "worse than the disease." The optimal treatment option for endometrial cancer is therefore one that treats the disease completely whilst not significantly affecting the relatively normal level of functioning that these women possess. Since 2008 at Singapore's National University Hospital, the standard treatment for endometrial cancer has been robot-assisted surgery, which allows women to have complete treatment of the disease without the effect of open surgery on their function and well-being.[3–5]

Endometrial cancer, if detected early and managed appropriately, should not involve debilitating treatments or result in morbidity and loss of function.

Adjuvant Treatment

Endometrial cancer that has spread outside of the uterus is usually treated with pelvic radiation therapy. If there is evidence of disease spread beyond the treatment boundaries of radiation therapy, then chemotherapy might have to be considered. These treatments take place in addition to surgery, or after surgery and surgical staging, and so are called adjuvant treatments.

Other Treatment Options

Women with endometrial cancer who are unfit for surgery may be given the option of hormonal therapy. This is usually in the form of oral megesterol acetate (Megace).

Prognosis by Stage in Endometrial Cancer

TABLE 45.4 5-Year Survival Rates in Endometrial Cancer by FIGO Stage

I	80%
II	70%
III	50%
IV	20%

References

1. National Registry of Diseases Office. (2014) *Annual Registry Report. Trends in Cancer Incidence in Singapore 2009–2013*. Singapore Cancer Registry, Health Promotion Board, Singapore.
2. ASTEC study group, Kitchener H, Swart AM, *et al.* (2009) Efficacy of systematic pelvic lymphadenectomy in endometrial cancer (MRC ASTEC trial): a randomised study. *Lancet* **373**(9658):125–136. doi:10.1016/S0140-6736(08)61766-3.
3. Mok ZW, Yong EL, Low JJ, Ng JS. (2012) Clinical outcomes in endometrial cancer care when the standard of care shifts from open surgery to robotics. *Int J Gynecol Cancer* **22**(5):819–825. doi: 10.1097/IGC.0b013e31824c5cd2.
4. Berek JS, Hacker NF. (2014) *Berek & Hacker's Gynecologic Oncology*, 6th edn.
5. Philip J, Saia D, Creasman WT. (2012) *Clinical Gynecologic Oncology*, 8th edn. Elsevier.

46

CARCINOMA OF THE OVARY

A. Ilancheran

Introduction

Ovarian carcinoma is the fifth most frequent cancer in females in Singapore and the second most common gynaecological malignancy in Singapore. The age standardised incidence rate (ASR) is 12.5 per 100,000 person years in 2009–2013. It is often known as the "Silent Killer," as the disease is insidious in the early stages and often patients are in an advanced stage when they present with symptoms.[1]

Pathology

Ovarian cancer can arise from any of the three layers of the ovary, viz: the epithelium, stroma or the germ cells. Epithelial ovarian cancers (EOCs) account for more than 85% of malignancies. About 10% of cancers arise from the germ cells and the rest from the stromal elements.

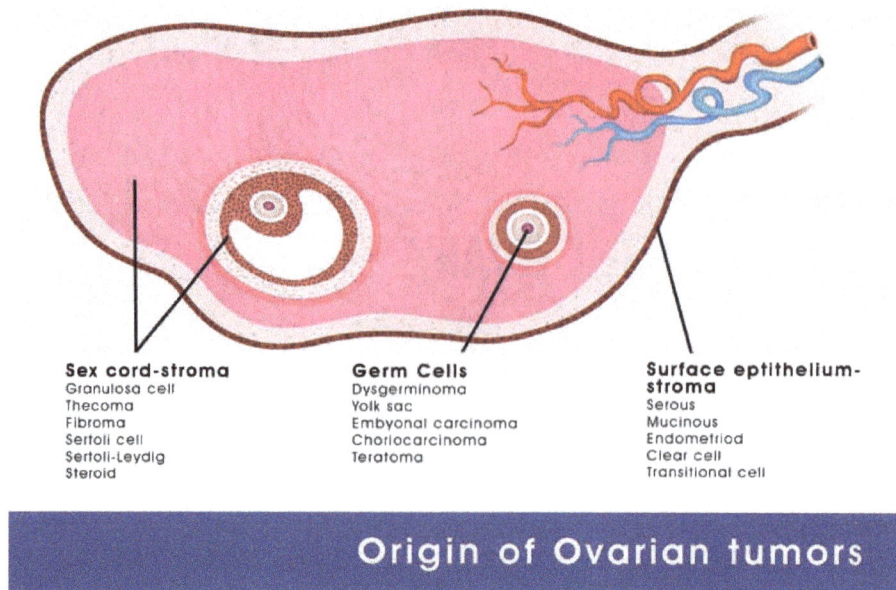

Sex cord-stroma
Granulosa cell
Thecoma
Fibroma
Sertoli cell
Sertoli-Leydig
Steroid

Germ Cells
Dysgerminoma
Yolk sac
Embyonal carcinoma
Choriocarcinoma
Teratoma

Surface epithelium-stroma
Serous
Mucinous
Endometriod
Clear cell
Transitional cell

Origin of Ovarian tumors

FIGURE 46.1 ■ Origin of ovarian tumours.

Classification of Ovarian Malignancies

Primary Ovarian Cancer

(a) Epithelial ovarian carcinomas (EOCs) e.g. serous carcinoma, mucinous adenocarcinoma clear cell adenocarcinoma, endometroadenocarcinoma, mixed adenocarcinoma, and undifferentiated carcinoma.
(b) Malignant germ cell tumours e.g. immature teratoma, dysgerminoma, yolk sac tumour, mixed malignant germ cell tumour, embryonal carcinoma, choriocarcinoma of the ovary. Granulosa cell tumour is the most common form of stromal tumours.
(c) Borderline ovarian tumour e.g. serous borderline tumour, and mucinous borderline tumour.

Metastatic Ovarian Cancer (where the Primary Site of Origin is not the Ovary)

(a) Gynaecological primary e.g. uterine cancer, cervical cancer
(b) Non-gynaecological primary e.g. colorectal cancer, gastric cancer

Aetiology

The strongest risk factor for EOC is related to reproductive factors such as the number of ovulatory cycles. High parity, use of the combined oral contraceptive pill, late menarche, early menopause and early age at first pregnancy, all reduce the risk.

About 5–10% of all EOCs are hereditary. There are three clinical genetic manifestations:

- "Site-specific" ovarian cancer
- Hereditary breast-ovarian cancer syndrome

Both of these are associated with mutations in the BRCA1 and BRCA2 tumour suppressor genes, which are present in about 90% of hereditary cases.

- Hereditary non polyposis colorectal cancer (HNPCC and Lynch II)

Ovarian cancer caused by BRCA mutations tend to occur in younger women. The lifetime risk is about 35–45% and 15–25% for the BRCA1 and BRCA2 gene mutations respectively. These cancers generally tend to be more aggressive.

Women with Lynch syndrome have a 10–12% risk of developing ovarian cancer and 40–60% risk of developing an endometrial cancer.

Other risk factors may include exposure to asbestos and talc, endometriosis and pelvic inflammatory disease.

Screening

Women at Average Risk

There are currently no proven screening methods for these women. Routine screening with either CA 125 or pelvic ultrasound is NOT recommended. The emphasis should be on educating women to be aware of early symptoms of ovarian cancer, such as bloating, abdominal girth change, change in bowel habits, or abdominal or pelvic discomfort.

Women with Strong Family History or a Proven Gene Mutation

Annual screening with CA 125 and transvaginal ultrasound should be offered (the limitations should be fully explained). Women with BRCA mutations should be offered prophylactic salpingo-oophorectomy after completion of the family, and those with HNPCC should have a hysterectomy with bilateral salpingo-oophorectomy.[2]

Diagnosis

Early stage EOC is insidious in onset. Hence more than 70–80% of EOC are diagnosed in advanced stage (III or IV) at presentation. Many patients are referred to other specialists other than gynaecologists. The main presenting symptoms of primary ovarian cancer include: abdominal swelling, abdominal pain/pressure, gastrointestinal symptoms, fatigue, vaginal bleeding and frequency.

Abdominal exam may reveal the presence of a mass arising from the pelvis, or in about 20–30%, clinically detectable ascites. Other evidence of advanced disease may be the presence of pleural effusion, enlarged inguinal or supraclavicular nodes or skin nodules.

Pelvic exam may reveal a solid, fixed, irregular adnexal mass. Characteristics to be noted on physical exam are given in Table 46.1:

TABLE 46.1 Physical Characteristics of Ovarian Tumours

	Benign	Malignant
Location	Unilateral	Bilateral
Mobility	Mobile	Fixed
Consistency	Cystic	Solid or firm
Cul-de-sac	Smooth	Nodular

Investigations in suspected ovarian cancer include blood tests and imaging. The best characterized tumour marker in EOC is CA 125, which is a serum glycoprotein. However, it is not a very specific tumour marker. Other than ovarian cancer (especially serous types), it can be raised in other malignancies such as colon, pancreas, breast and endometrial cancers. It is often raised in benign conditions such as endometriosis, leiomyoma or pelvic inflammatory disease, although rarely above 200 IU/ml. It is more valuable in postmenopausal women. It is important to remember, a normal CA 125 does NOT exclude a diagnosis of cancer.[3]

The most useful imaging modalities in the diagnosis of ovarian cancer are pelvic ultrasound and CT scans. The ultrasonographic features that may aid in the differentiation between benign and malignant adnexal masses are given in Table 46.2:

TABLE 46.2 Ultrasound Features of Ovarian Tumours

Benign	Malignant
Simple cyst, <10 cm in size	Solid or both solid and cystic
Septations <3 mm in thickness	Multiple septations <2 mm
Unilateral	Bilateral
Calcification, especially teeth	Ascites
Gravity-dependent layering of cyst contents	

CT scans of the thorax, abdomen and pelvis are taken to assess the extent of the disease.

Where investigations suggest ovarian cancer, the patient should be referred to a centre with a gynaecological-oncology multidisciplinary team. Evidence suggests that treatment in cancer centres improves the prognosis.

Management

The management of any gynaecological cancer involves staging followed by appropriate treatment. Staging in ovarian cancer is done surgico-pathologically. That is, the final stage is only arrived at after surgery to conform the diagnosis and extent of the spread, and the disease has been proven histologically. Table 46.3 lists the current staging. The treatment of the patient depends on:

- Stage of disease
- Tumour type and grade of differentiation
- Co-morbidities

TABLE 46.3 FIGO Staging of Ovarian Cancer

IA	Tumour limited to one ovary, capsule intact, no tumour on surface, negative washings.
IB	Tumour involves both ovaries, otherwise like IA.
IC Tumour limited to one or both ovaries	
IC1	Surgical spill
IC2	Capsule rupture before surgery, or tumour on ovarian surface.
IC3	Malignant cells in the ascites or peritoneal washings.
IIA	Extension and/or implants on the uterus and/or fallopian tubes
IIB	Extension to other pelvic intraperitoneal tissues

(Continued)

TABLE 46.3   (*Continued*)

IIIA (Positive retroperitoneal lymph nodes and/or microscopic metastasis beyond the pelvis)

IIIA1   Positive retroperitoneal lymph nodes only

  IIIA1(i)   Metastasis ≤ 10 mm

  IIIA1(ii)   Metastasis > 10 mm

IIIA2   Microscopic extrapelvic (above the pelvic brim) peritoneal involvement ± positive retroperitoneal lymph nodes

IIIB   Macroscopic, extrapelvic, peritoneal metastasis > 2 cm ± positive retroperitoneal lymph nodes. Include extension to capsule of liver/spleen.

IIIC   Macroscopic, extrapelvic, peritoneal metastasis > 2 cm ± positive retroperitoneal lymph nodes. Includes extension to capsule of liver/spleen.

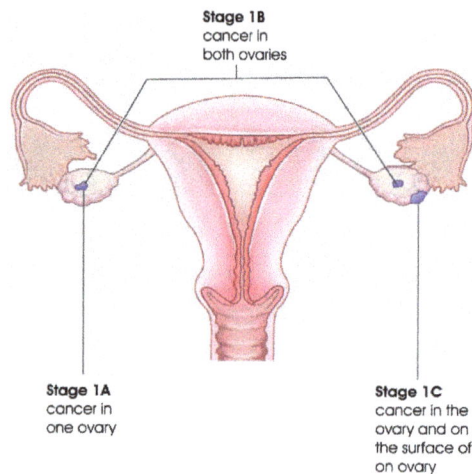

FIGURE 46.2 ■ Stage I — growth limited to ovaries.

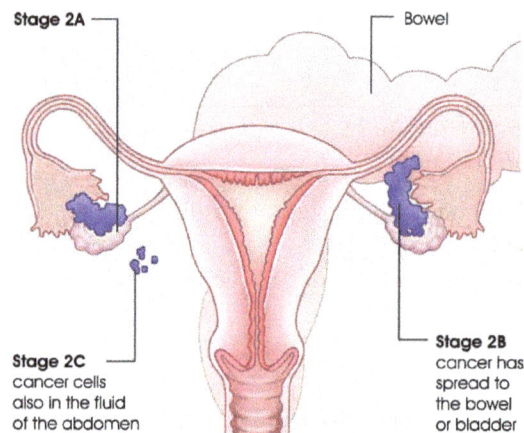

FIGURE 46.3 ■ Stage II — growth involving one or both ovaries with pelvic extension.

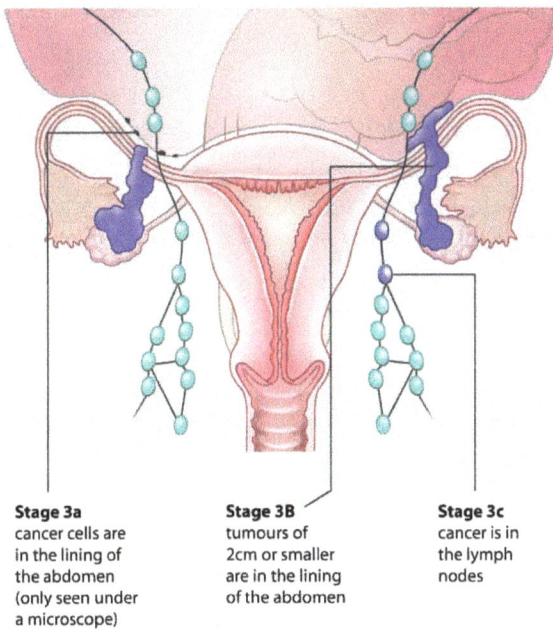

Stage 3a
cancer cells are
in the lining of
the abdomen
(only seen under
a microscope)

Stage 3B
tumours of
2cm or smaller
are in the lining
of the abdomen

Stage 3c
cancer is in
the lymph
nodes

FIGURE 46.4 ■ Stage III — tumour involving one or both ovaries with peritoneal extension.

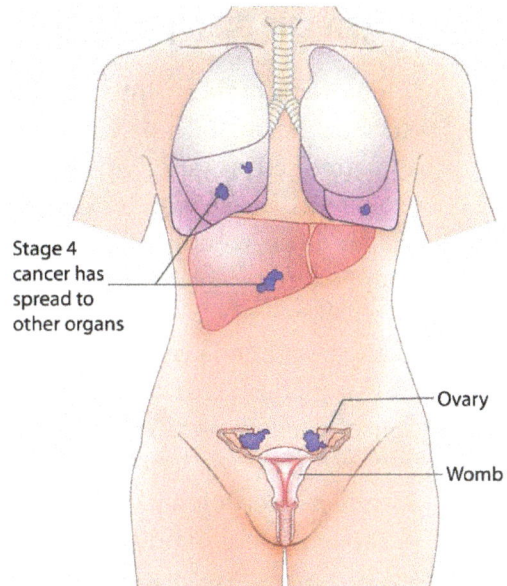

Stage 4 cancer has spread to other organs

Ovary

Womb

FIGURE 46.5 ■ Stage IV — tumour involving one or both ovaries with distant metastasis, pleural effusion, parenchymal liver metastases.

Surgery

The mainstay of treatment in ovarian cancer. It serves several functions: confirms diagnosis, is curative in early stage ovarian cancer, and most importantly, allows accurate staging of the cancer. It has also been shown that optimal cytoreductive surgery (CRS) to microscopic levels gives the best survival advantage for these patients. The main components of the surgery will include a total hysterectomy, bilateral salpingo-oophorectomy, omentectomy and removal of any other bulky disease with peritoneal washings. Occasionally, in young patients with early stage (IA) disease, unilateral salpingo-oophorectomy with fertility preservation may be justified.

Unfortunately, the majority of patients with ovarian carcinoma present with advanced disease (FIGO stage 2 and above). For patients with macroscopically advanced disease, survival depends on removing as much visible disease as possible. This is known as tumour debulking or cytoreduction. A total hysterectomy, bilateral salpingo-oophorectomy, omentectomy and complete resection of all macroscopic tumour nodules (optimal cytoreduction or optimal debulking) portends a better prognosis for the patients compared to "suboptimal" debulking, where large residual disease is left behind.[4,5]

• Systemic therapy

Chemotherapy is an integral part of the management of ovarian cancer except in early stage[1] well-differentiated ovarian cancer. It is most commonly given in an adjuvant setting after optimal CRS. However, in patients deemed to have very extensive disease which may preclude optimal CRS, chemotherapy can be administered in a neoadjuvant setting. In this instance, 3 cycles of chemotherapy is administered (to "chemically debulk" the tumour), followed by interval CRS and then followed by another 3 cycles of chemotherapy. The most widely used chemotherapy regime in ovarian cancer consists of a doublet, carboplatin and paclitaxel. Chemotherapy is usually administered as an intravenous infusion. There is evidence to show that intravenous and intra-peritoneal administration of chemotherapy can lead to better survival outcomes compared to intravenous administration alone. However, there are greater adverse effects with the intra-peritoneal route of administration.

In specific instances, there is also a role for angiogenesis inhibitors such as bevacizumab (concurrently with chemotherapy or as maintenance for patients with high risk of recurrence), and oral poly adenosine diphosphate-ribose polymerase (PARP) inhibitors such as olaparib (especially in women with known BRCA mutations).

For malignant germ cell tumour, the active chemotherapy agents are Bleomycin, Etoposide and Cisplatin which is used in all malignant cell tumours except for stage 1 pure dysgerminoma and grade 1 immature teratoma.

• Radiotherapy

This has a very limited role in ovarian cancer. Hormonal therapy may be used in chemoresistant or recurrent disease in a palliative setting.

Prognosis by Stage in Ovarian Cancer

Ovarian Carcinoma — Five Year Survival Rates

Stage 1a — almost 100%
Stage 1b/1c — 75%
Stage 2 — 65% to 70%
Stage 3 — 40% to 50%
Stage 4 — 20%

Malignant Germ Cell Tumours

These tumours are commonest in the first 2 decades of life and, fortunately, are exquisitely chemo-sensitive. Fertility sparing surgery is indicated even in advanced disease, followed by chemotherapy. The prognosis is excellent in stage 1 patients, and up to 75% in advanced stages.

Borderline Ovarian Tumours

These are a form of epithelial ovarian malignancy characterised by epithelial multilayering and malignant appearance but without stromal invasion. They tend to occur 1–2 decades younger than patients with ovarian carcinoma. The majority of these tumours present in early stage. For patients desirous of childbearing, fertility-sparing surgery with surgical staging (resection of the tumour with omental biopsy and peritoneal washings) is appropriate. Pelvic clearance is indicated in those who have completed family. Borderline tumours are indolent and generally not chemo-sensitive. The prognosis in most cases is excellent. However, they are prone to late relapses, even beyond 10 years.

References

1. Singapore Cancer Registry Interim Annual Report. (2015) Trends in Cancer Incidence in Singapore 2010–2014. National Registry of Diseases Office (NRDO).
2. Berchuck A, Cirisano F, Lancaster JM, *et al.* (1996) Role of *BRCA1* mutation screening in the management of familial ovarian cancer. *Am J Obstet Gynecol* **175**:738–746.
3. Goff BA. (2012) Ovarian cancer- screening and early detection. *Obstet Gynecol Clin N Am* 183–194.
4. Burger R. (2012) Advances in ovarian disease control. *Gynecol Oncol* **124**:5–9.
5. Engelen MJA, Kos HE, Willemse PHB, *et al.* (2006) Surgery by consultant gynecologic oncologists improves survival in patients with ovarian carcinoma. *Cancer* **106**:589–598.

INDEX

www.ingramcontent.com/pod-product-compliance
Lightning Source LLC
Chambersburg PA
CBHW081215220326
41598CB00037B/6791